Second Edition
# Dermatological Differential Diagnosis
### and Pearls

Second Edition

# Dermatological Differential Diagnosis

### and Pearls

**H. Eliot Y. Ghatan** MD, FRCPC

Brooklyn Veteran's Administration Hospital
New York

# The Parthenon Publishing Group

International Publishers in Medicine, Science & Technology

A CRC PRESS COMPANY
BOCA RATON     LONDON     NEW YORK     WASHINGTON, D.C.

**Library of Congress Cataloging-in-Publication Data**

Data available on request

**British Library Cataloguing in Publication Data**

Eliot, H.

   Dermatological differential diagnosis and pearls.
   – 2nd ed.

   1. Skin – Diseases – Diagnosis – Handbooks, manuals, etc.

   2. Diagnosis, Differential – Handbooks, manuals, etc.

   I. Title II. Ghatan, Y.

   616' .075

ISBN 1842141252

Published in the USA by
The Parthenon Publishing Group
345 Park Avenue South
10th Floor
New York, NY 10010, USA

Published in the UK and Europe by
The Parthenon Publishing Group
23–25 Blades Court, Deodar Road
London SW15 2NU, UK

Copyright © 2002
The Parthenon Publishing Group

First edition published 1994

Typeset by AMA DataSet, Preston, UK

Printed and bound by
Antony Rowe Ltd, Chippenham, UK

# Contents

## PART ONE    *Differential diagnosis*

### Section One    Primary eruptions

### Section Two    Secondary eruptions

## Section Three    Morphologic eruptions

## Section Four    Regional eruptions

## Section Five    Pediatric differential diagnosis

# PART TWO   *Dermatological pearls*

## Section One   Associations of skin disorders and other disorders

## Section Two   Body systems and skin disorders

## Section Three    Diseases and their features

## Section Four    Common Drug-Related Diseases

## Section Five    General dermatological and dermatopathological pearls

## Section Six    Malignancies associated with skin disorders

## Section Seven    Special states and skin

## Section Eight    Dermatological Trivial Pursuit

xiii

# Acknowledgements

It is with deep pleasure and humility that I wish to express my gratitude to The Providence. He has always been there for me and without Him this work and none of my other undertakings would ever have blossomed.

Three major institutions had a great impact in my life, and my career in particular. My undergraduate college, Yeshiva University (New York); my medical school, Albert Einstein College of Medicine of Yeshiva University (Bronx, NY); and my residency training affiliated hospitals of McGill University (Montreal, Quebec, Canada). My deepest gratitude is due to my teachers and to my mentors who made my career aspirations possible.

Two sets of couples had a major role over the three trying years of my training; they watched over our family interests, and they tied all the loose ends together: my in-laws, Dr Marvin and Mrs Sandra Sontag, whose dedication, guidance, and friendship have always been an inspiration, and their selflessness exemplary; my sister, Mrs Sarah Kohenteb and her husband, Mr Nadar Kohenteb, who were there when we needed them.

One teacher and friend requires special recognition, Dr Manfred Fulda. He has not only been an inspiring teacher, but also has served as a close and trusted friend of the family whose guidance and help have been most valuable.

Last, but not least, my parents have been the major source of encouragement, inspiration, and support throughout all the years of my formal education.

Many people became involved with this work one way or another. It was this collective involvement that made this work possible.

Dr Edward M. Young, Jr was gracious enough to read the entire manuscript and provided many helpful suggestions to improve this work. He was also kind enough to help me and guide me in publishing this book.

Dr Denise Sassville, a most knowledgeable dermatologist, cared to review the initial drafts of the manuscript and provided many helpful hints and corrections. I applaud his help.

Dr Robin C. Billick, a memorable teacher and friend, was kind enough to review the manuscript, and also to assist me in its publication.

I thank Dr William Gerstein and Dr Sammy Hutman for their review of the manuscript and their feedback.

Dr David Friedman, Dr Alfred Balbul, Dr Lawrence Frank and Dr Yelva Lynfield, though not directly involved with this book, provided an invaluable friendship that fostered this work.

# Introduction

Dermatology is a very privileged specialty, mainly due to the tremendous contribution of highly dedicated physicians and scientists. Over the past decade the scope of this specialty has continuously increased, with voluminous material published to keep up with the rapid pace of advancement. This volume provides a taxonomy of diagnostic material for the professional dermatologist and the inexperienced resident.

A rose is a rose is a rose is a rose,
although a rash is something else again.

In this book the author endeavors to highlight the essentials of 'every rash', its diagnosis and its differential diagnosis in many different ways.

Dermatological Differential Diagnosis – and Pearls is divided into two parts. In order to facilitate ease of use as a reference, alphabetical order has been used throughout the book.

Part one is concerned with the differential diagnosis. Part two, 'Pearls', is a listing of important concepts and factual material that should be available to every dermatologist.

Part One, the differential diagnosis, follows a simple, logical pattern. Within the traditional classification of the lesions, i.e. primary, secondary, etc., skin diseases are further subclassified into vascular, infectious, traumatic, etc. (see below), in the order spelled out by the mnemonic, VITAMIN HC:

Vascular
Infectious
Traumatic (foreign body, physical agents)
Allergic (eczematous)
Medications/metabolic
Idiopathic
Neoplastic
Hematologic
Congenital (heritable/familial: mode of inheritance is usually denoted, e.g. AD, AR, XR, etc.)

If the differential diagnosis is not extensive, an alphabetical system is used instead of the above-mentioned mnemonic. In this context, differential diagnosis is presented according to:

(1) The morphologic approach ('appearance of the lesion', primary lesion, secondary lesion)
(2) The regional approach ('address' of the lesion, e.g. hand, lip, palms, etc.)

The clinician may choose one of the approaches alone, or both approaches together, to arrive at a particular diagnosis. Even though in some cases a very exhaustive differential diagnosis listing may be encountered, the clinician may still narrow down his differential by considering other pertinent clinical information, together with some clues that are at times mentioned in conjunction with a particular diagnosis (e.g. characteristic feature, rare or common eruption, etc.)

A separate section on pediatric differential diagnosis (infants and children) is also included; a morphologic approach to diagnosis is used in this section.

Part Two, Dermatological Pearls, is another approach to characterize different diseases. It consists of eight sections, some of which are organized according to the same VITAMIN HC mnemonic described above.

Section 1, Associations, lists a number of dermatological diseases and their association with other systemic disorders.

Section 2 is a review of skin findings in various systemic disorders, e.g. diabetes, hyperthyroidism, kidney diseases, etc.

Section 3, Diseases and Their Features, has many subsections. One will find a listing of diseases, their etiology, their incubation periods, their vectors. Also, diseases with triad, tetrad, or pentad features are cited, and features of contact dermatitis and fungal diseases. Helpful diagnostic tests form another subsection.

Section 4 is a fairly comprehensive listing of dermatological disorders caused by various medications.

Section 5, General Dermatological Pearls, gives specific findings in different diseases or states (e.g. in which diseases one finds angioid streaks, leonine facies, etc.)

Section 6 is an extensive listing of malignancies that may be found in association with various dermatological disorders.

Section 7, Special States and Skin, deals with skin findings, for example, in old age, in pregnancy, etc.

Section 8, Dermatological Trivial Pursuit, is divided into two subsections. In the first subsection, morphologic and/or other features highly characteristic and/or diagnostic of different eruptions are alphabetically presented. Although this subsection may be commonplace for a seasoned clinician, a clinical neophyte may find it especially useful in conjunction with Part One of this book.

The second subsection is meant for those who like to challenge their knowledge of the rarer conditions which one is less apt to find in the daily dermatologic practice. It also serves to present pathognomonic or characteristic diagnostic findings of different eruptions.

# Abbreviations

| | |
|---|---|
| AD autosomal dominant | XR X-linked recessive |
| AR autosomal recessive | * most common |
| F female | + high incidence |
| HIV human immunodeficiency virus | ++ very high incidence, almost certain |
| M male | # most characteristic |
| XD X-linked dominant | |

# PART ONE

**Differential diagnosis**

# SECTION ONE

## Primary eruptions

# Macule and patch

## Infectious
leprosy
secondary syphilis (anetodermi
tertiary syphilis (cicatricial)
tuberculosis

## Traumatic
photoaging
radiodermatitis
scar

## Medicinal
post-steroid application or injection

## Idiopathic
acrodermatitis chronica atrophicans
anetoderma
atrophic lichen planus
atrophoderma of Pasini and Perini (a variant of
    morphea)
dermatomyositis
lichen sclerosis et atrophicus
macular atrophy
malignant atrophic dermatosis (Degos' disease)
morphea
necrobiosis lipoidica diabeticorum
poikiloderma atrophicans vasculare
sarcoidosis
scleroderma
striae
systemic lupus erythematosus

## Neoplastic
*Benign*
    atrophic seborrheic keratosis
    nevus lipomatosis

*Malignant*
    extramammary Paget's disease
    morphea-like basal cell carcinoma

## Congenital
aplasia cutis congenita
focal dermal hypoplasia (Goltz–Gorlin
    syndrome) (XR)
follicular atrophoderma
poikiloderma congenitale progeria (AR)
xeroderma pigmentosum (AR)
Werner's syndrome (AR)

## Vascular
progressive pigmentary purpura (capillaritis,
    Gougerot and Blum's dermatosis, Majocchi's
    disease, Schamberg's dermatosis)
stasis dermatitis

## Infectious
erythrasma
pinta
tinea nigra palmaris
tinea versicolor
kala azar (systemic leishmaniasis)

## Traumatic
erythema ab igne
postinflammatory hyperpigmentation
radiodermatitis

## Allergic

berloque dermatitis (psoralen-containing perfumes, cosmetics, fruits, e.g. figs, lemons, limes; plants containing furocoumarins, e.g. dill, parsley, rotten celery, weeds)
phytophotodermatitis

## Medicinal

adriomycin, argyria, arsenic, bleomycin, busulfan, chloroquine, chlorpromazine, clofazimine, 5-fluorouracil, gold, hydroxyurea, minocin, mustard (topical), psoralen, tar melanosis (melanodermatitis toxica), tetracycline
*Fixed drugs*
 barbiturates
 phenacetin
 phenolphthalines
 salicylates

## Metabolic

ACTH (adrenocorticotropic hormone) administration
Addison's disease
adrenalectomy
B₁₂ deficiency
biliary cirrhosis
hemochromatosis
hypercortilism
hyperthyroidism
niacin deficiency (pellagra)
melasma (idiopathic, oral contraceptive pills, progestin, pregnancy)
MSH (melanocyte-stimulating hormone) administration
pituitary hyperplasia
porphyria cutanea tarda
sprue
Whipple's disease

## Idiopathic

acanthosis nigricans
acromelanosis
amyloidosis (lichen, macular)
café au lait spots
erythema dyschromicum perstans
parapsoriasis
systemic sclerosis

## Neoplastic

Becker's nevus
ephelides
junctional nevus
lentigo maligna/simplex/senilis
mongolian spots
nevus of Ito/Ota/spilus
seborrheic keratosis
urticaria pigmentosa

## Congenital

ataxia telangiectasia (AR)
Bloom's syndrome (AR)
centrofacial lentiginosis (AD)
Cronkhite–Canada syndrome
dyskeratosis congenita (XR)
Fanconi's syndrome (AR)
incontinentia pigmenti (XD)
LEOPARD syndrome (multiple lentigines syndrome) (AD), *L*entigines, *E*KG conduction abnormalities, *O*cular hypertrolism, *P*ulmonary stenosis, *A*bnormal genitalia, *R*etarded growth, *D*eafness)
Peutz–Jegherts' syndrome (AD)
Moynahan's syndrome (multiple lentigines, congenital mitral stenosis, dwarfism, mental deficiency, genital hypoplasia)
POEMS syndrome (*P*olyneuropathy, *O*rganomegaly, *E*ndocrinopathies, *M* protein, *S*kin manifestations)
Tay syndrome
tuberous sclerosis (AD)
neurofibromatosis (AD)
xeroderma pigmentosum (AR)

## BLUE/SLATE GREY

## Infectious

maculae cerulae (secondary to louse bite)

## Traumatic

erythema ab igne
tattoo

## Medicinal

amiodarone
bismuth

chloroquine
fixed drug eruption
gold
hydroxychloroquine
mercury
minocin
phenothiazine
silver-containing nose drops

## Metabolic
ochronosis

## Idiopathic
erythema dyschromica perstans
hemochromatosis
Riehl's melanosis

## Neoplastic
blue nevus
malignant melanoma
mongolian spot
nevus of Ito
nevus of Ota (50% are congenital)

## DUSKY BLUE

## Vascular
acrocyanosis
Burger's disease
chilblain
embolic (cholesterol, septic, thrombus)
Raynaud's phenomenon

## Traumatic
frostbite

## Idiopathic
amyloidosis
cold agglutinin
cryoglobulinemia
lupus anticoagulant
protein C deficiency
reflex sympathetic dystrophy

## RED

## Infectious
cellulitis
erysipelas
*exanthems*
    brucellosis
    cytomegalovirus
    echovirus
    enterovirus
    erythema infectiosum
    infectious hepatitis
    infectious mononucleosis
    measles
    mucocutaneous lymph node syndrome
        (Kawasaki disease)
    rat bite fever
    rocky mountain spotted fever
    roseola infantum
    rubella
    scarlet fever
    syphilis (congenital or secondary)
    toxoplasmosis
    typhoid fever
    typhus

## Traumatic
first degree burn
intertrigo

## Medicinal
drug induced

## Idiopathic
cholinergic urticaria
collagen vascular disease
erythromelalgia
*Flushing syndromes*
    carcinoid syndrome
    ingestion of alcohol/food/drug (amyl
        nitrate,   nicotinic acid)
    menopause
    nervous system disorders
    pheochromocytoma
    Raynaud's phenomenon
    urticaria pigmentosum
rheumatic fever (erythema marginatum)
Still's disease (juvenile rheumatoid arthritis)

transient erythemas of newborn (erythema of
the newborn, erythema toxicum
neonatorum, incontinentia pigmenti)
urticaria

## WHITE (Hypomelanosis)

### Vascular
nevus anemicus
nevus oligemicus

### Infectious
*Fungal*
    tinea versicolor
*Bacterial*
    leprosy (tuberculoid)
*Spirochaetal*
    pinta
    syphilis
    yaws

### Traumatic
burn
thermal injury
ultraviolet
X-ray

### Allergic
postinflammatory (arsenic, chemical
    depigmentation, kwashiorkor, leprosy, pinta,
    sarcoidosis)

### Medicinal
azelaic acid
hydroquinones
mercaptoamines
phenols
physostigmine
sulphydryl

### Metabolic
amino acid disorders
hypopituitarism
thyroid disease

### Idiopathic
atrophic lichen planus
idiopathic guttate hypomelanosis
lichen sclerosis et atrophicus (scarring)
lupus erythematosus
morphea
pityriasis alba
psoriasis
sarcoidosis
scleroderma
Tietze's syndrome
vitiligo

### Neoplastic
amelanotic melanoma
halo nevus
mycosis fungoides

### Congenital
*Generalized*
    albinism (AD, AR)
    Chédiak–Higashi syndrome (AR)
    phenylketonuria (AR)
*Localized*
    ataxia telangiectasia (AR)
    Darier's disease (AD)
    dyskeratosis congenita (XR)
    incontinentia pigmenti achromicus
        (hypomelanosis of Ito, present at birth or
        early infancy)
    nevus depigmentosus
    piebaldism (AD)
    tuberous sclerosis (AD)
    Waardenburg's syndrome (AD)
    xeroderma pigmentosum (AR)

## YELLOW (Carotenemia)

### Infectious
viral hepatitis

### Medicinal
carotenoid
quinacrine

**Metabolic**
biliary obstruction
diabetes mellitus (10%)
hypothyroidism (10%)
increased bilirubin
ingestion of large amount of carrots, green
    vegetables, oranges

# Papule

## BLUE-BLACK

**Traumatic**
foreign body

**Idiopathic**
lichen planus

**Neoplastic**
*Benign*
    angiokeratoma
    blue nevus
    comedo (blackhead)
    giant comedo
    osteoma cutis
*Malignant*
    leukemia
    lymphoma
    malignant melanoma
    mycosis fungoides
    pigmented basal cell carcinoma

## BROWN

**Infectious**
*Fungal*
    deep fungal
    tinea versicolor
*Bacterial*
    mycobacterial

*Parasitic*
    leishmaniasis
*Spirochetal*
    syphilis
    yaws
*Viral*
    cat scratch fever

**Traumatic**
foreign body

**Idiopathic**
lichen amyloidosis
sarcoidosis

**Neoplastic**
dermatofibroma
histiocytosis X
nevi
seborrheic keratosis
basal cell carcinoma
malignant melanoma
urticaria pigmentosa (juvenile)

## FLESH-COLORED

**Infectious**
*Fungal*
    cryptococcosis
    histoplasmosis

*Viral*
   condyloma acuminata
   flat wart
   molluscum contagiosum

**Idiopathic**
amyloidosis
granuloma annulare
lichen amyloidosis
lichen nitidus
lymphangioma circumscriptum
pretibial myxedema
sarcoidosis

**Neoplastic**
*Benign*
   acrochordon
   colloid degeneration (colloid milium)
   comedo (closed)
   connective tissue nevi
   cylindroma
   dermatofibroma
   hidradenoma papilliferum
   histiocytosis (generalized eruptive)
   keloid
   knuckle pad
   milia
   multicentric reticulohistiocytosis
   neurofibroma
   nevi
   papular mucinosis
   steatocystoma multiplex
   syringoma
   trichilemmoma
   trichoepithelioma
   xanthogranuloma
   xanthoma
   malignant atrophic papulosis (Degos'
   disease)
*Malignant*
   amelanotic melanoma
   basal cell carcinoma
   merkel cell tumor
   metastasis

**Congenital**
Hunter's syndrome (XR)

**GROUPED**

*Annular grouping*
**Infectious**
syphilis (secondary, tertiary)

**Allergic**
contact dermatitis

**Idiopathic**
elastosis perforans serpiginosa
erythema elevatum diutinum
granuloma annulare
lichen planus
lymphocytic infiltrate of Jessner
Miescher's granuloma
necrobiosis lipoidica diabeticorum
sarcoidosis

**Neoplastic**
alopecia mucinosa
basal cell carcinoma
leiomyoma
leukemia
lymphocytoma cutis
lymphoma
mastocytoma

*Irregular grouping*
**Infectious**
folliculitis
herpes simplex
herpes zoster

**Traumatic**
insect bites
miliaria

**Allergic**
contact dermatitis

**Idiopathic**
focal dermal hypoplasia (Goltz's syndrome)

*Linear*
**Infectious**
herpes zoster
molluscum contagiosum
verruca

**Traumatic**
self-induced
trauma

**Allergic**
contact dermatitis

**Idiopathic**
focal dermal hypoplasia
granuloma annulare
incontinentia pigmenti
lichen planus
lichen striatus
linear porokeratosis
psoriasis
sarcoidosis

**Neoplastic**
epidermal nevi
ichthyosis hysterix (extensive epidermal nevi)
leiomyoma (multiple, cutaneous)
nevus unius lateralis (unilateral epidermal
    nevus)
nevus verrusocus
papular mucinosis

**Congenital**
Darier's disease (AD)

*Zosteriform*
herpes zoster
inflammatory linear verrucous nevus
Koebner's phenomenon
lichen planus
lichen striatus
nevus unius lateralis

## HYPERKERATOTIC

**Infectious**
*Fungal*
    fungal (and deep fungal)
*Bacterial*
    tuberculosis
*Viral*
    verruca plana/vulgaris

**Traumatic**
callus
corn

**Medicinal**
arsenic
lithium

**Metabolic**
phrynoderma (vitamin A deficiency)

**Idiopathic**
confluent reticulate papillomatosis
    (Gougerot–Carteaud), epidermal nevus,
    follicular lichen planus, keratosis pilaris,
    keratosis punctata, lichen spinulosus, lichen
    striatus, localized epidermolytic
    hyperkeratosis
*Perforating disorders*
    elastosis perforans serpiginosa
    Kyrle's disease
    perforating folliculitis
pityriasis rubra pilaris

**Neoplastic**
actinic keratosis
cutaneous horn
keratoacanthoma
seborrheic keratosis

**Congenital**
acrokeratosis verruciformis of Hopf (AD)
Darier's disease (AD)

## LICHENOID

**Infectious**
molluscum contagiosum
syphilis (secondary)
tuberculid (lichen scrofulosorum)
verruca plana

**Traumatic**
frictional (in atopics)

**Allergic**
lichen simplex chronicus

**Medicinal**
lichenoid drug

**Idiopathic**
lichen amyloidosis
lichen myxedematosus
lichen nitidus
lichen planus
lichen ruber moniliformis
lichen sclerosis et atrophicus
lichen spinolosus
lichen striatus
papular granuloma annulare
sarcoidosis

## PAINFUL

See Nodule and tumor (other, painful)

## PAPULONECROTIC

**Vascular**
polyarteritis nodosa
vasculitis
Wegener's granulomatosis

**Infectious**
atypical tuberculosis
gonococcus
meningococcus
papulonecrotic tuberculoid
sporotrichosis
tularemia
varicella

**Traumatic**
facticial
insect bite

**Idiopathic**
Degos' disease
lymphomatoid papulosis
pityriasis lichenoides et varioliformis acuta
pyoderma gangrenosum

## RED

**Vascular**
angiokeratoma, angioma, cholinergic urticaria,
hemangioma, pyogenic granuloma, vasculitis,
venous lake

**Infectious**
*Fungal*
deep fungal disease
*Bacterial*
cat scratch disease
erysipelas
folliculitis
leprosy
mycobacteria
*Parasitic*
leishmaniasis
scabies
*Spirochetal*
syphilis (secondary)
*Viral*
herpes simplex/zoster

**Traumatic**
burns (chemical, heat, ultraviolet)
cutis anserina (goose bumps, secondary to cold)
insect bite

foreign body
miliaria

## Allergic
autoeczematization
contact dermatitis
polymorphous light eruption

## Medicinal
drug eruption
fixed drug eruption

## Idiopathic
acne
erythema annulare centrifigum
erythema elevatum diutinum
erythema gyratum repens
erythema multiforme
erythroplasia of Queyrat
granuloma annulare
granulosis rubra nasi
juvenile rheumatoid arthritis
lichen planus
pityriasis lichenoides et varioliformis
pityriasis rosea
rosacea
sarcoidosis
systemic lupus erythematosus

## Neoplastic
Kaposi's sarcoma
leukemia
lymphoma
malignant angioendothelioma
metastasis
mycosis fungoides

## Congenital
blue rubber bleb nevus syndrome
Fabry's disease (XR)

## RED, ACUTE, GENERALIZED

bacterial sepsis
drug eruption

eruptive xanthomas
folliculitis
guttate psoriasis
lymphomatoid papulosis
miliaria profunda/rubra
papular urticaria
pityriasis lichenoides chronica
pityriasis lichenoides et varioliformis acuta
pityriasis rosea
scabies
viral eruption

## SYMMETRICAL

## Infectious
tinea versicolor
secondary syphilis

## Allergic
atopic dermatitis
keratosis pilaris
seborrheic dermatitis

## Medicinal
drug eruption

## Idiopathic
lichen amyloidosis
lichen myxedematosus
lichen planus
pityriasis rosea
pityriasis rubra pilaris
psoriasis

## Congenital
Darier's disease (AD)

## WART-LIKE AND SCALY

actinic keratosis
Darier's disease
elastosis perforans serpiginosa
epidermal nevus
keratoacanthoma (multiple)
lichen amyloidosis

lichen myxedematosus
lichen planus
lupus erythematosus
Kyrle's disease
pemphigus foliaceus
perforating collagenosis
perforating folliculitis
pityriasis rubra pilaris
prurigo nodularis
psoriasis
seborrheic keratosis
verruca

## WAXY

Darier's disease
lichen amyloidosis
lipoid proteinosis (hyalinosis cutis et mucosae, AR)
papular mucinosis (lichen myxedematosus)
pretibial myxedema

## YELLOW

**Infectious**
lupus vulgaris
**Idiopathic**
necrobiosis lipoidica diabeticorum

**Neoplastic**
eruptive xanthomas
nevus lipomatosis
nevus sebaceous
sebaceous hyperplasia
xanthogranuloma
xanthoma

**Congenital**
focal dermal hypoplasia (XD)
pseudoxanthoma elasticum (AD, AR)

# Plaque

## ANNULAR

**Vascular**
urticaria

**Infectious**
*Fungal*
fungal
deep fungal
*Bacterial*
erysipeloid
erythema chronica migrans
leprosy
lupus vulgaris
*Parasitic*
cutaneous larva migrans
*Spirochetal*
secondary syphilis

**Allergic**
eczema (nummular)
lichen simplex chronicus
polymorphous light eruption
seborrheic dermatitis

**Medicinal**
fixed drug eruption

**Idiopathic**
actinic granuloma (Miescher's granulomatosis)
alopecia mucinosa
discoid lupus
erythema annulare centrifugum
erythema multiforme
granuloma annulare
granuloma faciale
Jessner's lymphocytic infiltrate

lichen planus
lichen myxedematosis (papular mucinosis)
lichen sclerosis et atrophicus
morphea
necrobiosis lipoidica diabeticorum
parapsoriasis
pityriasis rosea (Herald's patch)
psoriasis
sarcoidosis

**Neoplastic**
*Benign*
    lymphocytoma cutis
*Premalignant*
    Bowen's disease
*Malignant*
    basal cell carcinoma
    leukemia
    lymphoma
    mycosis fungoides

**Congenital**
porokeratosis of Mibelli (AD)

## INFILTRATED

**Allergic**
polymorphous light eruption

**Medicinal**
lichenoid drug eruption

**Idiopathic**
Jessner's lymphocytic infiltrate
lichen planus
lupus erythematosus

**Neoplastic**
leukemia
lymphoma
metastasis

## RED

**Infectious**
*Fungal*
    fungal
*Bacterial*
    leprosy
    lupus vulgaris
*Parastitic*
    leishmaniasis

**Allergic**
contact dermatitis
polymorphous light eruption
seborrheic dermatitis

**Medicinal**
fixed drug eruption

**Idiopathic**
alopecia mucinosa
discoid lupus erythematosus
erythema elevatum diutinum
eosinophilic granuloma
granuloma annulare
granuloma faciale (red–brown or violaceous
    color)
Jessner's lymphocytic infiltrate
psoriasis
sarcoidosis
Sweet's syndrome
rosacea

**Neoplastic**
*Benign*
    lymphocytoma cutis
*Premalignant*
    actinic keratosis
    Bowen's disease
*Malignant*
    leukemia
    lymphoma
    malignant angioendotheliomatosis
    mycosis fungoides

15

# Pustule

**Infectious**

*Fungal*
   dermatophyte
   deep fungal (blastomycosis, sporotrichosis)
   candidiasis

*Bacterial*
   actinomycosis
   anthrax
   atypical mycobacteria
   carbuncle
   cellulitis
   ecthyma
   erysipelas
   erysipeloid
   folliculitis
   furuncle
   gonococcemia
   impetigo of Bockhart
   impetigo contagiosa
   meningococcemia
   rhinoscleroma
   staphylococcal scalded skin syndrome
      (Ritter's disease)
   sycosis barbe

*Parasitic*
   myiasis
   scabies
   swimmer's itch

*Viral*
   cowpox
   herpes simplex/zoster
   vaccinia
   varicella
   variola

**Traumatic**
insect bites
pustular miliaria

**Allergic**
contact dermatitis secondarily infected

**Medicinal**
bromide
iodide
lithium
mercury
steroid acne

**Idiopathic**
acne
eosinophilic folliculitis
erythema toxicum neonatorum
impetigo herpetiformis
pustular psoriasis
pyoderma gangrenosum
subcorneal pustular dermatosis
Sweet's syndrome
transient neonatal pustular melanosis

**Congenital**
acrodermatitis enteropathica (AD)

# Vesicle and bulla

**Vascular**
lymphangioma circumscriptum

**Infectious**
*Fungal*
dermatophyte
*Bacterial*
bullous impetigo
gas gangrene
rickettsial pox
toxic epidermal necrolysis
*Viral*
hand, foot, and mouth disease
herpes simplex/zoster
Kaposi's varicelliform eruption
milker's nodule
orf
smallpox
vaccina
varicella

**Traumatic**
burn
insect bites

**Allergic**
dyshidrosis

**Medicinal**
drugs
bullous fixed drug eruption
toxic epidermal necrolysis

**Idiopathic**
herpes gestationis
lichen planus

lichen sclerosis et atrophicus
pemphigus
pityriasis lichenoides et varioliformis acuta
porphyria cutanea tarda
systemic lupus erythematosus

**Neoplastic**
urticaria pigmentosa

**Congenital**
Darier's disease (AD)
epidermolysis bullosa dystrophic/letalis/simplex
incontinentia pigmenti (XD)

## ASYMMETRICAL

**Infectious**
*Fungal*
dermatophyte infection
*Parasitic*
cutaneous larva migrans
scabies

**Traumatic**
insect bites

**Allergic**
contact dermatitis
nummular eczema

**Idiopathic**
bullous pemphigoid

## GROUPED

### Infectious
herpes simplex/zoster

### Allergic
dermatitis venenata

### Idiopathic
bullous pemphigoid
dermatitis herpetiformis
epidermolysis bullosa simplex
pemphigus vulgaris

### Neoplastic
lymphangioma circumscriptum

## HEMORRHAGIC

### Infectious
*Bacterial*
   gonococcemia
   meningococcemia
*Viral*
   herpes simplex
   herpes zoster
   smallpox

### Idiopathic
erythema multiforme

## SYMMETRICAL

autoeczematization
contact dermatitis
dermatitis herpetiformis
erythema multiforme
vasculitis

## UMBILICATED

eczema herpeticum
herpes simplex
herpes zoster
milker's nodule
orf
smallpox
vaccina
varicella

# Nodule and tumor

## BLUE–PURPLE

### Vascular
hemangioma

### Neoplastic
angiosarcoma
hemangioendothelioma
Kaposi's Sarcoma
leukemia
lymphoma
malignant melanoma
mycosis fungoides

## CYST

bronchogenic cyst
cutaneous ciliated cyst

dermoid
epidermal
eruptive vellus hair cyst
ganglion
median raphe cyst of penis
milia
parasitic
pilar
steatocystoma multiplex
thyroglossal cyst

## Cyst, Calcified
calcified epidermal/pilar cyst
calcinosis cutis in association with collagen
    vascular diseases
metastatic calcification
osteoma cutis
primary calcification
pilomatricoma

## FLESH-COLORED TO RED, PAINFUL

### Vascular
polyarteritis
temporal arteritis
thrombophlebitis

### Infectious
*Fungal*
    deep fungal
    systemic mycosis
*Bacterial*
    carbuncle
    cat scratch fever
    lymphogranuloma venereum
    mycobacterial disease

### Traumatic
cold
insect bite
trauma

### Idiopathic
erythema induratum
erythema nodosum

hidradenitis suppurativa
panniculitis (with pancreatic disease)
Weber–Christian disease

### Neoplastic
leiomyoma

## FLESH-COLORED TO RED, PAINLESS

### Vascular
angiokeratoma
arteriovenous malformation
hemangioma
hemangiopericytoma
periarteritis nodosa
pyogenic granuloma
vasculitis

### Infectious
*Fungal*
    deep fungi
    systemic mycosis
*Bacterial*
    anthrax
    atypical mycobacteria
    bacterial abscess
    leprosy
    rheumatic fever
    rhinoscleroma
    tularemia
*Parasitic*
    leishmaniasis
    myiasis
    nematodes
    nodular scabies
*Spirochetal*
    syphilis
    yaws
*Viral*
    milker's nodule
orf
verruca

### Traumatic
foreign body granuloma
hypertrophic scar

keloid
phlebolith

**Allergic**
prurigo nodularis

**Idiopathic**
calcinosis cutis
erythema elevatum diutinum
granuloma annulare
gouty tophi
juvenile xanthogranuloma
morphea
multicentric reticulohistiocytosis
rheumatoid arthritis
sclerema neonatorum
subcutaneous granuloma annulare
Sweet's syndrome
systemic lupus erythematosus
subcutaneous fat necrosis of the newborn

**Neoplastic**
*Benign*
    atypical fibroxanthoma
    hibernoma
    keratoacanthoma
    leiomyoma
    lipoma
    Spitz nevus
    tumors (of adnexal appendages, blood
        vessels, elastic fibers, fat, histiocytes,
        lymphocytes, melanocytes, muscle,
        nerve)
*Appendageal tumors*
    adenoma sebaceum
    clear-cell acanthoma/hidradenoma
    cylindroma
    eccrine poroma/spiradenoma
    hydrocystoma
    nevus sebaceous
    pilomatricoma
    sebaceous adenoma/epithelioma
    syringoma
    trichoepithelioma
    trichofolliculoma
    trichilemmoma
*Histiocytic tumors*
    dermatofibroma
    dermatofibrosarcoma protuberans

    eruptive xanthoma
    fibrous histiocytoma
    histiocytosis X
    sclerosing hemangioma
*Other non-X histiocytic tumors*
    benign cephalic histiocytosis
    juvenile xanthogranuloma
    progressive nodular histiocytosis
    xanthoma disseminatum
*Neural tumors*
    neurofibroma
    neurilemmoma
    neuroma
*Premalignant*
    actinic keratosis
    Bowen's disease
    cutaneous endometriosis
*Malignant*
    angiosarcoma
    basal cell carcinoma
    Kaposi's sarcoma
    leukemia
    lymphoma
    nodular malignant melanoma
    metastasis
    soft tissue sarcomas
    squamous cell carcinoma

## INFECTIOUS ASCENDING

*Fungal*
    blastomycosis (primary inoculation)
    sporotrichosis
*Bacterial*
    atypical mycobacteria
    cat scratch disease
    mycobacteria (primary inoculation)
    nocardia
    pseudomonal infections (glanders:
        *Pseudomonas mallei*; melioidosis:
        *P. pseudomallei*)
    rat bite fever (sodoku, caused by *Spirillum*
        *minus*)
    tularemia

## OTHER, PAINFUL

(Mnemonic = C/O BENGAL)
Cutaneous endometriosis
Osteoma cutis

Blue rubber bleb nevus
Eccrine spiradenoma
Neurilemmoma, Neuroma
Glomus tumor
Angiolipoma
Leiomyoma

connective tissue nevus
eruptive vellus hair cyst (yellowish to reddish
    brown color)
lipoma
pseudoxanthoma elasticum
steatocystoma multiplex
xanthoma

# Telangiectasia

## Vascular
angiokeratoma
angiomata
capillaritis
nevus araneus
nevus flammeus (essential,
    Klippel–Trenaunay–Weber syndrome,
    Sturge–Weber syndrome)
telangectasia macularis eruptiva perstans
varicose veins
venous lake

## Traumatic
actinic damage
aluminum foundry workers
postsurgery (in suture line under tension)
radiodermatitis
trauma

## Metabolic
Cushing's syndrome
diabetes mellitus
liver disease
pregnancy

## Medicinal
estrogens
topical steroids

## Idiopathic
Degos' disease
diffuse neonatal hemangiomatosis
essential telangectasia
mixed connective tissue disease
necrobiosis lipoidica diabeticorum
poikiloderma vasculare atrophicans
rosacea
scleroderma
systemic lupus erythematosus
unilateral nevoid telangiectatic syndrome
xeroderma pigmentosum

## PERIUNGUAL

CREST syndrome
dermatomyositis
Raynaud's syndrome
rheumatoid arthritis
scleroderma
systemic lupus erythematosus

## POIKILODERMATOUS DISEASES

Bloom's syndrome
Cockayne's syndrome
dyskeratosis congenita

21

poikiloderma atrophicans vasculare
Rothmund–Thomson syndrome
pseudoxanthoma elasticum
xeroderma pigmentosum

## SPIDER TELANGIECTASIA

carcinoid syndrome
Cushing's disease
hepatic disease
physiological
polycythemia vera
pregnancy
rosacea

**Neoplastic**
basal cell carcinoma
mastocytoma
metastases (carcinoma telangiectasia)

**Congenital**
ataxia telangectasia (AR)
Osler–Weber–Rendu syndrome (hereditary
    hemorrhagic telangectasia, AD)

# Purpura

## NON-INFLAMMATORY (flat) PURPURA

**Thrombocytopenic (decreased platelets)**
*Primary*
congenital amegakarocytosis
hereditary
idiopathic thrombocytopenic purpura

*Secondary*
*Immunologic*
    drug hypersensitivity
    post-transfusion
*Non-immunologic*
    disseminated intravascular coagulation
    hemangioma
    physical
    prosthetic heart valves
    radiation
    thrombotic thrombocytopenic purpura
    uremia

*Decreased platelet formation*
aplastic anemia
bone marrow injury
vitamin deficiency
Wiskott–Aldrich syndrome

*Platelet sequestration*
hypothermia
splenomegaly

*Functional disorders of platelets*
Bernard–Soulier syndrome
Glanzmann's thrombocytopenia
storage pool disease
Von Willebrand's disease

*Infections*
bacterial
fungal
rickettsial
viral

**Non-thrombocytopenic**
**Vascular**
capillary fragility
fat and/or tumor-induced embolism
orthostatic purpura
platelet embolism (secondary to
    thrombocythemia as in amyloidosis,
    autoerythrocyte sensitization, and scurvy)

**Infectious**
purpura fulminans (gangrenosa, usually following
    meningococcal meningitis, scarlet fever,
    varicella)
various infections (bacterial, fungal, viral)

**Traumatic**
actinic (senile, solar) purpura

factitious purpura
mechanical purpura
orthostatic (stasis) purpura
toxic venoms
traumatic purpura (raised intravascular
   pressure – coughing, vomiting)

## Allergic
cold allergy
food allergy

## Medicinal
anaphylactoid purpura (allopurinol, aspirin,
   cephalosporins, hydralazine, gold,
   non-steroidal anti-inflammatory drugs,
   penicillin, phenytoin, quinidine, sulfonamides,
   thiazides)
cocaine
corticosteroids
coumadin necrosis

## Metabolic
Cushing's syndrome
diabetes mellitus
scurvy
uremia

## Idiopathic
amyloidosis
autoerythrocyte sensitization
   (Gardner–Diamond syndrome)
cachectic purpura
Henoch–Shönlein purpura
postcardiotomy syndrome
purpura simplex

### *Pigmentary purpuric eruptions*
Doucas and Kapetenakis (itching) purpura
Gougerot and Blum syndrome (pigmented
   purpuric lichenoid dermatitis)
Majocchi's disease (purpura annularis
   telangiectodes)

Schamberg's disease (progressive pigmentary
   dermatitis)
## Hematologic
disseminated intravascular coagulation
dysproteinemic purpura (purpura
   cryoglobulinemia and cryofibrinogenemia)
purpura secondary to clotting disorders
Waldenström's macroglobulinemia

## Congenital
Ehlers–Danlos syndrome

## INFLAMMATORY (palpable purpura, leukocytoclastic vasculitis)

## Vascular
cholesterol emboli
polyarteritis nodosa (chronic or cutaneous)
Takayasu's disease
temporal arteritis

## Infectious
*Bacterial*
   gonococcemia
   group A hemolytic *Streptococcus*
   leprosy
   meningococcemia
*Staphylococcus aureus*
   tuberculosis
*Spirochetal*
   secondary syphilis
*Viral*
   hepatitis
   mononucleosis

## Medicinal
aspirin
chloroquine
indocin
iodides
penicillin
phenothiazines
phenylbutazone
quinidine
sulfa
thiazides

**Idiopathic**

*Collagen vascular disease*
dermatomyositis
polymyositis
rheumatoid arthritis
Sjögren's syndrome
systemic lupus erythematosus
*Other*
acute febrile neurophilic dermatosis
(Sweet's syndrome)
allergic granulomatosis (Churg–Strauss
syndrome)
Behçet's syndrome
erythema elevatum diutinum
erythema nodosum
Gougerot–Ruiter
granuloma faciale
Henoch–Shoenlein purpura
inflammatory bowel disease
lymphomatoid granulomatosis
serum sickness (urticarial eruptions)
Wegener's granulomatosis

**Neoplastic**

carcinoma of bowel/lung
leukemia
lymphoma
multiple myeloma

**Hematologic**

cold agglutinins
cryofibrinogens
hypocomplementemic vasculitis
mixed cryoglobulinemia

## PETECHIAE

**Infectious**

*Bacterial*
bacterial endocarditis
*Viral*
coxsackie
echovirus
infectious mononucleosis
rubella

**Medicinal**

drug eruption

**Idiopathic**

Wiskott–Aldrich syndrome

**Hematologic**

thrombocytopenia

# Urticaria (/angioedema)

Individual lesions last 12–24 h by definition
Acute urticaria: recurrent episodes last < 6
  weeks
Chronic urticaria: recurrent episodes last > 6
  weeks

## GENERAL CLASSIFICATION

1. Idiopathic (70% of cases)
2. Immunologic
     Complement-mediated
     IgE-dependent (e.g. erythema nodosum)
3. Non-immunologic
     Alteration in arachidonic acid
     metabolism
     Direct mast-cell release (e.g. contrast
     dye, venom)

**Infectious**

focus of infection (cholecystitis, cystitis, dental
  abscess, fungal infection, otitis, pharyngitis,
  rheumatic fever, sinusitis, vaginitis)
intestinal parasites
viral infections (Epstein–Barr, infectious
  hepatitis, etc.)

## Traumatic

contactants: cosmetics (e.g. hair spray, nail polish, etc.) mouthwash, silk, soap, toothpaste, wool
inhalants: animal danders, pollen
insect bites
physical urticaria: aquagenic, cholinergic, cold, dermographism, heat, pressure, solar (light), vibratory
venoms

## Allergic

atopic diathesis (controversial if there is increased incidence of urticaria)
blood products
cheese
eggs
food additives (dyes and tartrazine)
fruits (bananas, berries, grapes, tomatoes, etc.)
fish
milk
mold
nuts
radiocontrast dye
seafood
serum sickness

## Medicinal

antibiotics
aspirin*
azo-dyes
benzoates
cocaine
curare
dextran
menthol
nonsteroidal anti-inflammatory drugs
opiates
penicillin* (even trace amounts in food, may produce urticaria in a patient with a positive intracutaneous test for penicillin)
pilocarpine
polymyxin B
quinine
sulfa

## Metabolic

diabetes mellitus
hyperthyroidism
menstruation
pregnancy

## Idiopathic

dermatomyositis
idiopathic
necrotizing vasculitis
rheumatoid arthritis
Sjögren's syndrome
systemic lupus erythematosus
underlying fatigue/stress/tension

## Neoplastic

leukemia
lymphoma
underlying cancer

## Congenital

complement cascade component deficiencies
hereditary angioedema

# Ulcer

(May be a primary or a secondary eruption)

## Vascular

arteriosclerosis
bacterial emboli
cholesterol emboli
consumption coagulopathy
cryoglobulinemia
decubitus
diabetes mellitus
giant-cell arteritis

hypertensive cardiovascular disease
pernio
polyarteritis
Raynaud's disease
stasis (varicose veins)
thromboangiitis obliterans
thrombotic thrombocytopenic purpura

## Infectious
*Fungal*
   deep fungi (blastomycosis,
   chromoblastomycosis, coccidiomycosis,
   cryptococcoses, histoplasmosis,
   sporotrichosis)
*Bacterial*
   actinomycosis
   anthrax
   botryomycosis
   cat-scratch fever
   chancroid
   diphtheria
   ecthyma
   glanders
   granuloma inguinale
   leprosy
   lupus vulgaris
   melioidosis
   mycobacteria (and atypical mycobacteria,
     *M. ulcerans*)
   pasteurella multocida
   plagueprogressive bacterial synergistic
     gangrene
   pseudomonas
   scrofuloderma
   tularemia
*Parasitic*
   amebiasis
   leishmaniasis
*Spirochetal*
   syphilis
   tropical phagedena
   yaws

## Traumatic
animal bite
burn (actinic, chemical, electrical, thermal)

factitial
insect bite (brown recluse spider)
trauma (pressure)

## Metabolic
hyperparathyroidism

## Idiopathic
erythema induratum
gout
pyoderma gangrenosum
rheumatoid vasculitis
scleroderma
systemic lupus erythematosus
Wegener's granulomatosis

## Neoplastic
calcinosis cutis
basal cell carcinoma
metastasis
mycosis fungoides
squamous cell carcinoma

## Hematologic
cold agglutinins
hemoglobinopathy
hemolytic anemia (congenital)
polycythemia vera
sickle cell disease

## Congenital
prolidase deficiency (AR)
Werner's syndrome (AR)

## Painless ulcer
diabetes mellitus
leprosy
necrotizing fasciitis
polyneuropathy
tabes dorsalis
syringomyelia

# SECTION TWO

## Secondary eruptions

# Erosion/excoriation

## Infectious
*Fungal*
candidiasis
dermatophytosis
*Parasitic*
insect bite
lice
scabies
swimmer's itch

## Allergic
atopic dermatitis
neurodermatitis
prurigo nodularis
stasis dermatitis

## Medicinal
drug eruption
steroids (systemic or topical)

## Metabolic
diabetes mellitus
liver disease
pregnancy
renal failure
secondary hyperparathyroidism

## Idiopathic
central nervous system disease
delusional parasitosis

dermatitis herpetiformis
epidermolysis bullosa
ichthyosis
intertrigo
lichen planus
neuropathy
pemphigus
porphyria cutanea tarda
psychosis
sarcoidosis
senile skin
toxic epidermal necrolysis

## Neoplastic
Hodgkin's disease
leukemia
lymphoma
mycosis fungoides

## Hematologic
polycythemia vera

## Congenital
bullous ichthyosiform erythroderma
    (epidermolytic hyperkeratosis, AD)
Ehlers–Danlos
epidermolysis bullosa
Hailey–Hailey disease (AD)

# Granuloma formation

**Infectious**
*Fungal*
  aspergillus
  blastomyces
  coccidioides
  cryptococcus
  histoplasma
  sporothrix
*Bacterial*
  BCG vaccine
  brucella
  lymphogranuloma
  toxoplasma
*Spirochetal*
  cat scratch
  treponema

**Traumatic**
beryllium
radiotherapy
sea urchin
silica
starch
zirconium

**Allergic**
bird fanciers'
coffee bean
farmer's lung
mushroom workers'

**Medicinal**
chemotherapy

**Idiopathic**
chronic granulomatous disease of childhood

Churg–Strauss allergic granulomatosis
Crohn's disease
giant-cell arthritis
hepatic granulomatous disease
histiocytosis X
hypogammaglobulinemia
immune complex disease
lymphomatoid granulomatosis
Melkersson–Rosenthal syndrome
panniculitis
Peyronie's disease
primary biliary cirrhosis
sarcoidosis
systemic lupus erythematosus
Wegener's granulomatosis
Whipple's disease

**Neoplastic**
carcinoma
dermoid cyst
sebaceous cyst

## LYMPHEDEMA

**Primary or Idiopathic:**
Congenital (Milroy's disease)
Lymphedema of Praecox

**Secondary:**
Filariasis
Inflammation
Irradiation
Lymphangitis
Neoplasms
Recurrent cellulites
trauma

# Necrosis

**Vascular**
arteriosclerosis
Buerger's disease
emboli (atheroma, fat, thrombus)
hypertensive ulcer
Kasbach–Merritt syndrome
polyarteritis
Raynaud's phenomenon
temporal arteritis
Wegener's granulomatosis

**Infectious**
*Fungal*
blastomycosis
cryptococcoses
histoplasmosis
mucormycosis
sporotrichosis
*Bacterial*
actinomycosis
anthrax
atypical mycobacteria
diphtheria
nocardia
*Pseudomonas*
Rocky Mountain spotted fever
*Streptococcus*
typhus
*Parasitic*
amebiasis
*Spirochetal*
bejel
syphilis
yaws

*Viral*
herpes zoster
vaccina

**Traumatic**
cold electrical injury
heat
iatrogenic (accidental) intra-arterial injection
pressure
radiation
trauma
venoms

**Medicinal**
chemotherapeutic agents (bleomycin, etc.)
coumarin
ergot
heparin
norepinephrine
(any) vasoconstrictive agent

**Metabolic**
diabetes mellitus

**Idiopathic**
*Collagen vascular disease*
rheumatoid arthritis
systemic lupus erythematosus
*Other*
pyoderma gangrenosum
disseminated intravascular coagulation

**Hematologic**
cryofibriginemia
cryoglobulinemia

## NECROSIS OF DISTAL EXTREMITIES

arteriosclerosis
calciphylaxis
carcinoma
cholesterol emboli

CREST syndrome
mixed connective tissue disease
myeloid metaplasia
polyarteritis nodosa
scleroderma
septic emboli
Sjögren's syndrome
systemic lupus erythematosus

# Scaling

**Infectious**
dermatophytosis
scarlet fever

**Allergic**
asteatotic eczema (and other eczematous
    eruptions)
seborrheic dermatitis

**Medicinal**
arsenic ingestion
drug eruption

**Idiopathic**
acanthosis nigricans

exfoliative dermatitis
Kawasaki's disease
pityriasis rubra pilaris
postdermatosis
psoriasis
xerosis

**Neoplastic**
carcinoma
lymphoma
mycosis fungoides

**Congenital**
epidermolytic hyperkeratosis
keratodermas

# Sclerosis

**Infectious**
leprosy
lymphogranuloma venereum
filariasis
poststreptococcal (recurrent)

**Traumatic**
radiation fibrosis
surgical trauma
trauma of drug (L-tryptophan, polyvinylchloride,
  toxic oil, vitamin K injection)

**Medicinal**
bleomycin

**Metabolic**
acromegaly
myxedema

**Idiopathic**
amyloidosis
carcinoid syndrome
graft versus host disease
porphyria cutanea tarda
scleromyxedema

**Neoplastic**
infiltrating carcinoma
urticaria pigmentosa

**Congenital**
ataxia telangiectasia (AR)
congenital generalized fibromatosis
erythropoietic protoporphyria (AR)
Hunter's syndrome (XR)
Hurler's syndrome (AR)
lipoid proteinosis (AR)
phenylketonuria (AR)
progeria (AR)
Werner's syndrome (AR)

# Sinus formation

## AXILLAE

hidradenitis suppurativa

## ANOGENITAL

**Infectious**
amebic colitis

deep fungi
lymphogranuloma venerum

**Idiopathic**
Crohn's disease, hidradenitis suppurativa
pilonidal cyst
diverticulitis (of sigmoid colon)
ulcerative colitis

**Neoplastic**
colonic carcinoma

## BACK, BUTTOCK, CHEST

acne conglobata

## BONE

osteomyelitis

## EAR

hidradenitis suppurativa (retroauricular area)

## FACE

*Congenital*
   lip sinus
   midline of nose
   periauricular
*Acquired*
   acne conglobata
   actinomycosis
   dental sinus
   nocardia infection
   pyoderma faciale

## FEET

mycetoma

## FINGER (toe) WEB

caused by penetration of hair

## NECK

actinomycosis
bronchial cleft cyst
dental sinus
scrofuloderma
thyroglossal duct cyst

## ORAL

dental sinus

## OTHER

botryomycosis

## RECTAL

carcinoma of bowel
inflammatory bowel disease

## SCALP

perifolliculitis capitis abscedes et suffodiens

# SECTION THREE

## Morphologic eruptions

# Acneiform

**Infectious**
folliculitis (including *Demodex* and *Pityrosporum* folliculitis)
secondary syphilis
herpes gladiatorum

**Traumatic**
acne aestivalis
acne detergicans
acne mechanica

**Medicinal**
acne cosmetica
acne medicomentosa
bromoderma
chloracne

iododerma
occupational acne (coal tar derivatives, oil)
pomade acne
steroid acne

**Idiopathic**
acne conglobata
acne fulminans
acne miliaris necrotica (acne varioliformis)
acne vulgaris
lupus miliaris disseminatus faciei
nevus comedonicus
perioral dermatitis
pyoderma faciale
rosacea
trichostasis spinulosa

# Annular (erythema)

**Vascular**
urticaria

**Infectious**
*Fungal*
dermatophytosis (tinea circinata, tinea corporis, tinea cruris, tinea versicolor)
*Bacterial*
impetigo contagiosa
leprosy (borderline)
lupus vulgaris

*Spirochetal*
Lyme disease (erythema chronicum migrans)
secondary syphilis

**Traumatic**
insect bite

**Allergic**
nummular eczematous dermatitis
seborrheic dermatitis

**Medicinal**
fixed drug eruption

**Idiopathic**
bullous pemphigoid
dermatitis herpetiformis
discoid lupus erythematosus
erythema annulare centrifugum
erythema dyschromicum perstans
erythema gyratum repens
erythema marginatum
erythema multiforme
granuloma annulare
granuloma faciale
Jessner's lymphocytic infiltrate
lichen planus
necrolytic migratory erythema

pemphigus vulgaris
pityriasis rosea
porokeratosis
psoriasis
subacute lupus erythematosus
purpura annulare telangiectodes (benign
    pigmented purpura)
sarcoidosis

**Neoplastic**
mycosis fungoides
urticaria pigmentosa

**Hematologic**
familial annular erythema

# Desquamative

**Infectious**
scarlet fever
staphylococcus scalded skin syndrome
viral exanthems

**Traumatic**
fever
sunburn

**Medicinal**
benzoyl peroxide
retinoic acid derivatives
salicylic acid

**Metabolic**
kwashiorkor
pellagra

**Idiopathic**
erythroderma desquamativum (Leiner's disease)
exfoliative dermatitis (see also erythrodermic
    eruptions)
Kawasaki's disease
keratolysis exfoliativa (lamellar dyshidrosis)
normal desquamation in the newborn
Stevens–Johnson syndrome
toxic epidermal necrolysis
toxic erythemas

**Congenital**
acrodermatitis enteropathica
continuous peeling skin syndrome
ichthyoses

# Eczematous

asteatotic eczema (eczema craquele)
atopic dermatitis
chronic acral dermatitis
dyshidrotic eczema (pompholyx)
hyperkeratotic palmar dermatitis
juvenile plantar dermatosis
lichen simplex chronicus

### Eczema associated with systemic diseases
acrodermatitis enteropathica (AR)
ahistidinemia
Hartnup's syndrome (AR)
Hurler's syndrome (AR)
phenylketonuria (AR)
X-linked agammaglobulinemia
Wiskott–Aldrich syndrome (XR)

neurodermatitis
nummular (discoid) eczema
pityriasis alba
seborrheic dermatitis
stasis (gravitational) dermatitis
Sulzberger's syndrome (exudative discoid and
   lichenoid dermatitis)

allergic contact dermatitis
dermatophytid ('-id reaction')
eczematous dermatophytosis
eczematous drug eruption
eczematous polymorphous light eruption
infectious eczematoid dermatitis
irritant contact dermatitis
photoallergic contact dermatitis

# Erythrodermic (exfoliative dermatitis)

*Definition*: > 75% of skin involved
*Rule of thumb*:
4 eczema 40%
3 psoriasis 30%
2 drug 20%
1 malignancy 10%

### Infectious
*Fungal*
   dermatophytosis
*Bacterial*
   scarlet fever
   staphylococcal scalded skin syndrome

*Parasitic*
   scabies

### Traumatic
immersion burn

### Allergic
atopic dermatitis
contact dermatitis
neurodermatitis
seborrheic dermatitis
stasis dermatitis

39

**Medicinal**
drugs

sclerema neonatorum
toxic epidermal necrolysis

**Idiopathic**
dermatomyositis
graft versus host disease
idiopathic
lichen planus
pemphigus foliaceus
pityriasis rosea
pityriasis rubra pilaris
psoriasis

**Neoplastic**
leukemia
lymphoma
mycosis fungoides
other malignancies

**Congenital**
congenital ichthyosiform erythroderma

# Hyperkeratotic

**Infectious**
deep fungal
dermatophytosis
leprosy
Norwegian scabies

ichthyosis (and its variants)
pityriasis lichenoides chronica
pityriasis rosea
pityriasis rubra pilaris
porokeratosis
psoriasis
sarcoidosis

**Allergic**
atopic dermatitis
chronic stasis dermatitis
lichen simplex chronicus
seborrheic dermatitis
prurigo nodularis
xerosis

**Neoplastic**
*Benign*
   epidermal nevi
   ichthyosis hystrix (extensive epidermal nevi)
*Premalignant*
   actinic keratosis
   Bowen's disease
*Malignant*
   Hodgkin's disease
   intestinal malignancies
   Kaposi's sarcoma
leukemia
mycosis fungoides

**Medicinal**
clofibrate
nicotinic acid

**Metabolic**
thyroid disorders

**Congenital**
Darier's disease (AD)
erythrokeratoderma variabilis
palmo plantar keratodermas
porokeratosis (AD)

**Idiopathic**
acanthosis nigricans
hyperkeratosis lenticularis perstans (flegel)
hypertrophic lichen planus
parapsoriasis

# Linear pattern

beaded lines (in trunk of black persons)
coccidiodomycosis
epidermal nevus
factitial
incontinentia pigmenti
larva currens
lichen planus
lichen striatus
linear acantholytic dermatosis
linear contact dermatitis
linear granuloma annulare

linear rheumatoid nodules
linear scleroderma
molluscum contagiosum
Mondor's disease
periarteritis nodosa
plane wart
porokeratosis of Mibelli
psoriasis
temporal arteritis
thrombophlebitis

# Livedo reticularis pattern

**Vascular**
acrocyanosis
arterial disorder (livedo racemosa)
atrophie blanche
cerebrovascular disease (Sneddon's syndrome)
embolic phenomenon
hypertension
panarteritis
vasculitis

**Infectious**
meningococcemia
pneumococcal sepsis
rheumatic fever
syphilis
tuberculosis

**Traumatic**
exposure to cold (cutis marmorata)

**Medicinal**
amantadine

drug reactions

**Metabolic**
hypercalcemia
hyperviscosity states
oxalosis
pancreatitis
pheochromocytoma

**Idiopathic**
*Collagen vascular disease*
    dermatomyositis
    rheumatoid arthritis
    scleroderma
    systemic lupus erythematosus
*Other*
    anticardiolipin antibody syndrome
    decompression sickness
    neurogenic disease
    primary and secondary Raynaud's
    phenomenon
    Sneddon–Wilkinson syndrome

**Neoplastic**
leukemia
mycosis fungoides

**Hematologic**
cryoglobulinemia
polycythemia vera
thrombocytopenic purpura (idiopathic or
    thrombotic)

# Morbilliform

**Infectious**
*Bacterial*
    meningococcemia
    Rocky Mountain spotted fever
    scarlet fever
    secondary syphilis
    typhus
*Parasitic*
    toxoplasmosis
*Viral*
    echovirus
    coxsackie virus
    dengue
    erythema infectiosum

infectious hepatitis
roseola
rubella
rubeola

**Medicinal**
drugs (ampicillin*)

**Idiopathic**
graft versus host disease
juvenile rheumatoid arthritis
pityriasis rosea

# Papulosquamous

**Infectious**
dermatophytosis
secondary syphilis

**Allergic**
asteatotic dermatitis
atopic dermatitis
contact dermatitis
lichen simplex chronicus
seborrheic dermatitis

**Medicinal**
drug eruption

**Idiopathic**
discoid lupus erythematosus
erythema annulare centrifigum
lichen planus
lichen striatus (and other lichenoid eruptions)
parapsoriasis
pityriasis lichenoides chronica
pityriasis rosea
pityriasis rubra pilaris
psoriasus

# Scarred

**Infectious**

*Fungal*
deep fungus blastomycosis (cribriform scar),
(mycetoma, Madura foot)

*Bacterial*
atypical mycobacteria
dissecting cellulitis
erythema induratum
kerion
lymphogranuloma venereum
lupus vulgaris
papulonecrotic tuberculid
tuberculosis due to BCG vaccination

*Parasitic*
leishmaniasis

*Spirochetal*
tertiary syphilis

*Viral*
herpes zoster
varicella

acne vulgaris
ainhum
anetoderma
atrophic lichen planus
cicatricial pemphigoid
Ehlers–Danlos syndrome
epidermolysis bullosa acquisita
folliculitis decalvans
hidradenitis suppurativa
lichen sclerosis et atrophicus
lupus miliaris disseminata faciei
mid-dermal elastolysis
morphea
poikiloderma vasculare atrophicans
porphyria cutanea tarda
pseudopelade
pyoderma gangronosum
sarcoidosis
systemic lupus erythematosus
ulerythema ophryogenes

**Traumatic**
brown recluse spider bite
chloracne
factitial
radiodermatitis (chronic)
thermal burn

**Idiopathic**
acne conglobata
acne keloidalis nuchae
acne vermoulante

**Neoplastic**
extramammary Paget's disease
morpheaform basal cell carcinoma
Paget's disease of breast

**Congenital**
Degos' disease
Ehlers–Danlos syndrome
epidermolysis bullosa dystrophica
Hailey–Hailey disease (AD)

# Serpiginous

**Vascular**
urticaria

**Infectious**
*Fungal*
dermatophytosis (tinea corporis*)
*Bacterial*
granuloma inguinale
*Parasitic*
cutaneous larva migrans
*Spirochetal*
secondary and tertiary syphilis

**Traumatic**
erythema ab igne
marine organism stings

**Allergic**
contact dermatitis
phytophotodermatitis

**Idiopathic**
elastosis perforans serpiginosa
erythema gyratum repens
granuloma annulare
variegate parapsoriasis

**Congenital**
epidermal nevi (and the generalized form, ichthyosis hystrix)
erythrokeratoderma variabilis (AD)
ichthyosis linearis circumflexa (AR)
incontinentia pigmenti (XD)
porokeratosis (AD)

# Verrucous

**Infectious**
*Fungal*
blastomycosis
chromoblastomycosis
*Bacterial*
atypical mycobacteria (*Mycobacterium marinum*)
tuberculosis verrucosa cutis
*Parasitic*
Norwegian scabies
*Viral*
condyloma
epidermodysplasia verruciformis
verruca vulgaris

**Traumatic**
halogenoderma

**Allergic**
lichen simplex chronicus
prurigo nodularis

**Idiopathic**
acanthosis nigricans
dermatitis (pyoderma) vegetans (blastomycosis-like pyoderma)
Kyrle's disease

lichen striatus
rupioid psoriasis

### Neoplastic
calcinosis cutis
dermatosis papulosis nigra
linear epidermal nevus (and the generalized
    form, ichthyosis hystrix)
nevus sebaceus
nevus verrucosus
seborrheic keratosis
syringocystadenoma papilliferum

verrucous carcinoma
warty dyskeratoma

### Congenital
Darier's disease (AD)
ichthyosis linearis circumflexa (AR)
incontinentia pigmenti (XD, third stage)
localized congenital ichthyosiform
    erythroderma
pachyonychia congenita (AD)
palmar and plantar keratoderma
porokeratosis (AD)

# Zosteriform (dermatomal)

### Vascular
Beckwith–Wiedemann syndrome
Cobb syndrome
Klippel–Trenaunay syndrome
lymphangioma circumscriptum
Sturge–Weber syndrome

### Infectious
cellulitis
herpes simplex
herpes zoster
lymphangitis
syphilis

### Idiopathic
granuloma annulare
keratosis pilaris
lichen aureus
lichen planus
lichen striatus
pseudolymphoma
psoriasis
sarcoidosis
vitiligo

### Neoplastic
*Benign*
    Becker's nevus
    blue nevus
    connective tissue nevus
    epidermal nevus
    melanocytic nevus
    Spitz nevus
    syringocystadenoma papilliferum
    trichoepithelioma
    xanthoma
*Malignant*
    angiosarcoma
    basal cell carcinoma
    Kaposi's sarcoma
    leukemia
    lymphoma
    metastatic

### Congenital
neurofibromatosis (AD)
porokeratosis (AD)

# SECTION FOUR

## Regional eruptions

Specific body regions are listed alphabetically

# Acral purpura

antiphospholipid antibody syndrome
atherosclerosis
cholestrol emboli
cryoglobulinemia
cryofibrinogenemia
gonococcemia
hepatitis C related cryoglobulinemia
hyperglobulinemic purpura
left atrial myxoma

leukocytoclastic vasculitis
polyarteritis nodosa
Rocky mountain spotted fever
sepsis
Sneddon syndrome
Subacute bacterial endocarditis
Systemic lupus erythematosus
Ttraumatic aneursmal emboli
Wegener granulomatosis

# Ankle edema

agenesis of venous valve
deep vein thrombosis
fluid retention
heart failure
hypoalbuminemia

kidney failure
Klippel–Trenaunay syndrome
lipodystrophy
lymphedema
venous obstruction

# Antecubital and popliteal fossae

atopic dermatitis
contact dermatitis

pseudoxanthoma elasticum

# Anus

**Vascular**
hemorrhoids

**Infectious**
*Fungal*
  candidiasis
  dermatophytosis
*Bacterial (may cause ulceration)*
  actinomycosis
  gonorrhea
  granuloma inguinale
  lymphogranuloma venereum
  tuberculosis cutis
*Parasitic*
  amebiasis
  pinworm (oxyuriasis)
*Spirochetal*
  syphilis (primary and secondary)
*Viral*
  condyloma acuminata
  cytomegalovirus (causes ulceration)
  herpes simplex
  molluscum contagiosum

**Allergic**
contact dermatitis
dermatitis medicomentosa
lichen simplex chronicus
seborrheic dermatitis

**Traumatic**
factitious
fissure
fistula
stricture
trauma

**Medicinal**
antibiotic-induced protitis (broad spectrum,
  tetracycline*)

**Metabolic**
hyperhidrosis

**Idiopathic**
Crohn's disease
hidradenitis suppurativa
hypo/hyper-pigmentation
lichen sclerosis et atrophicus
leukoplakia
lichen planus
psoriasis

**Neoplastic**
anal carcinoma
apocrine adenoma
extramammary Paget's disease
Kaposi's sarcoma
malignant melanoma

# Areolae (breast)

basal cell ca of nipples
contact dermatitis* (breast feeding, jogger's
    nipple)
erosive adenomatosis of the nipple
florid papillomatosis of the nipple
Fox–Fordyce disease
Hidradenitis suppurativa
Hyperkeratosis of nipple & areola
lymphadenosis benigna cutis
mamillary fistula
neurofibroma
neurofibromatosis
nevoid keratosis
Paget's disease
Painful nipple
psoriasis
scabies
seborrheic dermatitis
Seborrheic keratosis

Liver disease
thyrotoxicosis

*Medication induced*
    Alkylating agents
    Androgenetic steroids
    Antiretroviral agents
    Cimetidine
    Digitalis
    Estrogens
    heroin
    Marijuana
    Oral contraceptives
    Spironolactone

*Neoplastic*
    Adrenal tumors
    Hormone-producing neoplasm
    Reduced testosterone production or
    activation
    Testicular tumors

**Gynecomastia**
*Hormonal:*
Estrogen–Testosterone Imbalance:
    Congenital adrenal hyperplasia
    Hermaphroditism
    Increased estrogen secretion states
    Klinefelter's syndrome

*Increased peripheral conversion to estrogen*
Adrenal disease

**Nipple discharge**
Breast sarcoma
Ductal carcinoma insitu
Facticial disease
Invasive breast cancer
Paget's disease of brease
Papillary adenoma
Periductal mastitis

# Arms and forearms

**Infectious**
herpes zoster
insect bite

**Allergic**
contact dermatitis
exzematous dermatitis

**Idiopathic**
acne
achromia
dermatomyositis
granuloma annulare
keratosis pilaris
lichen planus
psoriasis
scleroderma

**Neoplastic**
fibroma
lipoma
nevi
nodular pseudosarcomatousfasciitis (arms, most
    commonly)

**Congenital**
xeroderma pigmentosum (AR)

# Axillae

**Infectious**
*Fungal*
    candidiasis
    dermatophytosis
*Bacterial*
    erythrasma
    furunculosis
    impetigo
    trichomycosis
    axillaris (lepothrix, *Corynebacterium tenuis*)
*Parasitic*
    lice
    scabies

*Other disorders*
    acanthosis nigricans (and pseudoacanthosis
    nigricans)
    cutaneous papillomatous (confluent and
        reticulated papillomatosis of Gougerot
        and Carteaud)
    Fox–Fordyce disease
    hidradenitis suppurativa
    postinflammatory hyperpigmentation
    psoriasis
    striae distensae
    reticulated pigmented dermatosis of the
    flexures (Dowling–Degos' disease)

**Allergic**
contact dermatitis
seborrheic dermatitis

**Neoplastic**
acrochordon
apocrine adenoma
axillary freckling (Von Recklinghausen's disease)
carcinoma of apocrine glands
epidermal nevus
eruptive xanthoma
fibroma
nevus
xanthoma disseminatum

**Metabolic**
alkaptonuria (ochronosis, color is brown)
chromhidrosis (color may be yellow*, black,
    blue, green)

**Idiopathic**
*Bullous disorders*
    bullous pemphigoid
    impetigo herpetiformis
    pemphigus vegetans
    subcorneal pustular dermatosis
        (Sneddon–Wilkinson disease)

**Congenital**
Darier's disease (AD)
Hailey–Hailey disease (AD)
lipoid proteinosis (hyalinosis cutis et
    mucosae, AR)
pseudoxanthoma elasticum (AD, AR)

# Back

acne
Becker's nevus
cutaneous papillomatosis
disseminated epidermolytic acanthoma
hibernoma
lichen spinulosis
macular amyloidosis
meningoceles

nevus anemicus
pleomorphic lipoma
seborrheic keratosis
spindle cell lipoma
superficial spreading melanoma *in situ* (especially in men)
transient acantholytic dermatosis (Grover's disease)

# Buttocks

**Infectious**

*Fungal*
blastomycosis
candidiasis
dermatophytosis

*Bacterial*
abscesses (fistula-in-ano, ischiorectal, pilonidal cyst)
furunculosis
lupus vulgaris

*Parasitic*
cutaneous larva migrans
insect bite
scabies

*Viral*
herpes simplex
herpes zoster

**Allergic**
contact dermatitis

**Idiopathic**
acne vulgaris
dermatitis herpetiformis
erythema elevatum diutinum
Gianotti–Crosti syndrome
parapsoriasis
psoriasis
striae distensae

**Neoplastic**
angiokeratoma circumscriptum
malignant fibous histiocytoma
nevus lipomatosus superficialis
smooth muscle hamartoma (lumbar region)

# Cheeks

**Infectious**

*Fungal*
tinea barbe
tinea faciei
tinea versicolor

*Bacterial*
erysipelas
impetigo contagiosum
leprosy
lupus vulgaris
sycosis

*Spirochetal*
syphilis

*Viral*
herpes simplex
herpes zoster
verruca plana

**Allergic**
atopic dermatitis
contact dermatitis
polymorphous light eruption
seborrheic dermatitis

**Medicinal**
fixed drug eruption

**Idiopathic**
achromia
acne
alopecia areata
folliculitis ulerythema reticulata
granuloma faciale
melasma
neurotic excoriation
pityriasis alba
rosacea
sarcoidosis
scleroderma
systemic lupus erythematosus
vitiligo

**Neoplastic**
actinic keratosis
basal cell carcinoma
cutaneous horn
epitheloid sarcomas
keratoacanthoma
malignant fibrous histiocytoma
melanoma
nevi
seborrheic keratosis
squamous cell carcinoma

**Congenital**
xeroderma pigmentosum (AR)

# Chest

**Infectious**
tinea versicolor

**Allergic**
seborrheic dermatitis

**Idiopathic**
acne
keloids
scars
transient acantholytic dermatitis (Grover's
    disease)

**Neoplastic**
eruptive velus hair cyst
eruptive xanthoma
eruptive syringoma
multiple leiomyomas/lipoma
nevus anemicus
steatocystoma multiplex
trichoepithelioma

**Congenital**
Darier's disease (AD)

# Chin

**Infectious**
actinomycosis
dental sinus
impetigo
sycosis
verruca plana

**Traumatic**
radiodermatitis

**Allergic**
contact dermatitis
eczema
fixed drug eruption

**Idiopathic**
acne
hypertrichosis
perioral dermatitis
pityriasis rosea

**Neoplastic**
basal cell carcinoma
neurofibroma
nevi
sebaceous cyst

# Ear

## EAR CANAL

ceruminoma (tumor of ceruminous glands)
dermatophytosis
furunculosis
Kimura's disease (periauricular location)
psoriasis
seborrheic dermatitis

## EAR LOBES

**Vascular**
angioedema
pyogenic granuloma

**Infectious**
*Fungal*
    otomycosis (blastomycosis,
    epidermophytosis, trichophytosis)
*Bacterial*
    actinomycosis
    borrelial lymphocytoma
    cellulitis
    impetigo contagiosum
    furunculosis
    leprosy
    lupus vulgaris
*Infestation*
    Chicherio ulcer of leishmaniasis
*Spirochetal*
    syphilis

**Traumatic**
acanthoma fissuratum
chondrodermatitis nodularis chronica helicis
frostbite (pernio)
radiation
seroma (pseudocyst of the auricle,
    posttraumatic)

**Allergic**
atopic dermatitis
contact dermatitis
eczematous (atopic, infectious dermatitis)
infectious eczema
seborrheic dermatitis

**Metabolic**
calcinosis
gouty tophi
ochronosis (alkaptonuria)

**Idiopathic**
elastotic nodule of the ear
granuloma annulare
hydroa vacciniforme
Jessner's lymphocytic infiltrate
lupus erythematosus
lymphadenosis benigna cutis
psoriasis
relapsing polychondritis
sarcoidosis

**Neoplastic**
*Benign*
    cutaneous horn
    lipoma
    sebaceous cyst
*Premalignant*
    actinic keratosis
    Bowen's disease

*Malignant*
    basal cell carcinoma
    Kaposi's sarcoma
    melanoma
    squamous cell carcinoma

## POSTAURICULAR

In chloracne, it is the most commonly affected
    site.
Lichen myxedematous

# Elbows and knees

contact dermatitis
dermatitis herpetiformis
erythema multiforme
gout
granuloma annulare
juxta-articular nodes (rheumatic diseases,
    syphilis, yaws)

lichen simplex chronicus
psoriasis
scabies
xanthoma tuberosum multiplex

# Eye

## ON EYELID in general

**Vascular**
angioedema

**Infectious**
chancriform pyoderma of the face
folliculitis
molluscum contagiosum
verruca

**Allergic**
contact dermatitis
dermatitis medicamentosa
seborrheic dermatitis

**Idiopathic**
amyloidosis

comedo
dermatomyositis
histiocytic syndromes
lichen planus
lupus erythematosus
sarcoidosis

**Neoplastic**
basal cell carcinoma
carcinoma of sebaceous gland (most common
    site)
hydrocystoma
keratoacanthoma
milia
multiple mucosal neuroma (thickening of
    eyelids)
necrobiotic xanthogranuloma
nevi
seborrheic keratosis
syringoma
xanthelasma

## AROUND EYE

acne
adenoma sebaceum
basal cell nevus syndrome (AD)
colloid degeneration (milium)
dermoid cyst
hidrocystoma
lipoid proteinosis (AR)(linear waxy papules on
    free edge of eyelid)
necrobiotic xanthogranuloma
periorbital papules & plaques
sarcoidosis
senile comedones (Favre and Racouchot
    syndrome)
syringoma
trichoepithelioma
tricholemmoma
xanthelasma

**Eyebrow (loss, madarosis)**
alopecia areata
atopic dermatitis
hypothyroidism

leprosy (lepromatous)
ulerythema ophryogenes

**Eyelashes, long**
*AIDS*
    cyclosporine
    Kala–Azar
    Leukocyte A interferon

**Eyelid (Yellow papule)**
atypical lymphoid infiltrate
diffuse planar xanthoma
Erdheim–Chester disease
juvenile xanthogranuloma
lipoid proteinosis
necrobiosis lipoidica
necrobiotic xanthogranuloma
orbital lipogranulomata
primary systematic amyloidosis
sarcoid
tuberous xanthomata
Wegener's granulomatosis
xanthelasma

# Face

## BROWN ERUPTIONS OF THE FACE

**Idiopathic**
granuloma faciale
melasma
postinflammatory hyperpigmentation
sarcoidosis

**Neoplastic**
*Benign*
    dermatosis papulosa nigra
    lentigo maligna (most common location)
    nevus
    seborrheic keratosis

*Malignant*
    pigmented basal cell carcinoma
    malignant melanoma

## DESTRUCTIVE MIDLINE ERUPTIONS OF THE FACE

**Vascular**
Wegener's granulomatosis

**Infectious**
*Fungal*
    paracoccidioidomycosis (S. American
    blastomycosis)
    rhinosporidiosis
    zygomycosis (phycomycosis)

*Bacterial*
  leprosy
  lupus vulgaris
  necrotizing fascitis
  noma
  rhinoscleroma
*Parasitic*
  leishmaniasis
  myiasis
*Spirochetal*
  bejel
  syphilis
  yaws

## Idiopathic
lethal midline granuloma
sarcoidosis

## Neoplastic
basal cell carcinoma
lymphoma (reticulum cell sarcoma)
nasal gliomas and dermoids
squamous cell carcinoma

## EDEMA OF THE FACE

## Vascular
angioedema
Sturge–Weber syndrome
superior vena cava syndrome

## Infectious
erysipelas
herpes zoster
leprosy
lupus vulgaris
mononucleosis
trichinosis

## Allergic
allergic contact dermatitis
photoallergy
phytotoxicity

## Medicinal
steroids

## Metabolic
hypothyroidism
myxedema
nephrotic syndrome
scleromyxedema

## Idiopathic
acne
amyloidosis
dermatomyositis
fat pads
granulomatous chelitis
Melkersson–Rosenthal syndrome
panniculitis
rosacea
sarcoidosis
systemic lupus erythematosus

## Neoplastic
angiosarcoma
Kaposi sarcoma
leukemia (chronic lymphocytic leukemia*)
lymphoma
lymphosarcoma
mycosis fungoides
myeloma

## Congenital
Aper's syndrome
facial hemihypertrophy
Hurler's syndrome (AR)
infantile cortical hyperostosis
McCune–Albright syndrome

## FLESH-COLORED ERUPTIONS OF THE FACE

## Infectious
lepromatous leprosy
molluscum contagiosum
verruca plana

**Traumatic**
keloid

**Idiopathic**
amyloidosis
lupus miliaris disseminatus faciei
papular granuloma annulare

**Neoplastic**
*Benign*
cylindroma
fibrous histiocytoma
juvenile xanthogranuloma
neurofibroma
nevus
nevus sebaceous
pilomatrichoma
syringoma
trichoepithelioma
trichofolliculoma
*Malignant*
basal cell carcinoma

## LUPUS-LIKE ERUPTIONS OF THE FACE

**Vascular**
telangiectasia macularis eruptiva perstans

**Allergic**
contact dermatitis
erythrosis pigmentata faciei (erythrose
   peribuccale pigmentaire of Brocq)
perioral dermatitis
phototoxicity
polymorphous light eruption
seborrheic dermatitis

**Medicinal**
fixed drug eruption
poststeroid atrophy

**Idiopathic**
dermatomyositis
discoid lupus erythematosus
granuloma faciale

Jessner's lymphocytic infiltrate
pemphigus erythematosus
rosacea
scleroderma
systemic lupus erythematosus

**Congenital**
Bloom's syndrome (AR)
Cockayne's syndrome (AR)
Rothmund–Thomson syndrome (AR)

## RED/BLUE ERUPTIONS OF THE FACE

**Vascular**
angiokeratoma
hemangioma
pyogenic granuloma
urticaria

**Infectious**
infected acne cyst
syphilis

**Allergic**
contact dermatitis
polymorphous light eruption

**Medicinal**
fixed drug eruption

**Idiopathic**
alopecia mucinosa
granuloma faciale
Jessner's lymphocytic infiltrate
lichen myxedematosus
lichen planus
rosacea
sarcoidosis
systemic lupus erythematosus

**Neoplastic**
*Benign*
angiolymphoid hyperplasia with eosinophils
   (Kimura's disease)

apocrine/eccrine hydrocystoma
blue nevus
eccrine poroma/spiradenoma
fibrous histiocytoma
juvenile xanthogranuloma
lymphocytoma cutis
nasal glioma
pilomatricoma
Spitz's nevus
urticaria pigmentosa
*Malignant*
angiosarcoma
leukemia
lymphoma
mycosis fungoides
pigmented basal cell carcinoma

## WHITE/YELLOW ERUPTIONS OF THE FACE

**Infectious**
lupus vulgaris
molluscum contagiosum

**Idiopathic**
amyloidosis
xanthoma
xanthelasma

**Neoplastic**
adenoma sebaceum
closed comedo
juvenile xanthogranuloma
milia
nevus sebaceous
Spitz's nevus
sebaceous adenoma
sebaceous hyperplasia
syringoma

## VESICULOBULLOUS ERUPTIONS OF THE FACE

**Infectious**
bullous impetigo
herpes simplex
herpes zoster
varicella

**Traumatic**
factitious
insect bites
miliaria crystallina
second-degree burn

**Allergic**
contact dermatitis
polymorphous light eruption

**Medicinal**
bullous fixed drug eruption

**Idiopathic**
Behçet's syndrome
bullous erythema multiforme
bullous lichen planus
bullous pemphigoid
dermatitis herpetiformis
hydroa vacciniforme
pemphigus
porphyria cutanea tarda
toxic epidermal necrolysis

**Neoplastic**
urticaria pigmentosa

**Congenital**
Hailey–Hailey disease (AD)

# Foot

**Vascular**
angioedema
pyogenic granuloma
urticaria

**Infectious**
coccidioidal granuloma
Madura foot
pitted keratolysis
plantar wart
pyoderma
scabies
secondary syphilis
tinea pedis
tuberculosis

**Traumatic**
calcaneal petechiae (black heel)
callus
corn (clavus)
immersion foot
pernio
surfer's nodules

**Medicinal**
fixed drug eruption

**Metabolic**
hyperhidrosis

**Allergic**
atopic dermatitis
contact dermatitis

juvenile plantar dermatosis
pompholyx

**Idiopathic**
ainhum
erythema multiforme
hyperkeratosis plantaris
keratoderma climacterium
lichen planus
mal perforans (neuropathic ulcer)
pustulosis plantaris
Reiter's disease
scleroderma
symmetrical lividities of palms and soles (plantar
    erythema)

**Neoplastic**
*Benign*
    arsenical keratoses
    digital fibroma
    eccrine poroma
    glomus tumor
    myxoid cyst
    nevi
    painful fat herniation (piezogenic papules)
*Malignant*
    epitheloid sarcoma
    Kaposi's sarcoma
    malignant melanoma

**Congenital**
epidermolysis bullosa
hyperkeratosis lenticularis perstans (Flegel's
    disease, AD)
keratoderma palmaris et plantaris

# Forehead

acne
actinic keratosis
basal cell carcinoma
contact dermatitis
eczematous dermatitis
herpes zoster

nevi
psoriasis
scleroderma (*Én coup de Sabre*)
seborrheic dermatitis
seborrheic keratosis

# Genital

## PENILE/SCROTAL ERUPTIONS

**Vascular**
angiokeratoma of Fordyce
hemangioma
lymphangioma
lymphedema
pyogenic granuloma
urticaria

**Infectious**
*Fungal*
candida
dermatophytes
histoplasmosis
sporotrichosis
tinea versicolor
*Bacterial*
actinomycosis
chancroid
diphtheria
erysipelas
erythrasma
Fournier's gangrene
furunculosis
gardnerella vaginalis
gonorrhea
granuloma inguinale

lymphogranuloma venereum
tuberculosis
*Parasitic*
amebiasis
pediculosis pubis
scabies
*Spirochetal*
chancre (syphilis)
condyloma latum
*Viral*
bowenoid papulosis
condyloma acuminatum
herpes simplex
molluscum contagiosum

**Traumatic**
erosive balanoposthitis (secondary to poor
hygiene)
factitious
lipogranulomatosis (silicon injection)
trauma

**Allergic**
atopic dermatitis
contact dermatitis (dermatitis venenata;
contraceptive jellies, poison ivy/oak, rubber
condoms)
seborrheic dermatitis

**Medicinal**
fixed drug eruption

**Metabolic**
necrolytic migratory erythema (glucagonoma
  syndrome)
verruciform xanthoma

**Idiopathic**
aphthae (Behçet's syndrome)
bullous pemphigoid
Crohn's disease
erythema multiforme
Henoch–Shönlein syndrome
lichen nitidus
lichen planus
lichen sclerosis et atrophicus (balanitis xerotica
  obliterans)
necrobiosis lipoidica diabeticorum
non-venereal sclerosing lymphangitis
pearly penile papule
pemphigus vulgaris
Peyronie's disease
pigmented penile papules
psoriasis
pyoderma gangrenosum
Reiter's syndrome
sclerosing lymphangitis (non-venereal)
Stevens–Johnson syndrome
Zoon's (plasma cell) balanitis

**Neoplastic**
*Benign*
  epidermal cyst
  leiomyoma
  nevus
  seborrheic keratosis
*Premalignant*
  cutaneous horn
  erythroplasia of Queyrat
  leukoplakia
*Malignant*
  basal cell carcinoma
  extramammary Paget's disease
  fibrosarcoma
  hemangioendothelioma
  Kaposi's sarcoma
  leiomyosarcoma
  malignant melanoma

metastases
rhabdomyosarcoma
sarcomas
squamous cell carcinoma

**Congenital**
acrodermatotis entropathica (AD)
angiokeratoma corporis diffusum
  (Fabry's disease, XR)
Hailey–Hailey disease (AD)
porokeratosis of Mibelli (AD)

## PENILE ULCER

aphthosis (Behçet's disease)
chancre (syphilis)
chancroid
gonorrhea
granuloma inguinale
herpes simplex (primary and recurrent)
tuberculosis
trauma
tumor
verruca

## VAGINA/VULVA ERUPTIONS

*Acute ulcer of vaginal area*
**Infectious**
*Bacterial*
  chancroid
  gonorrhea
  granuloma inguinale
  syphilis
*Viral*
  hand, foot and mouth disease
  herpes simplex/zoster

**Allergic**
contact dermatitis

**Medicinal**
fixed drug eruption

**Metabolic**
uremia

**Idiopathic**
cicatricial pemphigoid
Steven–Johnson syndrome

**Congenital**
dystrophic epidermolysis bullosa
Hailey–Hailey disease (AD)

**Chronic eruption or ulcer of vaginal area**
**Vascular**
angiokeratoma (of Fordyce)
elephantiasis of vulva
hemangioma
lymphangioma
pyogenic granuloma
telangiectasia of the vulva
thrombophlebitis of vulva
vulvar varicosities

**Infectious**
*Fungal*
  blastomycosis
  moniliasis
  tinea cruris
*Bacterial*
  actinomycosis
  Bartholin gland abscess
  chancroid
  follicullitis
  furunculosis
  gonorrhea
  granuloma inguinale
  lymphogranuloma venereum
  tuberculosis
*Parasitic*
  pediculosis
  pinworms
  scabies
  trichomoniasis
*Spirochetal*
  syphilis
*Viral*
  herpes simplex/zoster

**Traumatic**
factitious
hematoma secondary to trauma

**Metabolic**
diabetes mellitus

**Idiopathic**
acanthosis nigricans
acne (comedo)
aphthae
Behçet's syndrome
Crohn's disease
hidradenitis suppurativa
intertrigo
lichen planus
lichen sclerosis et atrophicus
pyoderma gangrenosum
ulcerative colitis

**Neoplastic**
*Benign*
  Bartholin gland cyst
  ectopic breast tissue
  endometriosis
  epidermal cyst
  fibroepithelial polyp
  fibroma
  Fox–Fordyce disease
  granular cell tumors
  hidradenoma papilliferum
  leiomyomas (fibroid)
  lipoma
  Muellerian cyst
  neurofibroma
  nevus
  sebaceous hyperplasia and tumors
  seborrheic keratosis
  syringoma
*Premalignant*
  Bowen's disease
*Malignant*
  basal cell carcinoma
  Bartholin's gland carcinoma
  extramammary Paget's disease
  Kaposi's sarcoma
  malignant melanoma

metastases
sarcoma
squamous cell carcinoma
verrucous carcinoma

psoriasis
seborrheic dermatitis
Zoon's vulvitis (vulvitis chronica
    plasmacellularis)

### Pruritus With Rash of Vaginal Area
associated with pruritus ani
candidiasis
contact dermatitis (allergic or irritant)
Crohn's disease
dermatophytosis
herpes simplex/zoster
lichen sclerosis et atrophicus
lichen simplex chronicus

### Pruritus Without Rash of Vaginal Area
diabetes mellitus
pediculosis
pinworms
psychogenic
scabies
vaginitis (atrophic vaginitis, candida, gardnerella,
    trichomonas)
vulvodynia

# Groin

### Infectious
candidiasis
erythrasma
tinea cruris

impetigo herpetiformis
pemphigus vegetans
subcorneal pustular dermatosis
    (Sneddon–Wilkinson disease)
*Other disorders*
    Dowling–Degos' disease (reticulate
        pigmented anomaly of the flexures)
psoriasis

### Traumatic
intertrigo

### Allergic
lichen simplex chronicus
seborrheic dermatitis

### Neoplastic
eruptive xanthoma
xanthoma disseminatum

### Idiopathic
*Bullous disorders*
    bullous pemphigoid
    chronic bullous disease of childhood

### Congenital
Darier's disease (AD, rare)
Hailey–Hailey disease (AD)

# Hair

## *Cicatricial (scarring)*

### Infectious
favus
kerion
leprosy
lupus vulgaris
perifolliculitis capitis abscedens et suffodiens
 (dissecting cellulitis of scalp)
pseudopelade of Brocq*
tertiary syphilis

### Traumatic
postnecrotic herpes zoster
trauma (burn, radiation, etc.)

### Idiopathic
*Bullous disorders*
 cicatricial pemphigoid
*Collagen vascular disease*
 dermatomyositis
 discoid lupus erythematosus*
*Other disorders*
 acne keloidalis nuchae
 alopecia mucinosa
 alopecia parvimacularis
 amyloidosis
 chronic late (sclerotic) graft versus host
 disease
 folliculitis decalvans
 keratosis folliculoris spinulosa decalvans
 lichen planopilaris*
 lichen sclerosis et atrophicus
 lipedematous alopecia
 morphea
 necrobiosis lipoidica diabeticorum
 sarcoidosis
 scleroderma
 ulerythema ophryogenes

### Neoplastic
epidermal nevus
other tumors (basal cell carcinoma, cylindroma,
 lymphoma, squamous cell carcinoma,
 metastases)

### Congenital
aplasia cutis congenita
Darier's disease (AD)

## *Non-cicatricial (non-scarring)*

### Infectious
dermatophytosis (tinea capitis)
folliculitis
herpes zoster
secondary syphilis

### Traumatic
friction alopecia
hair cosmetics
traction alopecia
trichotillomania

### Allergic
contact dermatitis (irritant/primary; especially
 hair dyes)
exfoliative dermatitis

### Medicinal
β-blockers
chemotherapeutic agents
coumarin
dilantin
nonsteroidal anti-inflammatory drugs
oral contraceptive pill

**Metabolic**
androgenetic alopecia
hyper/hypo-thyroidism

**Idiopathic**
alopecia areata
*anagen effluvium*
    antimitotic (cancer therapy) agents
    excessive X-ray irradiation to scalp
    ingestion of arsenic/bismuth/coumarin/lead/
       thallium
hair shaft abnormalities (bamboo hair,
    monilethrix, pili torti, trichorrhexis nodosa,
    trichothiodystrophy)
medications (allopurinol, amitriptyline, anabolic
    steroids, anticonvulsants (carbamazepine),
    coumarin, discontinuation of
    estrogen-dominanted oral contraceptive
    pills, doxepin, haldol, heparin, indocin,
    lithium, nitrofurantoin, probenecid,
    propranolol, sulfasalazine, thioureas, timolol,
    triparanol, valporic acid, vitamin A excess)
postpartum
severe chronic illness
severe infectious
severe psychologic stress
*telogen effluvium*
    crash diets
    high fever
    hyper/hypo-thyroidism
    major surgery
    malnutrition (poor protein uptake)

**Congenital**
ectodermal dysplasias
progeria (AR)

## HIRSUTISM

**Traumatic**
iatrogenic (adrenocorticotropic hormone and
    systemic steroid therapy, anabolic steroids,
    testosterone)

**Medication**
corticosteroids
diazoxide
minoxidil

phenothiazine
phenytoin

**Metabolic**
acromegaly
Cushing's syndrome
physiologic (menopause, precocious puberty,
    pregnancy, puberty)

**Idiopathic**
end organ hypersensitivity

**Neoplastic**
*Benign*
    adrenal adenoma
    polycystic ovarian syndrome*
*Malignant*
    adrenal carcinoma
    hypertrichosis lanuginosa acquisita
    non-endocrine malignancies producing
       ACTH-like substance
    ovarian carcinoma (arrhenoblastoma,
       granulosa-theca-cell tumor, hilus-cell
       tumor, metastatic ovarian carcinoma)

**Congenital**
congenital adrenal hyperplasia

## HYPERTRICHOSIS

**Traumatic**
burn
chronic rubbing
head injury
plaster cast
PUVA
radiation

**Medicinal**
adrenocorticotropic hormone
astezolamide
corticosteroids
cyclosporine
dANAZOL
diaxoxide (common in children, not in adults)

dilantin
DIPHENYLHYDANTOIN (MORE COMMON
　IN FEMALES, OCCURS IN 2–3 MONTHS)
hexachlorobenzene
minoxidil
oral contraceptive pill (progestational
　component)
penicillamine
PSORALENS
steroid drugs containing androgens
STREPTOMYCIN
tamoxifen

## Metabolic
acromegaly
Cushing's syndrome
FETAL ALCOHOL (In 40% of children of
　alcoholics)
Fetal hydantoin
hyperprolactinemia
hypothyroidism
porphyria (congenital porphyria, porphyria
　cutanea tarda)
starvation

## Central nervous system disorders
anorexia nervosa
hyperostotic internal craniopathy (Morgani's
　syndrome)
multiple sclerosis
postencephalitis
schizophrenia

## Idiopathic
acquired hypertrichosis lanuginosa
dermatomyositis

## Neoplastic
Becker's nevus
hamartoma (smooth muscle hamartoma)
nevus

## Congenital
bird-headed dwarfism of Seckel
Cornelia–De Lange's syndrome
Craniofacial dysostosis and patent arteriosus
Gingival hyperplasia & hypertrichosis

Hurler's syndrome
hypertrichosis lanuginosa (universalis)
Leprechaunism
Lipoatrophic diabete (Lawrence–Seip
　Syndrome)
Morquio (mucopolysaccharidosis with bone
　changes)
Rubenstein–Taylor
Schynzel–Giedier
Winchester
idiopathic gingival fibromatosis and
　hypertrichosis
trisomy E

## PIGMENTARY HAIR DISORDERS

albinism
canities
copper deficiency (Menke's kinky-hair disease)
drugs (bleaches, chloroquine,
　fluorobutyrophenone, triparanol)
homocystinuria
iron deficiency (severe)
phenylketonuria
poliosis
protein malnutrition (kwashiorkor)

## Hypomelanosis of hair
A-Diffuse pigment loss or decrease
Aging
Albinism
Book syndrome
Chediak–Higashi syndrome
Chronic protein deficiency
Copper deficiency
Cross–McKusick–Breen syndrome
Downs syndrome
Fanconi's syndrome
Fisch's syndrome
Hallerman–Streiff syndrome
Hermansky–Pudlak syndrome
Histidinemia
Homocystinuria
Malabsorption syndrome
　Acquired immunodeficiency syndrome
　(malnutrition)
　ulcerative colitis
　vitamin B12 deficiency

Medication
  bleomycin
  chloroquine
  haloperidol
  hydroxychloroquine
  mephenesin
  nafoxidine
  p-Aminiobenzoic acid
  valproic acid
Menkes' kinky hair syndrome
myotonia dystrophica
nephrosis
phenylketonuria
Pierre Robin syndrome
progeria
prolidase deficiency
Rothmund–Thomson syndrome
Seckel's syndrome("bird-headed"dwarfism)
Treacher–Collins syndrome
tyrosinuria
vitiligo
Waardenburg'syndrome
Werner's syndrome
Woolf's syndrome
Ziprkowski–Margolis syndrome

**B-localized pigment loss or decrease**
Alezzandrini's syndrome
alopecia areata
Burns (thermal,ultraviolet)
chloroquine
halo nevi
hydroxychloroquine
ionizing radiation
leukoderma acquisitum centrifugum
malignant melanoma
mephenesin
neurofibromatosis
piebaldism

postinflammatory
prolidase deficiency
trauma
tuberous sclerosis
vitiligo
Vogt–Koyanagi–harada syndrome
Waardeburg's syndrome
Woolf's syndrome

## STRUCTURAL HAIR SHAFT DISORDERS

*Associated with increased fragility*
Menkes' kinky-hair syndrome (XR)
monilethrix (AD, rarely AR)
Netherton's syndrome (trichorrhexis
  invaginata, AR)
pili torti (AD)
Pohl–Pinkus constriction (equivalent of Beau's
  line on nails)
trichomalacia
trichoptilosis
trichorrhexis nodosa (most common)
trichothiodystrophy (AR)

*Not associated with increased fragility*
pili annulati (ringed hair, AD)
pili multigemini (multiple of terminal hairs)
spun glass hair syndrome (uncombable hair
  syndrome)
straight hair nevus (similar to woolly hair
  syndrome, seen in Blacks)
trichonodosis
trichostasis spinulosa (retention of multiple
  vellus hairs)
woolly hair syndrome

# Hand

**Vascular**
pyogenic granuloma

**Infectious**
*Fungal*
  deep fungal infection (sporotrichosis)
  dermatophytosis
*Bacteria*
  anthrax
  atypical mycobacteria
  erysipeloid
  furuncle
  leprosy
  primary inoculation tuberculosis
  tularemia
*Parasitic*
  scabies
*Spirochetal*
  syphilis
*Viral*
  cowpox
  molluscum contagiosum
  orf
  verruca vulgaris

**Traumatic**
calluses
foreign body granuloma
radiodermatitis

**Allergic**
contact dermatitis
dermatitis medicamentosa
dyshidrotic eczema
eczematous dermatitis
'-id reaction'

**Metabolic**
calcinosis
gout
pellagra

**Idiopathic**
disseminated lupus erythematosus

erythema multiforme
granuloma annulare
hyperhidrosis
keratoderma
pityriasis rubra pilaris
lichen planus
porphyria cutanea tarda
psoriasis
scleroderma
vitiligo

**Neoplastic**
*Benign*
  giant-cell tumor of tendon sheaths
  glomus tumor
  keratoacanthoma
  myxoid cyst
  synovial cysts
  xanthoma
*Premalignant*
  actinic keratosis
*Malignant*
  basal cell carcinoma
  melanoma
  squamous cell carcinoma

**Congenital**
acrokeratosis verruciformis (of Hopf, AD)
xeroderma pigmentosum (AR)

## HAND DERMATITIS

**Endogenous**
atopic dermatitis
psoriasis

**Exogenous**
contact dermatitis (allergic, irritant)
infections: bacterial, hand/foot/mouth disease,
  herpes simplex, scabies, tinea manum

# Hands and feet

## Infectious
*Fungal*
 dermatophyte
*Bacterial*
 bullous impetigo
*Parasitic*
 scabies
*Viral*
 hand, foot, and mouth disease
 herpes simplex

## Traumatic
friction blister
insect bites
second degree burn

## Allergic
contact dermatitis
dyshidrotic eczema
photoallergic drug eruption
polymorphous light eruption

## Medicinal
bullous fixed drug eruption

## Metabolic
diabetic bullae

## Idiopathic
acrodermatitis perstans (acrodermatitis
 continua, dermatitis repens)
bullous lichen planus
bullous pemphigoid
discoid lupus erythematosus
erythema elevatum diutinum
erythema multiforme
hydroa vacciniforme
porphyria cuatnea tarda
Sweet's syndrome
vesicular '-id reaction'

## Congenital
acrokeratoelastoidosis of Costa (AD)
epidermolysis bullosa
Weber–Cockayne syndrome (AR)

# Inframammary

acrochordon
candidiasis
contact dermatitis
cutaneous papillomatosis
intertrigo
lichen nitidus
psoriasis

reticulated pigmented dermatosis of the
 flexures
seborrheic dermatitis
subcorneal pustular dermatosis
 (Sneddon–Wilkinson's disease)
tinea versicolor

72

# Leg

**Vascular**
angiokeratoma circumscriptum
Burger's disease
Churg–Strauss syndrome (allergic
　granulomatosis)
embolic nodule
leukocytoclastic vasculitis
nodular vasculitis
polyarteritis nodosa
superficial thrombophlebitis
Wegener's granulomatosis

**Infectious**
*Fungal*
　deep fungi (sporotrichosis)
　nodular granulomatous perifolliculitis
　Majocchi's granuloma
*Bacterial*
　staphylococcal infections
*Parasitic*
　cutaneous myiasis

**Idiopathic**
erythema induratum
erythema nodosum
sarcoidosis
subcutaneous fat necrosis
Sweet's syndrome
Weber–Christian disease

**Neoplastic**
Kaposi's sarcoma
metastases

**Vascular**
arterial claudication
lymphedema
spinal claudication
thrombophlebitis
varicose veins
venous claudication

**Infectious**
osteomyelitis

**Traumatic**
achilles tendonitis or tear
meniscial tear

**Idiopathic**
myalgia
osteoarthritis
peripheral neuropathy
rheumatoid arthritis

angioleiomyoma
angiolipoma
cold panniculitis (and other panniculitides)
erythema induratum
erythema nodosum
eccrine poroma
hematoma
Kaposi's sarcoma
leiomyoma
localized myxedema
lupus profundus
myositis
polyarteritis nodosa
sarcoma

superficial thrombophlebitis
trichinosis

## ULCER OF LEG

### Vascular
arteriovenous malformation
arteriosclerosis obliterans
atheromatous emboli
atrophie blanche
Burger's disease (thromboangiitis obliterans)
hypertensive ischemic ulcer
Klippel–Trenaunay–Weber syndrome
leukocytoclastic vasculitis
livedo reticularis
lymphedema
necrotizing angiitis
postphlebitis syndrome
septic emboli
stasis ulcer (varicose veins)

### Infectious
*Fungal*
blastomycosis
chromoblastomycosis
coccidiomycosis
cryptococcosis
histoplasmosis
mycetoma
sporotrichosis
*Bacterial*
actinomycosis
anthrax
atypical mycobacteria (and tuberculosis)
ecthyma
ecthyma gangrenosum
furuncle
leprosy
Meleney's gangrene (peptostreptococcus)
nocardia
tropical phagedenic ulcer (*Bacillus fusiformis*,
    *Spirochaeta vincenti*)
*Pseudomonas aeruginosa*
tularemia
*Parasitic*
leishmaniasis
*Spirochetal*
pinta
syphilis (tabes dorsalis)
yaws

### Traumatic
bites
burns (chemical, electrical)
chilblains (pernio)
facticious
frostbite
radiation dermatitis
traumatic

### Medicinal
barbiturate
ergot
halogens
methotrexate

### Metabolic
calcinosis cutis
diabetes mellitus
Gaucher's disease
gout
porphyria cutanea tarda
prolidase deficiency (AR)

### Idiopathic
acrodermatitis chronica atrophicans
epidermolysis bullosa
lichen planus
necrobiosis lipoidica diabeticorum
pancreatic fat necrosis
panniculitis
pyoderma gangrenosum
rheumatoid arthritis
Sjögren's syndrome
Weber–Christian disease

### Neoplastic
angiosarcoma
basal cell carcinoma
Kaposi's sarcoma
leukemia
malignant angioendothelioma
malignant melanoma
metastases
mycosis fungoides
squamous cell carcinoma
syringomyelia

**Hematologic**
coagulopathies
Cooley's anemia
cryoglobulinemia
Felty's syndrome
hereditary spherocytosis
microthrombotic angiopathy
paraproteinemia
polycythemia rubra vera
sickle cell anemia
thalassemia

amyloidosis
angioma serpiginosum
bromoderma
clear-cell acanthoma
lichen planus
lichen simplex chronicus
spitz nevus
stucco keratosis
superficial spreading melanoma *in situ* (especially in women)

# Lip

**Infectious**
candida

**Traumatic**
lip smacking
trauma

**Allergic**
contact dermatitis (allergic/primary irritant; cigarette holders, citrus fruits, chewing gum, cosmetics, dentifrices, mango, mouthwash, nail polish, sunscreen)
xerosis

**Medicinal**
deficiency of vitamin A/biotin/thiamine
hypervitaminosis A

**Metabolic**
accutane
etretinate

**Vascular**
angioedema
angioma
pyogenic granuloma
venous lake

**Infectious**
angular cheilitis (perlèche, candidiasis)
herpes simplex
syphilis (chancre, gummas)
verruca

**Traumatic**
angular cheilitis (secondary to ill-fitting dentures)

**Allergic**
cheilitis exfoliativa (seborrheic dermatitis)

**Medicinal**
drug-induced ulcer (chlorpromazine,
    methyldopa, phenobarbital, phenylbutazone,
    thiazides)

**Metabolic**
vitamin deficiencies

**Idiopathic**
cheilitis glandularis
elephantiasis
erythema multiforme
lichen planus
lupus erythematosus

**Neoplastic**
actinic cheilitis
basal cell carcinoma
Fordyce's spots
Leukoplakia
Microcystic adnexal carcinoma (upper lip)
mucocele
pilar sheath acanthoma (seen in the upper lip of
    adults)
plasma cell cheilitis
squamous cell carcinoma

**Congenital**
multiple mucosal neuromas

## SWELLING OF LIP

**Vascular**
angioedema
hemangioma
hematoma
lymphangioma

**Infectious**
dental abscess
granulomatous infections

**Idiopathic**
Ascher's syndrome
Crohn's disease
Fabry's disease
sarcoidosis

**Neoplastic**
leukemic infiltrate
neurofibroma

# Mouth

see Oral

# Nail

## ANONYCHIA

Coffin–Siris Syndrome
congenital ectodermal defect
ichthyosis

lichen planus
maternal hydantoin ingestion
nail-patella syndrome
Raynaud's phenomenon
severe allergic contact dermatitis

severe exfoliative disease
severe infection
trauma

## ARREST OF NAIL MATRIX

acrodermatitis enteropathica
amelogenesis imperfecta
antibiotics
bullous disorders
cytotoxic agents
high fever
hypoparathyroidism
Kawasaki's disease
local trauma or inflammation
radiation therapy
retinoid therapy
Stevens–Johnson syndrome
syphilis

## BEAU'S LINES

Transverse furrows that start in the matrix and
   progress distally with nail growth

acute hypocalcemia
Asian flu
carpal tunnel syndrome
chronic eczema
chronic glomerulonephritis
chronic paronychia
combined chemotherapy
coronary thrombosis
cuticle damage due to nervous habits
dapsone
diabetes mellitus
dysmenorrheae
exposure to severe cold
flurosis
gout
hand and wrist trauma
high fever
hydrochloride
hypertension
hyperthyroidism
hypoparathyroidism
hypopituitarism
intrauterine distress
local inflammation

malaria
mechlorethamine
measles
metoprolol
mucocutaneous and lymph node syndrome
mumps
mustine hydrochloride
myelomatosis
overzealous manicuring
pemphigus vulgaries
pneumonia
prednisone
procabazine
pustular psoriasis and telogen effluvium
Raynaud's disease
Retinoids
Severe seziures
Steven–Johnson syndrome
vincristine
Zinc deficiency

### Bilateral Beau's lines
seen with systemic disease

### Unilateral Beau's lines
seen with vascular abnormalities or trauma

## CHANGES IN COLOR OF NAIL

### Black
cyclophosphamide
doxorubicin
gangrene
gold salts
hemorrhage
malignant melanoma
nevocellular nevi
saprophytic onychomycoses
tar

### Blue
**Vascular**
cyanosis
Klippel–Trenaunay syndrome

**Traumatic**
ink

**Medicinal**
antimalarials
bleomycin
minocin
phenolphthalein
phenothiazines

**Idiopathic**
argyria
Wilson's disease

**Neoplastic**
glomus tumor

**Congenital**
congenital pernicious anemia

*Brown*
**Infectious**
syphilis

**Traumatic**
nail enamel
nail hardeners
post trauma
radiotherapy

**Medicinal**
adrenocorticotropic hormone
actinomycin D
anthralin
arsenic
bleomycin
busulfan
cyclophosphamide
doxycycline
iodine
ketoconazole
melphalan
methotrexate
minocin
nitrogen mustard

psoralen
sulfonamides
tetracycline

**Metabolic**
adrenal disease
malnutrition
pregnancy
vitamin B$_{12}$ deficiency

**Idiopathic**
normal racial pigmentation
Peutz–Jeghers' syndrome

**Neoplastic**
malignant melanoma
metastatic breast carcinoma
nevus

*Green*
*Aspergillus*
epidermophyton floccosum
*Pseudomonas*

*Grey*
formaldehyde
hydroquinone
silver nitrate

*Orange*
anthralin

*Orange–brown*
**Traumatic**
nail hardeners
nail polish

**Medicinal**
hydroxyquinone
mercury
vioform

**Metabolic**
Addison's disease
hemochromatosis
hyperthyroidism

**Pale**
anemia

**Purple**
coumarin
gentian violet

**Red**
angiomas
carbon monoxide
cardiac fialure
enchondromas
glomus tumor
lymphogranuloma venereum
polycythemia
rheumatoid arthritis
systemic lupus erythematosus

**Salmon–orange**
psoriasis

**White (leukonychia)**
acrokeratosis verrciformis
alopecia areata
cirrhosis
Darier disease
exfoliative dermatitis
hypoalbuminemia
leprosy
leukonychia punctata
leukonychia striata
pellagra
thiazides
zinc deficiency

**Yellow**
amphotericin B
carotene
diabetes mellitus
jaundice
lymphedema

nicotine
onychomycosis
penicillamine
tar
tetracycline

**Yellow–brown**
*Candida albicans*

## CLUBBING OF NAIL

Most commonly seen with cardiopulmonary
diseases

**Bilateral**
seen with systemic disease

**Unilateral**
seen with vascular abnormalities or trauma
bronchogenic carcinoma
bronchopulmonary disease
carcinoma of colon, esophagus, stomach
chronic active hepatitis
congenital heart disease
congestive heart failure
endocarditis
familial
hypervitaminosis A
idiopathic
malnutrition
polycythemia
sarcoidosis
subacute bacterial endocarditis
systemic lupus erythematosis
ulcerative colitis

## DYSTROPHY OF NAIL

**Acquired**
alopecia areata
Darier's disease
eczematous dermatitis
iron deficiency (koilonychia)
lichen planus
onychomycosis
paronychia
psoriasis

trauma
tumor
twenty nail syndrome

### Congenital
congenital ectodermal dysplasia
dyskeratosis congenita (XR)
epidermolysis bullosa
nail–patella syndrome (AD)
pachyonychia congenita (AD)

## HALF-AND-HALF NAIL (Lindsay's nails)

chronic renal failure

## HAPALONYCHIA (soft nail)

drugs (etretinate)
leprosy
malnutrition
myxedema
radiodermatitis
Raynaud's phenomenon

## HYPERKERATOTIC CUTICLES AND PROMINENT PERIUNGUAL TELANGIECTASIA

dermatomyositis
overlap syndrome
progressive systemic sclerosis
systemic lupus erythematosus

## KOILONYCHIA (spoon nail)

acanthosis nigricans
congenital
coronary artery disease
hemochromatosis*
iron deficiency anemia*
Plummer–Vinson syndrome*
Polycythemia
Repeated trauma (chemical or physical)
Syphilis

## LUNULA

**Blue lunula-**
Argyria
Chemotherapy
Exlax
Hemoglobin M disease
Hereditary acrolabial telangiectases
Wilson's disease
Zidovudine

**Brown lunula-**
Antineoplastic agents
Zidovudine

**Red lunula-**
Collagen vascular disease
alcoholism
Alopecia areata
Carbon monoxide poisoning
Chronic obstructive pulmonary disease
Congestive heart failure
Darier's disease
Glomus tumor
Keratosis induced by ionizing radiation
Lymphogranuloma venereum
Rheumatoid arthritis
Tobacco abuse
Subungal arteriovenous tumor

**Spotted lunar dyschromia-**
Alopecia ateata
Psoriasis

**White lunula-**
Alopecia areata
Cirrhosis
Congestive heart failure
Darier's disease
Diabetes mellitus
Ischemia
Leprosy
Malabsorption
Thyrotoxicosis

**Yellow lunula-**
Insecticides & weed killers
Tetracycline

**Triangular (v-shaped) lunula-**
Nail-patella syndrome (hereditary
    osteoonychodysplasia)
Trauma
Trisomy 21

## MACROLUNULA – APPLICATION OF HYDROCORTISONE TO CUTICLE

Habit-tic deformity
Hyperthyroidism
Median nail dystrophy

## MICROLUNULA & ANOLUNULA

Acromegaly
Adipose-genital dystrophy
Atherosclerosis
Brachyonychia
Chronic obstructive pulmonary disease
Erythrooietic protoporphyria
Goltz syndrome (focal dermal hypoplasia)
HIV infection
Hyperthyroidism
hypopituitarism
Hypothyroidism
Iron deficiency anemia
leprosy
malnutrition
monosomia
multiple myeloma
nail-patella syndrome
nerve injury
pacyonychia congenita
penicillamine
porphyria cutanea tarda
renal failure
rheumatoid arthritis
scleroderma
trisomy 21

## MEES' LINES

Transverse white bands (single or multiple) in
    the *nail plate*

acute and chronic renal failure
arsenic ingestion*
dissecting aortic aneurysm
septicemia
thallium poisoning

## MELANONYCHIA

**Infectious**
*Fungal*
    blastomycosis
    candida
    hendresonula tourloidea
    *Trichophyton soudanese*
*Bacteria*
    *Proteus mirabilis*
*Spirochetal*
    pinta
    secondary syphilis
*Viral*
    AIDS
    verruca vulgaris

**Traumatic**
carpal tunnel syndrome
dye
foreign body
irradiation
postinflammatory hyperpigmentation
onychotillomania
trauma

**Medicinal**
antimalarials
arsenic
AZT
bleomycin
cyclophosphamide
gold
ketoconazole
ketotin
methotrexate
minocycline

phenolphthalein
phenthiazine
psoralen
sulfonamide
tetracycline
timolol

**Metabolic**
Addison's disease
Cushing's syndrome
hemosiderosis
hyperbilirubinemia
hyperthyroidism
malnutrition
porphyria
pregnancy
vitamin $B_{12}$ deficiency

**Idiopathic**
acanthosis nigricans
Laugier–Hunziker syndrome
lichen planus
lichen striatus
Peutz–Jeghers syndrome
racial (Black, Hispanic, Indian)

**Neoplastic**
basal cell carcinoma
Bowen's disease
breast carcinoma
lentigo
malignant melanoma
metastatic malignant melanoma
mucous cyst
nevus
subungual fibrous histiocytoma

## MUEHRCKE'S LINES

Narrow white transverse bands in *nail bed*

chemotherapy
hypoalbuminemia

## ONYCHAUXIS

Simple hypertrophy of nail

acromegaly
Darier's disease
pityriasis rubra pilaris
psoriasis
trauma

## ONYCHOLYSIS

Separation of nail plate from the nail bed

**Vascular**
peripheral ishemia

**Infectious**
dermatophytosis*
leprosy
paronychia
polio
syphilis (secondary & tertiary)

**Traumatic**
contact irritants*
different nail treatments
factitious
exposure to weed killers
photo-onycholysis
trauma* (chemical or physical)

**Allergic**
atopic dermatitis
eczematous dermatitis
id reaction

**Medicinal**
doxycycline
minocycline
tetracycline
thiazides

**Metabolic**
diabetes mellitus
hypo/hyperthyroidism
hyperhidrosis
pellagra
pregnancy
vitamin C deficiency

**Idiopathic**
alopecia universalis
amyloidosis
bronchiectasis
erythropoietic porphyria
eryhtropoietic protoporphyria
histiocytosis
pemphigus vulgaris
porphyria cutanea tarda
pseudoporphyria of hemodialysis
psoriasis*
Raynaud's disease
Reiter's syndrome
scleroderma
shell nail syndrome
systemic lupus erythematosus
yellow nail syndrome

**Neoplastic**
Cutaneous T-cell lymphoma
Multiple myeloma
Sezary syndrome

**Hematologic**
anemia

**Congenital**
Cronkhite–Canada syndrome
hidrotic ectodermal dysplasia

## ONYCHOMADESIS

Periodic idiopathic shedding of the nail,
   commencing at its proximal end

Darier's disease
epidermolysis bullosa
keratosis punctata palmaris et plantaris

leprosy
lichen planus
multicentric reticulohistiocytosis
penicillin allergy
vascular abnormalities

## PAINFUL NAIL

**Vascular**
Raynaud's phenomenon

**Infectious**
abscess
herpes virus (herpetic whitlow)
osteomyelitis (acute)
paronychia (acute)
subungual verruca vulgaris
tuberculosis verrucosa cutis

**Traumatic**
cold injury
crush injuries
splinter
sports injury

**Neoplastic**
corn
enchondroma
fibroma
glomus tumor
keratoacanthoma
leiomyoma
malignant melanoma
neuroma
osteoid osteoma
squamous cell carcinoma

## PARONYCHIA (Chronic)

acrodermatitis enteropathica
bacterial infectious
celiac disease
hypoparathyroidism
Reiter's syndrome
retinoids

## PITS AND GROOVES OF NAIL

alopecia areata*
Darier's disease
dermatitis of posterior nail fold
lichen planus*
median nail dystrophy
paronychia
pityriasis rosea
physiological (post-illness, Beau's lines)
psoriasis*
Reiter's syndrome
rheumatoid arthritis
sarcoidosis
secondary syphilis
trauma

## PLUMMER'S NAIL

Concave contour with distal onycholysis

**allergic contact dermatitis**
hyperthyroidism
hypothyroidism
psoriasis
traumatic injury

## PTERYGIUM UNGUIS (DORSAL PTERYGIUM)

atherosclerosis
burns
cicatricial pemphigoid
congenital
diabetic vasculopathy
dyskeratosis congenita
dystrophic epidermolysis bullosa
graft versus host disease
idiopathic atrophy of the nails
infection
lichen planus*
onychotillomania
pemphigus foliaceus
peripheral vascular disease
radiodermatitis
raynaud's phenomenon
sarcoidosis (of proxinail nail fold)

systemic lupus erythematosus
toxic epidermal necrolysis
trauma
type 2 lepra reaction

## PTERYGIUM INVERSUS UNGUIUM (VENTRAL PTERYGIUM)

causalgia of the median nerve
congenital
connective tissue diseases
formaldehyde-containing hardeners
lenticular atrophy of the palmar creases
leprosy
neurofibromatosis
paresis
peripheral vascular diseases
Raynaud's phenomenon
Scarring in the vicinity of the distal nail groove
Subungual exostosis
systemic lupus erythematosus
Systemic sclerosis

## SHELL NAIL SYNDROME

Nail resembles clubbing nail, but the nail bed is *atrophic*. Associated with *bronchiectasis*

## SPLINTER HEMORRHAGE & SUBUNGAL PURPURA

**Vascular**
Burger's disease
emboli
hypertension
Raynaud's phenomenon
vasculitis

**Infectious**
hepatitis
HIV
meningococcemia
onychomycosis
psittacosis
rheumatic fever
septicemia

subacute bacterial endocarditis
trichinosis

### Traumatic
poor hygiene
trauma

### Allergic
eczematous dermatitis
exfoliative dermatitis

### Medicinal
tetracycline

### Metabolic
cirrhosis
diabetes mellitius
dialysis (hemo/peritoneal)
glomerulonephritis
hemochromatosis
hypertension
hypoparathyroidism
kidney disease
lung disease
mitral stenosis
peptic ulcer disease
scurvy
thyrotoxicosis

### Idiopathic
Behçet's disease
collagen vascular disease
cystic fibrosis
histiocytosis X
multiple sclerosis
pemphigoid
pemphigus
periarteritis nodosa
porphyria
psoriasis
Raynaud's disease
rheumatoid arthritis
sarcoidosis
vasculitis
Wegener's granulomatosis

### Neoplastic
cutaneous T-cell lymphoma
leukemia
variety of malignancies

### Hematologic
cryoglobulinemia
thrombocytopenia

### Congenital
Darier's disease (AD)
Histiocytosis
Osler—weber—Rendu

## TERRY'S NAIL

Entire nail plate or proximal end is white, but
the distal 1–2 mm of the nail shows a
normal pink color

adult onset diabetes mellitus
chronic congestive heart failure
cirrhosis*
very old age
hypoalbuminemia

## TRACHYONCHIA

Rough surfaced, brittle nails, frayed at edges

alopecia areata
chronic eczema
ichthyosis vulgaris
IgA deficiency
psoriasis

## TUMORS OF NAIL AND NAIL SURROUNDINGS

### Infectious
molluscum contagiosum
verruca vulgaris

**Traumatic**
foreign body granuloma
keloid

**Idiopathic**
erythema elevatum diutinum
Gottron's papules

**Neoplastic**
*Benign*
    dermatofibroma
    eccrine poroma
    enchondroma
    epidermal cyst
    exostosis
    fibrokeratoma
    giant-cell tumor of tendon sheath
    glomus tumor
    granuloma

    keratoacanthoma
    Koenen's periungual fibroma
    mucous cyst
    neurofibroma
    neuroma
    nevus
    osteochondroma
    pyogenic granuloma
*Premalignant*
    actinic keratosis
    Bowen's disease
*Malignant*
    amelanotic melanoma
    basal cell carcinoma
    fibrosarcoma
    Kaposi's sarcoma
    lymphoma
    metastasis
    sarcoma
    squamous cell carcinoma

# Neck

## GENERAL NECK ERUPTIONS

lichen simplex chronicus
seborrheic dermatitis

**Infectious**
actinomycosis
coccidioidal granuloma
folliculitis
dental sinus
herpes simplex/zoster
impetigo contagiosum
scrofuloderma
sycosis barbae
tinea corporis
verrucae

**Allergic**
contact dermatitis
eczematous dermatitis

**Metabolic**
pellagra

**Idiopathic**
acanthosis nigricans
acne
elastosis perforans serpiginosa
impetigo herpetiformis
lichen sclerosis et atrophicus
pityriasis rosea
pityriasis rubra pilaris (sides of the neck)
poikiloderma of Civatte
Riehl's melanosis
scleredema
scleroderma

**Neoplastic**
acrochordon*
basal cell carcinoma
chondroid syringoma
epidermal cyst
squamous cell carcinoma
warty dyskeratoma

**Congenital**
bronchogenic cyst
cutis laxa (AD)
Darier's disease (AD)
Hailey–Hailey disease (AD)
pseudoxanthoma elasticum (AD, AR)
thyroglossal cyst
webbed neck (Noonan's syndrome, Turner's syndrome)
X-linked ichythyosis (XR)

## NAPE OF THE NECK ERUPTIONS

**Infectious**
pyoderma (carbuncle, folliculitis, furunculosis)
tinea corporis

**Traumatic**
dermatitis actinica

**Allergic**
contact dermatitis
lichen simplex chronicus
seborrhea nuchum

**Idiopathic**
acne keloidalis nuchae
acne vulgaris
cutis rhomboidalis nuchae
elastosis perforans serpiginosa
lichen planus
pityriasis rosea

**Neoplastic**
actinic keratosis
basal cell carcinoma
lipoma
sebaceous cyst
squamous cell carcinoma

## NECK – WEBBED

Noonan syndrome
Turner syndrome

# Nose

## CHRONIC INFECTIONS WITH PREDILECTION FOR NOSE

leishmaniasis
leprosy
syphilis
tuberculosis

## CONGENITAL MIDLINE NASAL MASSES

abscess
chondroma
chordoma
dermoid
encephalocele
epidermoid cyst
ethmoidal cyst
fibroma (or fibrous dysplasia)

ganglioneuroma
glioma
hemangioma
lacrimal duct cyst
nasal polyp
neurofibroma
olfactory neuroblastoma
pilomatricoma
rhabdomyosarcoma
teratoma

## ULCER OF NOSE

**Vascular**
Wegener's granulomatosis

**Infectious**
*Fungal*
    aspergillosis
    alternariosis
    blastomycosis
    coccidioidomycosis
    histoplasmosis
    mucormycosis
    paracoccidiodomycosis
    rhinosporidiosis
    sporotrichosis
*Bacterial*
    leprosy
    mycobacterial
    noma
    rhinoscleroma
*Parasitic*
    leishmaniasis
*Spirochetal*
    syphilis
    yaws
Viral
    cytomegalovirus
    herpes simplex virus

**Traumatic**
factitious
inhalation of cocaine
trauma

**Medicinal**
arsenic ingestion

**Idiopathic**
Churg–Strauss disease
collagen vascular disease (lupus)
Crohn's disease
lethal midline granuloma
pyoderma gangrenosum
relapsing polychondritis
sarcoidosis
trigeminal trophic syndrome
Wegener's granulomatosis

**Neoplastic**
adenocarcinoma
basal cell crcinoma
chondrosarcoma
lymphoma (sinonasal)
melanoma
squamous cell carcinoma

## OTHER NASAL ERUPTIONS

**Infectious**
impetigo contagiosum
perforating folliculitis

**Allergic**
contact dermatitis
seborrheic dermatitis

**Idiopathic**
acne
granulosis rubra nasi
hydroa aestivale
lupus erythematosus
pemphigus vegetans
rhinophyma
rosacea
trichostasis spinulosa

**Neoplastic**
actinic keratosis
adenoma sebaceum
basal cell carcinoma
Bowen's disease
fibrous papule of the nose
glioma
milia

multiple benign cystic epitheliomas
nevus
sebaceous trichofolliculoma

squamous cell carcinoma

Pits in and around the nose may indicate the presence of cerebrospinal fluid fistula

# Oral

## BUCCAL MUCOSA

aphthous ulcer
eosinophilic ulcer of oral mucosa
Fordyce's spots
galvanism
irritation fibroma
linea alba
lichen planus
white sponge nevus

## GINGIVA

### Cobblestone appearance of gingiva
Cowden's disease
Crohn's disease
Darier's disease
lipoid proteinosis

### Hyperplasia of gingiva
**Infectious**
atypical mycobacteria
mycobacteria

**Traumatic**
mechanical trauma

**Medicinal**
cyclosporine
diltiazam
erthromcycin
nifedipine
phenytoin
sodium valporate
verapamil

**Metabolic**
hyperparathyroidism
pregnancy
scurvy

**Idiopathic**
acute necrotizing ulcerative gingivitis
chronic marginal gingivitis
Ehlers–Danlos syndrome
inflammatory periodontal disease

**Hematologic**
hereditary fibromatosis
thrombocytopenia, thrombocytopathy

**Neoplastic**
leukemia (a characteristic feature in acute monocytic/myelomonocytic leukemia)
lymphoma
verrucous carcinoma

### Other gingival eruptions
epulis fissuratum
giant-cell epulis
peripheral giant-cell granuloma
peripheral odontogenic fibroma
pyogenic granuloma
verrucous carcinoma

## ORAL MUCOSA AND SKIN

**Infectious**
*Fungal*
candidiasis

*Bacterial*
mycobacteria
*Spirochetal*
syphilis
*Viral*
herpes simplex/zoster
varicella
verruca

**Medicinal**
fixed drug eruption

**Idiopathic**
cicatricial pemphigoid
erythema multiforme
lichen planus
lichen sclerosis et atrophicus
multiple mucosal neuromas
pemphigoid
pemphigus vulgaris
systemic lupus erythematosus

**Congenital**
epidermolysis bullosa

## ORAL MUCOSA COBBLESTONE

Cowden's disease
Crohn's disease
Darier's disease

## ORAL PAPULES/PLAQUES

**Vascular**
lymphangioma (around & within mouth)

**Infectious**
condyloma acuminata
hairy leukoplakia

**Traumatic**
trauma

**Metabolic**
verruciform xanthoma

**Idiopathic**
Crohn's disease
discoid lupus erythematosus
Fordyce's disease (spots)
lichen planus
psoriasis
pyostomatitis vegetans

**Neoplastic**
*Benign*
fibroma
focal epithelial hyperplasia (Heck's disease)
mucocele
*Premalignant*
Bowen's disease
*Malignant*
squamous cell carcinoma
verrucous carcinoma

**Congenital**
Darier's disease (AD)
dyskeratosis congenita (XR)
hereditary benign intraepithelial dyskeratosis
hereditary mucoepithelial dysplasia
pachyonychia congenita (AD)
white sponge nevus

## ORAL PIGMENTATION

**Traumatic**
exposure to heavy metals (arsenic, bismuth, brass, cadmium, chrome, copper, gold, manganese, mercury, silver, tin)
foreign body (amalgam tattoos, carbon, dyes, ink, lead pencil)
postinflammatory
trauma

**Medicinal**
amiodarone
antimalarials
chlorpromazine
minocycline

oral contraceptive pills
phenolphthalein

## Metabolic
acromegaly
Addison's disease
hemochromatosis
physiologic
porphyria

## Idiopathic
Albright's syndrome

## Neoplastic
Kaposi's sarcoma
malignant melanoma
nevi
oral melanotic macule

## Hematologic
bleeding diathesis
β-thalassemia

## Congenital
neurofibromatosis (AD)
Peutz–Jeghers syndrome (AD)
Wilson's disease (AR)

## ORAL ULCER

## Vascular
Wegener's granulomatosis

## Infectious
*Fungal*
   candidiasis
   blastomycosis
   cryptococcosis
   histoplasmosis
   sporotrichosis
*Bacterial*
   actinomycosis
   leprosy
   molluscum contagiosum

   noma (a form of fusospirially gangrenous
      stomatitis)
   tuberculosis
*Spirochetal*
   acute necrotizing ulcerative gingivitis
      (Vincent's angina)
   chancre
   secondary and tertiary syphilis
   yaws
*Viral*
   cytomegalovirus
   hand–foot–mouth disease
   measles
   mononucleosis
   mumps
   rubella
   smallpox
   vaccina
   varicella

## Traumatic
trauma (burn, dentures, food, lye, seizure,
   self-inflicted, radiation therapy)

## Medicinal
antiseptics
aspirin
chemotherapeutics
methotrexate
phenol
silver nitrate etc.

## Metabolic
acatalasemia
diabetes mellitus
porphyria
pregnancy
uremia
vitamin $B_{12}$ or folic acid deficiency

## Idiopathic
any of vesiculobullous diseases above
Crohn's disease
erosive lichen planus
midline lethal granuloma
necrotizing sialometaplasia
neurotropic ulcer
pyostomatitis vegetans

**Neoplastic**
leukemia
odontogenic and salivary gland tumors
squamous cell carcinoma

**Hematologic**
agranulocytosis
cyclic neutropenia
hereditary mucoepithelial dysplasia (red lesions)
macroglobulinemia
sickle cell anemia

**Congenital**
dyskeratosis congenita (XR)
epidermolysis bullosa

## ORAL VESICLES AND BULLAE

**Infectious**
*Fungal*
    candidiasis
    histoplasmosis
    mucormycosis
*Viral*
    hand, foot, mouth disease
    herpangina
    herpes simplex/zoster

**Allergic**
contact dermatitis

**Idiopathic**
aphthous stomatitis
Behçet's syndrome
lichen planus
Reiter's syndrome
bullous disorders: bullous pemphigoid,
    cicatricial pemphigoid, dermatitis
    herpetiformis, pemphigus vegetans/vulgaris
Stevens–Johnson syndrome (erythema
    multiforme major)
toxic epidermal necrolysis

**Congenital**
epidermolysis bullosa
Hailey–Hailey disease (AD)

## ORAL WHITE ERUPTIONS

**Infectious**
candidiasis
histoplasmosis
oral hairy leukoplakia
secondary syphilis
verrucae

**Traumatic**
trauma (burn, dentures, food, lye, seizure,
    self-inflicted, radiation therapy)

**Allergic**
contact dermatitis

**Medicinal**
antiseptics
aspirin
phenol
silver nitrate, etc.

**Idiopathic**
aphthous stomatitis
leukokeratosis
leukoplakia
lichen planus
lichen sclerosis et atrophicus
lupus erythematosus
pityriasis rubra pilaris
psoriasis
porokeratosis of Mibelli

**Neoplastic**
actinic cheilitis
Bowen's disease
epidermal nevus
erythroplakia
Fordyce spots
sideropenic dysphagia
stomatitis nicotina
submucous fibrosis
verrucous carcinoma (squamous cell
    carcinoma)

## Congenital
Darier's disease (AD)
dyskeratosis congenita (XR)
familial benign intraepidermal dyskeratosis (AD)
hereditary mucoepithelial dysplasia (AD)
pachyonychia congenita (AD)
white sponge nevus (AD)

## PALATE

candidiasis
inflammatory papillary hyperplasia
Kaposi's sarcoma
necrotizing sialometaplasia
nicotine stomatitis
torus mandibularis/palatinus
tumors of minor salivary gland

## TONGUE

### Atrophy of tongue
geographic tongue
iron deficiency
lichen planus
lichen sclerosis et atrophicus
squamous cell carcinoma
systemic lupus erythematosus
tertiary syphilis
various vitamin deficiencies

### Atrophic glossitis
pellagra
pernicious anemia
severe malabsorption states

### Black hairy tongue (overproduction of pigment by bacteria)
excessive smoking
medication (oral antibiotic, e.g. penicillin,
    tetracycline, methyldopa)
presence of candidiasis

### Burning tongue
cancerophobia
candidiasis
contact allergy
diabetes mellitus

dry mouth syndrome (xerostomia)
drugs
fisured tongue
geographic tongue
heat accumulation
inadequate oral cleaning
iron deficiency
menopause*
nutritional deficiencies (especially B vitamins)
oral cancer (early on)
psychological (anxiety, depression)
stress induced muscle activity
trauma (especially from dentures)

### Fissured tongue
Down's syndrome
Geographic tongue
Melkersson–Rosenthal syndrome

### Furred tongue
febrile illnesses
smoking

### General tongue eruptions
## Vascular
hemangioma
lymphangioma
venous lake (phlebectases)

## Infectious
*Fungal*
    candidiasis
    histoplasmosis
*Spirochetal*
    primary and secondary syphilis (chancre,
    condyloma latum)
*Viral*
    condyloma acuminata
    herpes simplex/zoster

## Traumatic
trauma

## Idiopathic
aphthous ulcer
Crohn's disease

93

eosinophilic ulcer of the tongue
lichen planus
median rhomboid glossitis
psoriasis

## Neoplastic
*Benign*
    fibroma
    granular cell tumor (granular cell
    myoblastoma)
*Premalignant*
    Bowen's disease
*Malignant*
    metastases
    squamous cell carcinoma

## Hematologic
Moeller's glossitis

## *Geographic tongue*
Manifestation of atopy or psoriasis. Isolated
    finding

## *Glossitis*
malabsorption syndromes
pellagra (niacin or tryptophan deficiency)
pernicious anemia

## *Glossodynia (painful tongue)*
## Infectious
candidiasis
syphilis

## Traumatic
trauma

## Medicinal
after treatment with antibiotics

## Metabolic
diabetes mellitus
hypothyroidism
nutritional deficiency (niacin or riboflavin)

## Idiopathic
geographic tongue
lichen planus
papillitis
systemic lupus erythematosus
xerostomia

## Hematologic
anemia

## *Macroglossia*
## Vascular
angioneurotic edema
hemangioma
lymphoangioma (circumscriptum)

## Infectious
actinomycosis
gummata
leprosy

## Metabolic
acromegaly
hypothyroidism

## Idiopathic
amyloidosis
Beckwith–Wiedemann syndrome
Melkerson–Rosenthal syndrome
sarcoidosis
superior vena cava syndrome

## Neoplastic
blockage of lymphatics with carcinoma of
    tongue
cystic hygroma
hemangioma
lymphangioma
squamous cell carcinoma

## Congenital
Down's syndrome
Hunter's syndrome
Hurler's syndrome
lipoid proteinosis (AR)

neurofibromatosis (AD)
thyroglossal duct cysts

## Congenital
lipoid proteinosis (AR)
Down's syndrome
neurofibromatosis (AD)
thyroglossal duct cysts

### Oral hairy leukoplakia
HIV-infected patients

### Scrotal tongue (lingua plicata)
Cowden's syndrome
Down's syndrome
Melkerson–Rosenthal syndrome

### Smooth Tongue (atrophy of filiform papillae)
anemia
malabsorption states (spruce {celiac disease or gluten sensitive enteropathy)
nutritional deficiencies
Riley–Day Syndrome
vitamin deficiency

### Strawberry tongue
Kawasaki disease
scarlet fever
toxic shock syndrome

## XEROSTOMIA (dry mouth)

## Infectious
*Bacterial*
  actinomycosis
  tuberculosis
*Spirochetal*
  syphilis
*Viral*
  mumps

## Traumatic
radiation
scar
sialolithiasis (stone)
stricture
trauma (nerve injury)

## Medicinal
anticholinergics
diuretics
ergotamine
opiates
sympathomimetics

## Metabolic
diabetes mellitus
hypothyroidism
vitamin deficiency (A, nicotinic acid, riboflavin)

## Idiopathic
*Collagen vascular disease*
  dermatomyositis
  mixed connective tissue disease
  scleroderma
  Sjögren's syndrome
  systemic lupus erythematosus
*Other*
  multiple sclerosis
  graft versus host disease

## Neoplastic
carcinoma
lymphoma

## Hematologic
iron deficiency anemia
pernicious anemia

## Congenital
ectodermal dysplasia, aplasia or hypoplasia of salivary glands

# Palms

## ERYTHEMA OF PALMS

acute graft versus host disease
chronic febrile disease
chronic leukemia
chronic liver disease
chronic lung disease
chronic polyarteritis
familial
healthy female
hyperthyroidism, thyrotoxicosis
pregnancy
rheumatoid arthritis
subacute bacterial endocarditis

## PITS OF PALMS

arsenic ingestion
basal-cell nevus syndrome
Cowden's disease
Darier's disease

## TUMORS OF PALMS

epidermal inclusion cyst
Dupuytren's contracture
giant-cell tumor of tendon sheath
glomus tumor
retinacular ganglion
trigger finger

# Palms and soles

## HYPERKERATOSIS OF PALMS AND SOLES

### Infectious
dermatophytosis (including tinea nigra)
Norwegian scabies
pitted keratolysis (soles only)
verruca vulgaris

### Traumatic
callus
corn

### Medicinal
chronic arsenic ingestion

### Idiopathic
acquired keratodermas
dermatitis repens (acrodermatitis continua or
    perstans)
lamellar dyshidrosis (keratolysis exfoliativa)
lichen planus
pityriasis rubra pilaris
psoriasis
Reiter's disease
symmetrical lividities

**Neoplastic**
Bowen's disease
eccrine poroma
verrucous carcinoma

**Congenital**
basal-cell nevus syndrome
congenital ichthyosiform erythroderma
Darier's disease (AD)
dyskeratosis congenita (XR)
hidrotic ectodermal dysplasia
inherited keratoderma
lamellar ichthyosis (AR)
pachyonychia congenita (AD)
Sjögren–Larsson syndrome
tyrosinemia II (AR, Richner–Hanhart)

## PURPURA OF PALMS AND SOLES

erythema multiforme
hand, foot and mouth disease

Rocky Mountain spotted fever
secondary syphilis
smallpox
vasculitis

## PUSTULES OF PALMS AND SOLES

acrodermatitis continua (acrodermatitis
    perstans, dermatitis repens)
acropustulosis (infantile)
dermatophyte infection (tinea manum and
    pedis)
dyshidrotic eczema
infectious dermatitis
milker's nodule
monkeypox
orf
psoriasis
pustular bacterid
Reiter's syndrome
scabies

# Scalp

**Vascular**
hemangioma
pyogenic granuloma
telangiectasia

**Infectious**
erosive pustular dermatosis
herpes zoster
kerion
pediculosis
pyogenic infections
syphilis
tinea capitis (including favus)
tuberculosis
verruca vulgaris

**Allergic**
contact dermatitis
eczematous dermatitis
prurigo nodularis
seborrheic dermatitis

**Idiopathic**
alopecia
cutis verticis gyrata
discoid lupus erythematosus
lichen planopilaris
psoriasis
seborrhea nuchum
subcutaneous granuloma annulare

**Neoplastic**

*Benign*

    angiolymphoid hyperplasia with eosinophilia

    atypical fibroxanthoma

    comedo

    cylindroma

    dermatofibroma

    epidermal cyst

    keratoacanthoma

    mastocytoma

    nevi

    nevus sebaceous

    nevus verrucosus

    pilar cyst

    proliferating trichilemmal cyst (90% on the scalp)

    Spitz nevus

    seborrheic keratosis

    syringocystadenoma papilliferum

    warty dyskeratoma

*Premalignant*

    actinic keratosis

    Bowen's disease

*Malignant*

    alopecia neoplastica (breast carcinoma metastases in females; lung or kidney carcinoma metastases in males)

    angiosarcoma

    basal cell carcinoma

    malignant melanoma

    meningioma

**Congenital**

Darier's disease (AD)

# Shin

diabetic dermopathy

erythema nodosum*

lichen amyloidosis

lipogranulomatosis subcutanea

necrobiosis lipoidica diabeticorum

nodular vasculitis

purpura

sporotrichosis

subcutaneous fat (associated with pancreatitis)

syphilitic gummas

Weber–Christian disease

# Thigh

## GENERAL ERUPTIONS OF THIGH

atopic dermatitis

contact dermatitis

herpes zoster

lipoma

liposarcoma

keratosis pilaris

malignant fibrous histiocytoma

pyodermas

sarcomas

## INNER ASPECT OF THIGH

acrochordons

candidiasis

chronic bullous disease of children

contact dermatitis

eczematous dermatitis

erythrasma
granuloma inguinale
hidradenitis suppurativa
hyperhidrosis
intertrigo
lichen planus

lichen sclerosis et atrophicus
nevus
striae distensae
syphilis
tinea cruris
verrucae

# Toe

## PURPLE TOE LESIONS

### Vascular
acrocyanosis
Burger's disease
chilblain/pernio
embolic phenomenon (atheroma, cholesterol, clot, septic)
leukocytoclastic vasculitis
polyarteritis
Raynaud's phenomenon

### Traumatic
frost-bite
occlusive mass (fibroma, glomus tumor)

### Idiopathic
collagen vascular disease
cryoglobulinemia
erythromelalgia
lupus anticoagulant syndrome
paraproteinemia
protein C deficiency
Waldenstrom's macroglobulinemia

### Neoplastic
multiple myeloma

### Hematologic
polycythemia vera
thrombocytosis

# Tongue

see under oral

# Trunk

## GENERAL ERUPTIONS ON TRUNK

### Vascular
angioma
urticaria

### Infectious
*Fungal*
blastomycosis
coccidioidal granuloma
tinea corporis
tinea versicolor
*Bacterial*
actinomycosis
cellulitis
leprosy
lichen scrofulosorum
tuberculosis
*Parasitic*
lice
scabies
*Spirochetal*
secondary syphilis
*Viral*
herpes simplex and zoster

### Traumatic
insect bite

### Allergic
atopic dermatitis
contact dermatitis
lichen simplex chronicus
prurigo nodularis
seborrheic dermatitis

### Medicinal
fixed drug eruption

### Metabolic
pellagra

### Idiopathic
acne
anetoderma
confluent and reticulated papillomatosis
   (greatest intensity of eruption is between
   breasts and in the periumbilical area)
dermatomyositis
erythema annulare centrifigum
granuloma annulare
keloid
lichen planus
lichen sclerosis et atrophicus
lupus erythematosus
parapsoriasis
pityriasis rosea
poikiloderma vasculare atrophicans
psoriasis
scleroderma
vitiligo

### Neoplastic
*Benign*
neurofibroma
nevus
sebaceous cyst
seborrheic keratosis
*Premalignant*
actinic keratosis
Bowen's disease
*Malignant*
dermatofibrosarcoma protuberans
lymphoma
melanoma
mycosis fungoides
sarcoma

## VESICLES AND BULLAE ON TRUNK

**Vascular**
lymphangioma
pressure urticaria

**Infectious**
*Fungal*
dermatophyte (tinea corporis)
*Bacterial*
bullous impetigo
*Parasitic*
scabies
*Viral*
herpes simplex/zoster
varicella
variola

**Traumatic**
factitious
insect bite
miliaria
second degree burn

**Allergic**
contact dermatitis
vesicular '-id reaction'

**Medicinal**
bullous fixed drug eruption

**Idiopathic**
*Bullous disorders*
bullous lichen planus
bullous pemphigoid
chronic bullous dermatosis of childhood
dermatitis herpetiformis
diabetic bullae
herpes gestationis
pemphigus
subcorneal pustular dermatosis
transient acantholytic dermatosis (Grover's disease)
*Other*
erythema elevatum diutinum
erythema multiforme
pyoderma gangrenosum
toxic epidermal necrolysis

**Neoplastic**
urticaria pigmentosa

**Congenital**
congenital erythropoietic porphyria (Gunther's disease, AR)
Hailey–Hailey disease (AD)
incontinentia pigmenti (XD)

# Umbilicus

**Vascular**
Fabry's disease
hemangioma

**Infectious**
chigger mites
scabies
*Pseudomonas*
tuberculosis granuloma

**Traumatic**
pilonidal granuloma

**Allergic**
seborrheic dermatitis

**Idiopathic**
exuberant granulation in the newborn
Fox–Fordyce disease
herpes gestationis
hidradenitis suppurativa
perforating pseudoxanthoma elasticum
pruritic urticarial papules and plaques of
    pregnancy
psoriasis

endometriosis
epidermal cyst
fibroepithelial polyp
granular-cell myoblastoma
keloid
lipoma
nevus
pyogenic granuloma
teratoma metastases (Sister Mary Joseph's
    nodules)

**Neoplastic**
Bowen's disease
dermatofibroma
desmoid tumor

**Congenital**
anomalies of Urachus
remnants of omphalomesenteric duct

# Wrist

contact dermatitis
epitheloid sarcoma
erythema multiforme

lichen planus
scabies

# SECTION FIVE

## Pediatric differential diagnosis

# NEWBORNS

## Primary eruptions

### MACULE AND PATCH

**Brown**
café-au-lait spot
freckle
junctional nevus
lentigo
mongolian spot
nevus of ota
postinflammatory hyperpigmentation

**White**
ash-leaf spot
hemangioma (early, precursor)
hypomelanosis of Ito
piebaldism (AD)
postinflammatory hypopigmentation

**Yellow**
carotenemia

### PAPULE/NODULE

**Brown**
acrochordon
congenital nevus

**Red**
acne neonatorum
candidiasis
congenital syphilis
epidermal nevus
erysipelas
erythema toxicum
furuncle
insect bite
urticaria pigmentosa

**Skin-colored**
*Keratotic (rough-surfaced)*
epidermal nevus
verruca

*Non-keratotic (smooth-surfaced)*
acrochordon
connective tissue nevus
dermoid cyst
lipoma
lymphangioma
microcomedones
milia
molluscum contagiosum
neurofibroma
nevus
pilomatricoma*

**White**
comedones
milia
molluscum contagiosum

**Yellow**
Goltz's syndrome
juvenile xanthogranuloma
mastocytoma
nevus lipomatosis
nevus sebaceous
sebaceous hyperplasia

### PUSTULE

acne (neonatal)
candidiasis
erythema toxicum
folliculitis
herpes gestationis
herpes simplex

impetigo
incontinentia pigmenti
infantile acropustulosis
miliaria (crystallina or rubra)
nevus comedonicus
pemphigus
perioral dermatitis
pustular psoriasis
staph scalded skin syndrome
transient neonatal pustular melanosis
varicella

## VASCULAR

### Blanchable
erythema toxicum
hemangioma (flat)
mottling
urticaria

### Non-blanchable (petechiae and purpura)
coagulopathies
congenital infections: cytomegalovirus,
    enterovirus, herpes simplex, rubella, syphilis,
    toxoplasma
epidermolysis bullosa
erythroblastosis fetalis
hypoprothrombinemia (vitamin K deficiency)
idiopathic thrombocytopenic purpura
Kasabach–Merritt syndrome
systemic lupus erythematosus
trauma (e.g. vertex delivery)
Wiskott–Aldrich syndrome

## VESICULOBULLOUS

### Vascular
lymphangioma

### Infectious
*Fungal*
    candidiasis (congenital)
*Bacterial*
    bacterial sepsis
    impetigo neonatorum
    staphylococcal scalded skin syndrome

*Parasitic*
    scabies
*Spirochetal*
    syphilis (congenital)
*Viral*
    cytomegalovirus
    herpes simplex
    varicella

### Traumatic
burn
friction blister
miliaria crystallina/rubra
sucking blister

### Allergic
dermatitis (acute)

### Idiopathic
*Bullous disorders*
    epidermolysis bullosa
    herpes gestationis
    infantile acropustulosis
    pemphigus vulgaris
*Other*
    acne neonatorum
    erythema toxicum neonatorum (up to 50%
        of term infants: smear shows
        predominance of eosinophils)
    pustular psoriasis
    transient neonatal pustular melanosis
        (predominantly in Black infants; smear
        shows predominance of neutrophils)

### Neoplastic
nevus comedonicus
urticaria pigmentosa

### Congenital
acrodermatitis enteropathica (AD)
aplasia cutis congenita
congenital ichthyosiform erythroderma
incontinentia pigmenti (XD)

# Secondary eruptions

## ECZEMATOUS

acrodermatitis enteropathica (zinc deficiency)
ataxia telangiectasia (usually after 30 days of life)
atopic dermatitis
candidiasis
contact dermatitis
diaper dermatitis
histiocytosis X
hypogammaglobulinemia (usually after 30 days of life)
Leiner's disease (erythroderma desquamativum)
multiple carboxylase deficiency
scabies
seborrheic dermatitis

severe combined immunodeficiency syndrome
Wiskott–Aldrich syndrome (usually after 30 days of life)

## PAPULOSQUAMOUS

candidiasis
chronic dermatitis
congenital rubella
congenital syphilis
epidermal nevus
ichthyosis
neonatal systemic lupus erythematosus
pityriasis rubra pilaris
psoriasis
tinea corporis

# Miscellaneous

## ACRAL BULLOUS OR PAPULOSQUAMOUS ERUPTIONS

acrodermatitis entropathica
atopic dermatitis
chronic mucocutaneous candidiasis
citrulinemia
epidermolysis bullosa
erythema multiforme
essential fatty acid deficiency
histiocytosis X
Maple syrup urine disease
Multiple carboxylase deficiency
Propionic & methylmalonic acidemia
Psoriasis
Seborrheic dermatitis

## BLISTERS OF EROSIONS OF MUCOSA

aphthous stomatitis
burn (chemical or thermal)
candidiasis
congenital syphilis
epidermolysis bullosa
geographic tongue
herpes simplex
varicella

## BLUEBERRY MUFFIN

congenital cytomegalovirus, rubella, toxoplasmosis

hemolytic disease of newborn
hereditary spherocytosis
Letterer–Swie syndrome
neuroblastoma
twin-twin transfusion syndrome

## CONGENITAL INFECTIONS

congenital syphilis
congenital toxoplasmosis
cytomegalic inclusion disease
intrauterine herpes
neonatal herpes simples
neonatal varicella
rubella
varicella-zoster

## ERUPTIONS IN DIAPER AREA

**Infectious**
*Fungal*
    candidiasis
    dermatophytosis
*Bacterial*
    bullous impetigo
    streptococcus perianitis
*Parasitic*
    scabies
*Spirochetal*
    syphilis
*Viral*
    condyloma acuminata
    hand/foot/mouth disease
    herpes simplex
    varicella
    viral exanthems

**Traumatic**
miliaria

**Allergic**
atopic dermatitis
contact dermatitis (allergic/irritant)
fecal irritation (perianal area)
seborrheic dermatitis (and Leiner's disease)

**Idiopathic**
granuloma gluteale infantum
histiocytosis X (Letterer–Siwe disease)
intertrigo
linear IgA dermatosis
psoriasis
vesiculobullous disease: bullous pemphigoid, chronic bullous dermatosis of childhood, dermatitis herpetiformis, epidermolysis bullosa
vesiculopustular disease: transient neonatal pustular melanosis

**Congenital**
acrodermatitis entropathica (AD)
incontinentia pigmenti (XD)
multiple carboxylase deficiency (AR)

## ERYTHRODERMA

**Infectious**
candidiasis (congenital)
staphylococcal scalded skin syndrome

**Traumatic**
boric acid poisoning

**Allergic**
erythroderma desquamativum (Leiner's disease)
graft versus host disease
seborrheic dermatitis
toxic epidermal necrolysis
transfusion allergic reaction

**Metabolic**
biotin deficiency
dysmaturity desquamation
essential fatty acid deficiency
physiologic desquamation

**Idiopathic**
ichthyosis
pityriasis rubra pilaris
psoriasis

**Congenital**

citrullinemia

ichthyosiform erythrodermas

maple syrup disease

multiple carboxylase deficiency

*Localized, congenital alopecia*

aplasia cutis congenita

Conradi's disease

epidermal nevus

hair follicle hamartoma

incontinentia pigmenti

Leiner's disease

nevus

nevus sebaceus

sutural alopecia of Hellerman–Streiff

triangular alopecia of frontal scalp

*Diffuse, congenital alopecia*

atrichia congenita

cartilage–hair hypoplasia

congenital hypothyroidism

ectodermal dysplasia

follicular atrophoderma

Marinesco–Sjögren syndrome

monilethrix

pili torti

progeria

trichorrhexis invaginata

trichorrhexis nodosa

*Atrophic or Thin Nails*

acrodermatitis enteropathica

anonychia with ectrodactyly

dyskeratosis congenita

ectodermal dysplasia

Ellis–Van Creveld syndrome

epidermolysis bullosa

focal dermal hypoplasia

incontinentia pigmenti

nail–patella syndrome

periodic nail shedding

trisomy 13/18

Turner's syndrome

# INFANTS AND CHILDREN

## Primary eruptions

*Brown*

Becker's nevus

café-au-lait spot

freckles

incontinentia pigmenti

lentigo

melasma

mongolian spot

nevus (junctional)

nevus of Ota

postinflammatory hyperpigmentation

tinea versicolor

underlying endocrine abnormalities

*White*

ash-leaf spot (of tuberous sclerosis)

lichen sclerosis et atrophicus

piebaldism (AD)

postinflammatory hypopigmentation
scleroderma
tinea versicolor
vitiligo

### Yellow
carotenemia
jaundice

## PAPULE AND NODULE

### Brown
acrochordon
blue nevus
dermatofibroma
juvenile xanthogranuloma
lentigo
melanoma
nevus (intradermal)
spitz nevus
urticaria pigmentosa
wart (flat)

### Red
### Vascular
urticaria, pyogenic granuloma

### Infectious
*Fungal*
   candidiasis
   dermatophytosis
*Bacterial*
   erythema marginatum
   furunculosis
   scarlet fever
*Spirochetal*
   secondary syphilis
*Viral*
   mononucleosis
   measles
   rubella

### Traumatic
insect bites
hypertrophic scar
keloid

### Idiopathic
acne
erythema multiforme
granuloma annulare
guttate psoriasis
keratosis pilaris
pityriasis rosea
shagreen patch

### Neoplastic
angiofibroma
neurofibroma

### Skin-colored

*Keratotic (rough-surfaced)*
callus
corn
epidermal nevus
keratosis pilaris
wart

*Non-keratotic (smooth-surfaced)*
angiolipoma
basal cell carcinoma
comedone
connective tissue nevus
epidermal cyst
eruptive vellus hair cyst
exostosis
granuloma annulare
lipoma
molluscum contagiosum
mucous cyst
neurofibroma
pilomatricoma
rheumatoid nodule
syringoma
trichoepithelioma

### White
comedone
keratosis pilaris
milia
molluscum contagiosum

### Yellow
Goltz's syndrome

juvenile xanthogranuloma
mastocytoma
necrobiosis lipoidica diabeticorum
nevus lipomatosis
nevus sebaceus
urticaria pigmentosa
xanthoma

## PUSTULE

acne
bacterial infections (gonococcemia,
    meningococcemia, etc.)
candidiasis
folliculitis
fungal infections (disseminated, deep fungal,
    coccidioidomycosis, cryptococcus,
    histoplasmosis)
infantile acropustulosis
perioral dermatitis
pustular psoriasis
rosacea
scabies

## VASCULAR

### Blanchable
angiofibroma
erythema multiforme
hemangioma
livedo reticularis
pyogenic granuloma
spider angioma
telangiectasia
urticaria

### Non-blanchable (petechiae and purpura)
**Infectious**
*Bacterial*
    gonococcemia
    meningococcemia
    Rocky Mountain spotted fever
    *Pseudomonas* sepsis
    staphylococcus sepsis
    subacute bacterial endocarditis
*Viral*
    atypical measles
    herpes simplex

**Traumatic**
trauma

**Idiopathic**
erythema nodosum
progressive pigmentary purpura

**Neoplastic**
leukemia

**Hematologic**
hemophilia
idiopathic thrombocytopenic purpura

## VESICULOBULLOUS

**Vascular**
lymphangioma
mastocytosis
**Infectious**
*Fungal*
    dermatophytosis (acute, including tinea
    pedis)
*Bacterial*
    bullous impetigo
    congenital syphilis
    impetigo contagiosum
    staphylococcal scalded skin syndrome
    toxic epidermal necrolysis
*Viral*
    hand, foot and mouth disease
    herpes simplex
    varicella-zoster

**Traumatic**
burn
friction blister
insect bite
miliaria

**Allergic**
acute dermatitis
polymorphous light eruption

**Medicinal**
fixed drug eruption

**Metabolic**
diabetic bullae

**Idiopathic**
*Bullous disorders*
    bullous pemphigoid
    cicatricial pemphigoid
    chronic bullous dermatosis of childhood
    dermatitis herpetiformis
    epidermolysis bullosa
    pemphigus vulgaris
*Other*
    erythema multiforme
    parapsoriasis (acute)
    porphyria

**Congenital**
acrodermatitis entropathica (AD)
congenital ichthyosiform erythroderma
Ehlers–Danlos syndrome (cutis hyperelastica)
incontinentia pigmenti (XD)

## URTICARIA IN CHILDHOOD

*Food*
    eggs
    milk
    peanuts
    seafood
*Infections*
    adeno-and enterovirus infections
    dental abscess
    hepatitis B
    infection mononucleosis
    influenza
    lyme borreliosis
    sinus disease
    streptococcus group B
*Insect stings*
    bee
    fire ant
    wasp
    yellow-jacket
*Medication*
    cephalosporins
    penicillin
    phenytoin
    sulfa
*Other*
    animal dander
    juvenile rheumatoid arthritis
    leukemia
    lymphoma
    mold spores
    systematic lupus erythematosus

# Secondary eruptions

## ECZEMATOUS

**Infectious**
candidiasis
dermatophytosis
scabies
staphylococcal scalded skin syndrome

**Traumatic**
sunburn

**Allergic**
atopic dermatitis
contact dermatitis
diaper dermatitis
juvenile plantar dermatosis

Leiner's disease (erythroderma desquamativum)
nummular eczema
polymorphous light eruption
seborrheic dermatitis

### Medicinal
drug eruption

### Metabolic
hyper/hypovitaminosis
### Idiopathic
dermatitis herpetiformis
histiocytosis X

### Congenital
acrodermatitis entropathica (AD, zinc
     deficiency)
agammaglobulinemia
ataxia telangiectasia (AR)

Hartnup's syndrome (AR)
Hurler's syndrome (AR)
phenylketonuria (AR)
Wiskott–Aldrich syndrome

## PAPULOSQUAMOUS

Darier's disease
dermatitis (chronic)
dermatophytosis
ichthyosis
keratosis pilaris
lichen planus
parapsoriasis
pityriasis rosea
pityriasis rubra pilaris
porokeratosis of Mibelli
psoriasis
scabies
secondary syphilis
systemic lupus erythematosus

# Miscellaneous

## BLISTERS OR EROSIONS OF MUCOSA IN INFANTS AND CHILDREN

aphthous stomatitis
bullous pemphigoid
burn (chemical or thermal)
candidiasis
erythema multiforme
epidermolysis bullosa
geographic tongue
hand, foot and mouth disease
herpes simplex
pemphigus vulgaris
varicella-zoster

## ERYTHRODERMA IN CHILDREN

burn
congenital ichthyosiform erythroderma
psoriasis
scarlet fever
sclerema neonatorum
staphylococcal scalded skin syndrome
toxic epidermal necrolysis

## FEVER AND RASH IN CHILDREN

### Infectious
acute hepatitis
acute infectious mononucleosis
erythema marginatum (rheumatic fever)
erysipelas

gonococcemia
Lyme disease
measles
meningococcemia
Rocky Mountain spotted fever
roseola
rubella
scarlet fever
smallpox
subacute bacterial endocarditis
typhoid
viral exanthem

**Idiopathic**
acute dermatomyositis
acute systemic lupus erythematosus
Henoch–Schönlein purpura
juvenile rheumatoid arthritis
Kawasaki's disease
leukocytoclastic vasculitis
serum sickness

## HAIR DISORDERS

*Localized, acquired alopecia*
**Infectious**
kerion
pyoderma
tinea capitis
varicella-zoster

**Traumatic**
burn (chemical or thermal)
physical including radiation injury or traction
    alopecia

**Idiopathic**
lichen planus
porokeratosis of Mibelli
systemic lupus erythematosus

**Congenital**
Darier's disease (AD)

*Diffuse, acquired alopecia*
**Medicinal**
antimetabolites
antithyroid therapy
coumarin
heparin
thallium poisoning

**Metabolic**
acrodermatitis enteropathica
androgenetic
diabetes mellitus
hypervitaminosis A
hypopituitarism
hypoparathyroidism
hypothyroidism
marasmus

## LINEAR CHILDHOOD LESIONS

incontinentia pigmenti
lichen striatus
linear Darier's disease
linear epidermal nevus
linear lichen planus
linear lichen simplex chronicus
linear morphea
linear porokeratosis
linear psoriasis
linear verruca plana/vulgaris

## NAIL DISORDERS

*Atrophic or thin nails*
congenital
drug-induced
erythema multiforme
lichen planus
Raynaud's phenomenon
trauma
twenty-nail syndrome
vascular disorders

*Paronychia*
acrodermatitis enteropathica
bacterial infection
fungal infection

histiocytosis X
mucocutaneous candidiasis
Reiter's syndrome
systemic retinoids

**Thick nails**
ectodermal dysplasia
lichen planus
Norwegian scabies
onychomycosis
pachyonychia congenita (AD)
psoriasis
twenty-nail syndrome

**Tumors of nail**
angiokeratoma
blue nevus
blue ruber bleb
enchondroma of Maffucci syndrome
exostoses
fibroma
hemangioma
incontinentia pigmenti (late verrucous stage)
neurofibroma
osteochondroma

## NECROTIC LESIONS IN CHILDREN

acute hemorrhagic edema
bacterial endocarditis
chronic leukocytoclastic vasculitis
cryoglobulinemia, cryofibrinogenemia
dermatomyositis
ecthyma gangrenosum (pseudomonas sepsis)
gonococcemia
Henoch–Shonlein purpura
Idiopathic purpura fulminans
meningococcemia
polyarteritis nodosa
protein C or S deficiency
pseuomonas sepsis & other sepsis
Rat-bite fever
Rocky Mountain spotted fever

## VULVAR DISORDERS

**Vascular**
hemangioma

**Infectious**
candidiasis
gonorrhea
herpes
molluscum contagiosum
other non-specific infections
pediculosis
pinworm
scabies
streptococcal infections
tinea cruris
verrucae

**Traumatic**
burn (chemical, thermal)
enuresis
foreign body
physical abuse
tights
trauma

**Allergic**
contact dermatitis (allergic or irritant)
seborrheic dermatitis

**Metabolic**
Crohn's disease
other systemic disease

**Idiopathic**
agglutination of labia minora
lichen sclerosis et atrophicus
perineal fissures
psoriasis

## VULVAR PRURITUS IN CHILDREN

allergic contact dermatitis
atopic dermatitis

candidiasis
chlamydia
condyloma acuminatum
gonorrhea
haemophilus influenzae
herpes genitalis
inadequate hygiene
irritant dermatitis
lichen planus
lichen sclerosis
lichen simplex chronicus
molluscum contagiosum
neisseria meningitides
pediculosis pubis

pinworm
psoriasis
psychogenic
scabies
seborrheic dermatitis
shigella
staphylococcus aureas
staphylococcus pneumoniae
streptococcus pyogenes (group A B-hemolytic
    streptococcus)
tinea cruris
trichomoniasis
yersinia

# PART TWO

## Dermatological pearls

# SECTION ONE

## Associations of skin disorders and other disorders

This section lists diseases or conditions seen in association with other diseases or medications

# Acanthosis nigricans

Addison's disease
Bloom's syndrome
Crouzon's syndrome (craniofacial dysostosis)
Cushing's syndrome
diethylstilbestrol
glucocorticoid
insulin-resistant diabetes mellitus
lupoid nephritis
nicotinic acid
obesity (pseudoacanthosis nigricans)
pinealoma
pituitary tumors
Rud's syndrome (epilepsy, hypogonadism,
   ichthyosis, mental deficiency)

Seip's syndrome (accelerated osseous
   maturation, lipodystrophy, muscular
   hypertrophy)
Stein–Leventhal syndrome (polycystic ovary
   disease)
Wilson's disease

MALIGNANT

adenocarcinoma of breast, lung (less often
   colon, esophagus, gallbladder, kidney, liver,
   ovary, pancreas, prostate, rectum, uterus)
intra-abdominal adenocarcinoma*
   (gastrointestinal tract, (60% stomach))
tumor of APUDoma group

# Acrochordons in children

may be presenting sign of Nevoid Basal Cell Ca
   Syndrome

# Actinic keratosis

mutation of p53

# Acquired angioedema I

B cell lymphoma
Chronic lymphocytic lymphoma

Monoclonal gammapathy
Waldenstrom macroglobulinemia

# Acquired ichthyosis

**Infectious**
leprosy

**Medicinal**
butyrophenone
cimetidine
clofazamine
isoniazid
nicotinic acid
phenothiazine
triparanol

**Metabolic**
essential fatty acid deficiency
hypothyroidism
kwashiorkor

malabsorption syndrome
panhypopituitarism
pellagra
vitamin A deficiency or excess

**Idiopathic**
chronic hepatic disease
chronic renal disease
sarcoidosis
systemic lupus erythematosus

**Neoplastic**
cancer (bronchogenic carcinoma, Hodgkin's
    disease, other lymphomas)

# Adrenal failure (primary)

mucocutaneous candidiasis

vitiligo

# Alopecia areata

adrenal disease
atopy
cytomegalovirus infection
diabetes mellitus
Down's syndrome*

Hashimoto's thyroiditis
lichen planus
pernicious anemia
vitiligo

# Amyloidosis

## PRIMARY AMYLOIDOSIS

multiple myeloma

## SECONDARY SYSTEMIC AMYLOIDOSIS

Beta-2-microglobulin-induced amyloidosis
dystrophic epidermolysis bullosa

hemodialysis-related amyloidosis
hidradenitis suppurativa
lepromatous leprosy
osteomyelitis*
psoriatic arthritis
rheumatoid arthritis*
stasis ulcer
tuberculosis

# Anemia

blue rubber bleb (AD)
dermatitis herpetiformis
dyskeratosis congenita (XR)

Osler–Weber–Rendu (AD)
psoriasis
scleroderma

# Angiokeratoma

aspartylglycosaminidase deficiency
B-galactosidase deficiency
B-mannosidase deficiency

Fucosidosis
Neuraminidase deficiency (sialidosis)

# Angiokeratoma circumscriptum

cavernous hemangioma
Cobb's syndrome

Klippel–Trenaunay–Weber syndrome
nevus flammeus

# Angiokeratoma of Fordyce

hernia
lymphogranuloma venereum
prostatitis

thrombophlebitis
tumors of the bladder or epididymis
varicocele

# Antiphospholipid antibodies

autoimmune hemolytic anemia
autoimmune thrombocytopenic purpura
bacterial infections {endocarditis, sepsis}
Bechet's disease
Chronic active hepatitis
dermatomyositis / polymyositis
giant cell arteritis
HIV infection
Hodgkins' disease/lymphoproliferative disorders
leprosy

leukemia
Lyme disease
lymphoproliferative disorders
medications (chlorpromazine, clozapine,
    hydralazine,phenothiazines, phenytoin,
    procainamide, quinidine, steptomycin)
migrane headache
mixed connective tissue disease
multiple myeloma
multiple sclerosis

myasthenia gravis
mycoplasma
mycosis fungoides
myelofibrosis
paraproteinemia
polyarteritis nodosa
polymyalgia rheumatica
rheumatoid arthritis (adult or juvenile)
Sjogren's disease
Sneddon's syndrome

Solid tumors
syphilis
Systemic lupus erythematosus
Systemic sclerosis
Tuberculosis
Viral infections (adenovirus, hepatitis a, measles, mononucleosis, mumps, parvovirus, varicella}
Von Willebrand's disease

# Arsenic exposure

Bowen's disease (rarely basal cell carcinoma)
diffuse truncal hyperpigmentation with discrete hypopigmented macules
increased risk of internal malignancy (particularly lung ca)

invasive squamous cell carcinoma
small wart-like keratoses on palms, soles and ears

# Atopy

allergic rhinitis
altered cell-mediated immunity:
    increased susceptibility to fungi (*T. rubrum*), molluscum and warts
    increased susceptibility to *Staphylococcus aureus* infections
    increased susceptibility to viral infections (herpes virus (Kaposi's varicelliform eruption), vaccina)
    lowered incidence of allergic contact dermatitis
anterior subcapsular cataracts
asthma
cheilitis
conjunctivitis
delayed blanch to cholinergic drugs
Dennie's (line)–Morgan (folds) (accentuated lines or grooves below the margin of the lower lids)

geographic tongue
hyperlinear palms
increased IgE levels
ichthyosis vulgaris (AD)
keratoconus (elongation of the corneal surface)
keratosis pilaris
lichenification (lichen simplex chronicus)
lowered threshold to pruritic stimuli
orbital darkening
pallor (especially about ears, mouth and nose)
perifollicular accentuation
personality traits (active, aggressive, irritable, restless)
pityriasis alba
urticaria
white dermatographism
wool (and acrylic) intolerance
xerosis (lackluster skin)

# Becker's nevus

smooth muscle hamartoma

# Blue rubber bleb nevus syndrome

angiomas of gastrointestinal tract

# Bullous pemphigoid

diabetes mellitus
lupus erythematosus
myasthenia gravis
pernicious anemia
polymyositis

primary biliary cirrhosis
rheumatoid arthritis
thymoma
thyroiditis
ulcerative colitis

# Chronic dermatophytosis

atopic dermatitis
chronic mucocutaneous candidiasis
collagen vascular disease
corticosteroid use
Cushing's disease
diabetes mellitus

immunodeficiency states
Kaposi's sarcoma
lymphoma
peripheral vascular disease
thymoma

# Chronic mucocutaneous candidiasis

alopecia totalis
candida esophagitis or laryngitis
chronic active hepatitis
circulating autoimmune antibodies
dental enamel dysplasia
diabetes mellitus
hypoadrenalism
hypoparathyroidism
hypothyroidism

iron deficiency
keratoconjunctivitis
KID syndrome (keratitis, ichthyosis, deafness)
malabsorption
myasthenia gravis
pernicious anemia
pulmonary fibrosis
specific T-cell deficiency
vitiligo

# Connective tissue nevus

hemihypertrophy
macrodactyly

osteopoikilosis (dermatofibrosis lenticularis
    disseminata, Buschke–Ollendorff
    syndrome, AD)
tuberous sclerosis (shagreen patches)

# Cryoglobulinemia

**Infectious**
cytomegalovirus
hepatitis B, hepatitis C
infectious mononucleosis
subacute bacterial endocarditis
toxoplasmosis

**Idiopathic**
Behçet's syndrome
leukocytoclastic vasculitis
rheumatoid arthritis
Sjögren's syndrome
systemic lupus erythematosus

**Neoplastic**
chronic lymphocytic leukemia
lymphoma
multiple myeloma
Waldenstrom's macroglobulinemia
TYPE I CRYOGLOBULINS: multiple myeloma,
    waldestrom's macroglobulinemia
TYPE II CRYOGLOBULINS: hepatitis B,
    rheumatoid arthritis, Sjogren's disease
TYPE III CRYOGLOBULINS: chronic infections,
    hepatitis B & C, systemic lupus
    erythematosus

# Cutaneous horn

adenoacanthoma
angiokeratoma
angioma
arsenical keratosis
basal cell carcinoma
benign lichenoid keratosis
bowen's disease
cutaneous leishmaniasis
cyst (epidermal inclusion)
dermatofibroma
discoid lupus erythematotus
epidermal nevus
epidermolytic acanthoma
fibroma
granular cell tumor
inverted follicular keratosis

kaposi's sarcoma
keratoacanthoma
keratotic and micacious pseudoepitheliomatous balanitis
organoid nevus
paget's disease of the breast
prurigo nodularis
pyogenic granuloma
renal cell carcinoma
sebaceous adenoma
seborrheic keratosis
solar keratosis
suamous cell carcinoma
trichilemmal horn
trichilemmoma
verruca vulgaris

# Cutis verticis gyrata

acromegaly
Aper's syndrome (acrocephalosyndactylia)
acanthosis nigricans (secondary to diabetes mellitus)
amyloidosis

leukemia
myxedema
syphilis
pachydermoperiostosis
tuberous sclerosis (AD)

# Cylindroma

trichoepithelioma

# Darier's disease

acrokeratosis verruciformis of Hopf

# Dermatitis herpetiformis

Addison's disease
diabetes mellitus
gluten-sensitive enteropathy
hypochlorhydria
increased incidence of intestinal lymphoma
pernicious anemia
Raynaud's phenomenon
rheumatoid arthritis
Sjögren's syndrome

systemic lupus erythematosus
thyroid diseases:
 Grave's disease
 Hashimoto's thyroiditis
 hyperthyroidism
 idiopathic hypothyroidism
ulcerative colitis
vitiligo

# Dermatitis vegetans (pyoderma vegetans, blastomycosis-like pyoderma)

ulcerative colitis

# Dermatofibroma (multiple, > 15)

systemic lupus erythematosus
systemic steroid use in treatment of collagen
 vascular diseases
?viral association

# Diffuse plane xanthoma

hyperlipoproteinemia type IIA, III or IV

multiple myeloma

# Dissecting cellulitis of scalp

acne conglobata
Fox Fordyce disease

Pilonidal cyst
spondyloarthropathy

# Down's syndrome

acrocyanosis
alopecia areata
atopic dermatitis
cheilitis / fissured lip
cutis marmorata
dermatophytosis (onychomycosis, tinea pedis / cruris)
elastosis perforans sepiginosa
fissured lips/cheilitis
folliculitis
keratosis palmaris et plantaris

keratosis pilaris (atypical)
lichen simplex chronicus
Norwegian scabies
onychomycosis
scrotal tongue
seborrheic dermatitis
syringomas
tinea pedis/tinea cruris
vitiligo
xerosis

# Dupuytren's contracture

alcoholic liver disease
chronic invalidism
diabetes mellitus
epilepsy

knuckle pads
Peyronie's disease
pulmonary tuberculosis

# Eczema craquele (generalized)

adenocarcinoma of stomach
angioimmunoblastic lymphadenopathy
Hodgkin's disease

myxedema
zinc deficiency

# Eczema herpeticum
# (Kaposi's varicelliform eruption)

atopic dermatitis*
benign familial pemphigus
congenital ichthyosiform erythroderma
Darier's disease
mycosis fungoides

neurodermatitis
pemphigus foliaceus
secondary to burn
seborrheic dermatitis
Wiskott–Aldrich disease

# Eczematous dermatitis

chronic granulomatous disease
selective IgM deficiency

Wiskott–Aldrich syndrome
X-linked hypogammaglobulinemia

# Elastosis perforans serpinginosa

**LESS COMMON**

Rothmund–Thomson syndrome
systemic sclerosis

acrogeria
morphea
penicillamine-induced

Down's syndrome
Enlerhs–Danlos syndrome, Type IV

Marfan's syndrome
osteogenesis imperfecta
pseudoxanthoma elasticum

# Epidermolysis bullosa acquista

amyloidosis
carcinoma
chronic lymphocytic leukemia
diabetes mellitus
dermatitis-herpetiformis
Ehlers–Danlos syndrome
impetigo
inflammatory bowel disease
medication (arsenic, penicillamine,
    sulfonamides)

Multiple Endrocinopathy syndrome
myeloma
porphyria
poison oak dermatitis
rheumatoid arthritis
scarlet fever
systemic lupus erythematosus
thyroiditis
tuberculosis

# Eruptive xanthomas

chronic pancreatitis
marked hypertriglyceridemia

# Erythema ab igne
# (over the epigastrium or lower thoracic spine)

chronic pancreatitis

# Erythema annulare centrifugum

dermatophytosis
drug allergy

internal malignancy (rare)

# Erythema elevatum diutinum

dermatitis herpetiformis
hematologic abnormalities (IgA monoclonal
   gammopathy*)

HIV infection
multiple agent chemotherapy for tuberculosis

# Erythema gyratum repens

benign breast hyperthrophy
bullous pemphigoid
CREST syndrome
ichtyosis

internal malignancy, 84% of cases; most
   commonly first lung, followed by esophagus
   & breast
palmoplantar hyperkeratosis
pityriasis rubra pilaris
tuberculosis (pulmonary)

# Erythema infectiosum
# (fifth disease, HPV b19, parvovirus)

aplastic crisis
hydrops fetalis

syndrome of subacute arthralgias in women

# Erythema nodosum

**Infectious**

*Fungal*
blastomycosis
coccidioidomycosis
histoplasmosis
trichophyton fungal infections

*Bacterial*
brucellosis
*Campylobacter jejuni*
cat-scratch fever
lepromatous leprosy
leptospirosis
lymphogranuloma venereum
streptococcal infections*
tuberculosis
tularemia
*Yersinia enterocolitica*

*Parasitic*
American leishmaniasis
toxoplasmosis

*Viral*
herpes simplex
infectious mononucleosis

**Medicinal**
bromides
estrogens
iodides
oral contraceptive pills*
penicillin
sulfonamides*
sulfones
vaccines

**Metabolic**
pregnancy

**Idiopathic**
Behçet's syndrome
Crohn's disease
sarcoidosis and hilar adenopathy (Loffler's
syndrome, most common disease)
ulcerative colitis

**Neoplastic**
Hodgkin's disease
leukemia

# Erythermalgia

AIDS
atherosclerosis
back trauma or surgery
carcinoma (abdominal, colon, thymoma,
    astrocytoma)
carpal tunnel syndrome
cholestrol crystal emboli syndrome
conversion disorder
diabetes mellitus
familial nephritis
frostbite
gout
hereditary spherocytosis
hypercholesterolemia
hypertension
iodide (contrast injection)
leukemia (chronic myeloid leukemia*)
medications: nifedipine, felodipine, nicardipine,
    bromocriptine, norophedrine, pergolide,
    ticlopidine
mercury poisoning

metabolic disorders
mixed connective tissue disorder
multiple sclerosis
myeloid metaplasia
neck and other trauma
neuropathies
pernicious anemia
polycythemia vera
postphlebitic varices
recurrent bacterial infection
rheumatoid arthritis
thrombocythrmia
sciatica (spinal cord disease)
Sjorgren's syndrome
syphilis
systematic lupus erythematous
thrombocythemia*
vaccines:influenza,hepatitis
vasculitis
venous insufficiency
viral infections

# Flagellate erythema

Bleomycin use

dermatomyositis

# Folliculitis ulerythema reticulata (atrophodermia vermiculata)

congenital heart block (and other cardiac
    abnormalities)
Down's syndrome

neurofibromatosis (AD)
oligophrenia

135

# Furunculosis

diabetes mellitus

low serum iron

# Generalized granuloma annulare

diabetes mellitus
Epstein–Barr virus

HIV infection

# Gianotti–Crosti syndrome (papular acrodermatitis of childhood)

coxsackievirus
cytomegalovirus

Epstein–Barr virus
hepatitis B virus (subtype ayw)

# Grover's disease

asteatotic eczema
allergic contact dermatitis

atopic dermatitis
bullous pemphigoid

# Halo nevus

malignant melanoma

vitiligo (most common associated condition)

# Hepatitis B antigenemia

erythema nodosum
essential mixed cryoglobulinemia
Gianotti's disease (papular acrodermatitis)
polyarteritis nodosa (up to 50% have
 hepatitis B)

serum sickness-like prodrome
urticaria
vasculitis

# Hepatitis C & autoimmune hepatitis

cryoglobulin associated vasculitis
erythema nodosum
leukocytoclastic vasculitis
lichen planus

necrolytic acral erythema
porphyria cutanea tarda
pyoderma gangronosum
Sjogren's syndrome

# Chronic perianal herpes

AIDS
Amyloidosis
burns
Chemotherapy patients
Congenital thymus disorder
Cutaneous T-cell Lymphoma

Leukemia
Lymphoma
Nephrotic syndrome
Renal transplantation
uremia

# Herpes simplex

acquired immunodeficiency syndrome
amyloidosis
ascending myelitis
cancer chemotherapy
cervical carcinoma
congenital thymus disorder
cutaneous T cell lymphoma
erythema multiforme

immunodeficiency
immunosuppressive therapy
leukemia\lymphoma
nephritic syndrome
renal transplantation
severe burns
squamous cell carcinoma
uremia

# Hidradenitis suppurativa

acne conglobata
dissecting cellulitis of scalp
Fox Fordyce Disease
interstitial keratitis

low grade anemia
pilonidal cyst
spondyloarthropathy

# Human immunodeficiency virus infection

acquired ichtyosis
acute HIV exanthema
aphtosis
bacillary angiomatosis
candidiasis (very common) (Penicillium
    Marneffei)
condyloma/warts (common)
cryptococcosis
cytomegalovirus
dermatophytosis and onychomycosis
drug eruption
eosinophilic pustular folliculitis (rare)
epitheliod angiomatosis (rare)
granuloma annulare

hairy leukoplakia (Epstein–Barr virus infection,
    common)
herpes simplex and zoster (common)
histoplasmosis
hyperpigmentation
Kaposi's sarcoma (30–40% incidence)
lipodystrophy
molluscum contagiosum (common)
photoeruptions
premature graying of hair (common)
pruritus
psoriasis (uncommon)
purpuric papular eruptions
Reiter's syndrome
scabies

seborrheic dermatitis (common)
staphylococcal infections
syphilis (Venereal Disease Research
  Laboratories test may be very high or
  negative; incubation period for neurosyphilis
  may be very short (few months))

telangiectasias of the anterior chest wall
thrombocytopenic purpura (common)
tinea versicolor
xerosis
yellow or dark-blue nails

# Hyperimmunoglobulinemia E syndrome (Buckley's syndrome)

asthma
chronic mucocutaneous candidiasis
chronic nasal discharge

ichthyosis
recurrent otitis media

# Hypoparathyroidism (primary)

chronic mucocutaneous candidiasis

# Ichthyosis (acquired)

AIDS
Autoimmune disease
Endocrine disease
Hodgkin's Lymphoma*

medication
Multiple myeloma
Mycosis fungoides

# Idiopathic thrombocytopenic purpura

chronic lymphocytic leukemia

systemic lupus erythematosus

# IgA deficiency

dermatomyositis
increased incidence of malignancy (adenoma of
   colon/esophagus/stomach; reticular cell
   sarcoma; squamous cell carcinoma of lung;
   thyoma)
lupoid hepatitis

pernicious anemia
pulmonary hemosiderosis
rheumatoid arthritis
systemic lupus erythematosus
thyroiditis

# IGA monoclonal gammopathy

erythema elevatum diutinum
pyoderma gangrenosum

subcorneal pustular dermatosis

# Inflammatory bowel disease

aphthous ulcers
bowel-associated dermatosis–arthritis
   syndrome
clubbing of fingernails
epidermolysis bullosa acquisita
erythema nodosum
erythema multiforme
fissure

fistulae
metastatic Crohn's disease
mucous membrane lesions
pyoderma gangrenosum
urticaria
vasculitis
vitiligo

# Interleukins

erythropetin : excess hair growth
Interferon-alfa : alopecia (most common
   toxicity)

Interleukin 2 : acral desqumation, erosions in
   healed surgical scar, psoriasis exacerbation,
   vitiligo
granulocyte colony stimulating factor: Sweet's
   syndrome

# Juvenile xanthogranuloma

childhood leukemia (xantholeukemia, most
  commonly chronic myelogenous leukemia)
epilepsy

neurofibromatosis type I
Nieman-Pick disease
Urticaria pigmentosa

# Kaposi sarcoma (immunosuppressed-related)

aplastic anemia
asthma
bullous pemphigoid
dermatomyositis
hemolytic anemia
idiopathic thrombocytopenic purpura
leukemia
lymphoma
myeloma

nephrotic syndrome
pemphigus vulgaris
polymalgia rheumatica
polymyositis
rheumatoid arthritis
systematic lupos erythmatosus
temporal arteritis
ulcerative colitis
Wegener's granulomatosis

# Keratosis pilaris

atopic dermatitis
keratosis pilaris rubra faciei

ulerythema ophryogenes

# Kimura's disease

renal disease (especially nephrotic syndrome)

# Knuckle pads

Dupuytren's contracture
esophageal cancer
hyperkeratosis

oral leukoplakia
pseudoxanthoma elasticum
Unna-Thost palmoplantar keratoderma

# Kyrle's disease

congestive heart failure
diabetes mellitus

hepatic insufficiency
renal disease

# Lentigo maligna

porphyria cutanea tarda
tyrosinase positive oculocutaneous albinism

Werner's syndrome
Xeroderma pigmentosum

# Leukocytoclastic vasculitis

**Infectious**
*Bacterial*
   Neisseria
   Streptococcus
*Viral*
   cytomegalovirus
   Epstein–Barr
   hepatitis B

**Traumatic**
food dyes or preservatives

**Medicinal**
allopurinol
non-steroidal anti-inflammatory drugs
phenothiazines
phenytoin
quinidine

radiocontrast dye
sulfonamides
sulfonylureas
thiazides

**Neoplastic**
leukemia
lymphoma
myeloma

**Idiopathic**
inflammatory bowel disease
lupus erythematosus
mixed connective tissue disease
rheumatoid arthritis
Sjögren's syndrome

**Hematologic**
cryoglobulinemia
gammopathies

# Lichen planus

alopecia areata
bullous pemphigoid
chronic active hepatitis
dermatitis herpetiformis
dermatomyositis
diabetes mellitus and abnormal glucose
    tolerance (increased incidence $\times$ 3)
Hashimoto's thyroiditis
Hepatitis C
hypertension (coincidental)
graft versus host disease
morphea
myasthenia gravis
pemphigus foliaceus/vulgaris
pernicious anemia

primary biliary cirrhosis
Sjögren's syndrome
systemic sclerosis
thymoma
ulcerative colitis
urolithiasis (increased incidence $\times$ 6–12)
vitiligo
HLA-DR-1 is seen in:
    80% of patients with generalized lichen
        planus
    56% of patients with drug-induced lichen
        planus
    54% of patients with localized lesions of
        lichen planus
    31% of patients with oral lichen planus

# Lichen planus, oral

amebiasis
Dental amalgam (& other metal)
hepatitis C
herpes simplex

HIV
Medication
syphylis

143

# Lichen planus, ulcerative type

Castleman disease
diabetes mellitus*

Sjögren's syndrome

# Lichen sclerosis et atrophicus

achlorhydria with or without pernicious anemia
alopecia areata
atopic dermatitis, eczema
borrelia burgdorferi infection
diabetes mellitus
fasciitis
lichen planus

lupus panniculitis
myositis
pernicious anemia
primary biliary cirrhosis
systemic lupus erythematosus
thyroid disease (Grave's disease)
vitiligo

# Lipodystrophy

diabetes mellitus
glomerulonephritis

HIV infected patient on Protease inhibitors

# Lymphedema

elephantiasis verrucosa nostras
intestinal lymphangiectasia
Noonan's syndrome

Pes cavus microcphaly
Turner's syndrome
Yellow nail syndrome

# Merkel cell ca (in younger patients)

B cell lymphoma
Cowden disease

Ectodermal dysplasia

# Multiple myeloma

angioedema (with C1 inhibitor deficiency)
cutaneous amyloidosis
cutaneous plasmacytoma
follicular hyperkeratosis
leukocytoclastic vasculitis
necrobiotic xanthogranuloma
POEMS syndrome

pyoderma gangrenosum
scleroderma
scleromyxedema
Sneddon–Wilkinson's disease (subcorneal
    pustular dermatosis)
Sweet's syndrome
xanthoma (plane)

# Mucocutaneous candidiasis

adrenal failure
AIDS
alopecia areata
autoimmune thyroid disease
chronic active hepatitis
diabetes mellitus
Di George's syndrome (congenital absence of
    thymus)
gonadal failure
hypothyroidism

melabsorption
Nezelof's syndrome (hypoplasia of thymus)
pernicious anemia
primary hypoparathyroidism (about 75% of
    patients)
Swiss type of agammaglobulinemia (hypoplasia
    of thymus and all lymphoid tissues)
thymoma
vitiligo

# Multicentric reticulohistiocytosis

cancer of breast,bronchus,cervix,colon,
   stomach & ovary
diabetes insipidus
diabtes mellitus

lymphoma
sarcoma
throid disorders
tuberculosis

# Neurovascular syndromes

ataxia telangiectasia
Cobb's syndrome
Fabry's disease (angiokeratosis diffusum
   corporis)
Klippel–Trenauney–Weber syndrome
   (dermatomal hemangiomatosis with spinal
   vascular malformation)

Lindau–Von Hippel disease (hemangioblastoma
   of cerebellum and retina)
Osler–Weber–Rendu disease
Sturge–Weber syndrome (craniofacial or
   trigeminocranial angiomatosis, cerebral
   calcification)

# Nevus anemicus

neurofibromatosis

# Occupation related diseases

British coal miners – trichophyton rubrum
Chinese rice farmers-schistosomiasis
confectioners – *Candida albicans*
construction workers – {contact dermatitis}
   chromium ( cement, leather boots), rubber,
   epoxy resin
fish porters – erysipeloid

hairdressers – {contact dermatitis}
   P-Phenylenediamine, formaldehyde,
   fragrences, glyceryl monothioglycolate
healthcare workers – {contact dermatitis}
   rubber, gluteraldehyde, preservatives
housekeepers – {contact dermatitis} rubber,
   fragrances, preservatives

Indian sand dredgers – Rhinosporidiosis
Kenyan shepherds – Rift Valley Fever
pet shop helpers – psittacosis
photographers – {contact dermatitis} color
developers

schoolteachers – oxyuriasis
speleologist – histoplasmosis
tripe scrapers – leptospirosis

# Pellegra

carcinoid
5-fluorouracil
Hatnup's disease
isoniazid

Niacin deficiency
6-mercaptopurine
sulfapyridine

# Pemphigus erythematosus/vulgaris

Castleman's disease (with pemphigus vulgaris)
lupus erythematosis
malignancy (colon*, hematopoietic*)

myasthenia gravis
thymoma

# Perifolliculitis capitis

acne conglobata
pilonidal cyst

portal occlusion skin diseases

# Pernicious anemia

Addison's disease
autoimmune thyroiditis
dermatitis herpetiformis

hypoparathyroidism
vitiligo

# Peyronie's disease

β-adrenergic blocking agents
diabetes mellitus
Dupuytren's contracture
fibrosis of the auricular cartilage

fibrosis of the endocardium and
    retroperitoneum in carcinoid syndrome
Weber–Christian disease

# Plummer–Vinson syndrome

cheilosis
iron-deficiency anemia

koilonychia
squamous cell carcinoma of the esophagus

# Porphyria cutanea tarda

cirrhosis
diabetes mellitus
hepatitis C

hepatomas
lupus erythematosus
lymphoma

# Primary biliary cirrhosis

CREST syndrome
familial

rheumatoid arthritis
thyroiditis

# Pseudoainhum

burn
congenital deformity
diabetes mellitus
frostbite
leprosy
morphea
pachyonychia congenita (AD)
parasitic disease
pityriasis rubra pilaris

Raynaud's disease
scleroderma
syphilis
syringomyelia
systemic sclerosis
trauma
Vohwinkel's disease (keratoderma hereditarum
    mutilans)

# Pseudoxanthoma elasticum

accelerated atherosclerosis
gastrointestinal hemorrhage during pregnancy
    (Gronbland–Strandberg syndrome)

sickle cell anemia

# Psoriasis

eczema (of hands in particular)
lichen planus

lichen simplex chronicus
seborrheic dermatitis

# Pyoderma gangrenosum

acne conglobata
Behçet's syndrome
chronic active hepatitis
Crohn's disease

diabetes mellitus
diverticulosis
hairy cell leukemia
hidradenitis suppurativa

Hodgkin's disease
myeloma
myelocytic leukemia
myelofibrosis
osteoarthritis
paraproteinemia
polycythemia vera
primary liver cirrhosis

rheumatoid arthritis
sarcoidosis
Sneddon–Wilkinson syndrome
Takayasu's disease
ulcerative colitis*
Wegener's granulomatosis
spondylitis

# Pyostomatitis vegetans

ulcerative colitis

# Reactive angioendotheliomatosis

cryoglobulinemia
paraproteinemia

systemic infections (especially bacterial
endocarditis)

# Reactive perforating collagenosis

acquired type with diabetes mellitus
chronic renal failure

retinopathy

# Reticulohistiocytosis

carcinoma
diabetes mellitus
hemoblastoses

thyroid disorders
tuberculosis

# Rheumatoid arthritis

bullous pemphigoid
cicatricial pemphigoid
dermatitis herpetiformis
epidermolysis bullosa acquisita
pemphigus foliaceus/vulgaris

overlap syndrome with dermatomyositis
scleroderma
systemic lupus erythematosus

alopecia areata
erythema elevatum diutinum
erythromelalgia
Felty's syndrome (granulocytopenia,
    rheumatoid arthritis, splenomegaly)
Mondor's disease
pyoderma gangrenosum
Sjögren's syndrome
subcorneal pustular dermatosis
vitiligo

# Sarcoidosis

cryptococcosis
Scabies, Norwegian
thyroid disease

underlying carcinoma
vitiligo

# Scleroderma

Diabetes mellitus
Monoclonal gammopathy (IgG Kappa or
    Lambda)

# Scabies, Norwegian

bacillary dysentery
Beriberi
Bloom's syndrome
Cerebrovascular accidents (with paralysis of
    extremity)
Connective tissue disorders
Diabetes mellitus
Down's syndrome
Immunosuppressive therapy
Kaposi's sarcoma

Leprosy
Lymphoreticular malignancies
Malnutrition
Parkinson's disease
Renal failure (chronic)
Syringomyelia
Systemic vasculitis
Tabes dorsalis
Tuberculosis
Vitamin A deficiency

# Seborrheic dermatitis

AIDS
Parkinson's disease

unilateral injury to facial innervation (unilateral
    seborrheic dermatitis)

# Sjögren's syndrome

chronic active hepatitis
chronic graft versus host disease
dermatitis herpetiformis
hepatitis C
necrotizing angiitis
periarteritis nodosa
polymyositis
primary biliary cirrhosis

rheumatoid arthritis*
scleroderma
splenomegaly
Sweet's syndrome
systemic lupus erythematosus
thrombotic thrombocytopenic purpura
thyroid enlargement
Waldenstrom's macroglobulinemia

# Sneddon's syndrome

Association of livedo reticularis, usually in a
   young to middle-aged adult who develops
   cerebrovascular problems

# Spider nevus

liver disease
oral contraceptive pills
pregnancy

rheumatoid arthritis
thyrotoxicosis
with estrogen treatment

# Steroid (topical) side-effects

acne
allergic contact dermatitis
atrophy*
conjunctival sac contamination
delayed wound healing
hypertrichosis
hypopigmentation (more common with
   intralesional steroids)

induction of glaucoma with periorbital
   application)
masking of skin infection (e.g. tinea incognito)
perioral dermatitis
provocation of erythema craquele
rosacea
striae
telangiectasia

# Subcorneal pustular dermatosis (Sneddon–Wilkinson)

IgA paraproteinemia
increase in IgA
multiple IgA myeloma

pyoderma gangrenosum
ulcerative colitis

# Sweet's syndrome
# (acute febrile neutrophilic dermatosis)

Behcet's disease
Benign monoclonal gammopathy
Chronic active hepatitis
Crohn's disease
cytomegalovirus
Fanconi's anemia
granulocyte colony-stimulating factor
hemoproliferative disease
histoplasmosis
HIV infection
leprosy
leukemia (acute myelogenous leukemia*)
mixed connective tissue disease
mycobacteria
oral contraceptives
other carcinomas
pregnancy

rheumatoid arthritis
salmonellosis
sepsis
Sjogren's syndrome
thyroiditis
tonsillitis
toxoplasmosis
transient myeloid proliferation
typhus
Trimethoprim sulfamethoxazole
Tuberculosis
Ulcerative colitis
upper respiratory tract infection (typically precedes it by 1–3 weeks)
ureaplasmosis
vulvovaginal infection
yersiniosis

# Thyroid disease

acanthosis nigricans
alopecia areata
bullous pemphigoid
chronic angioedema/urticaria
Cowden's disease
dermatitis herpetiformis
dermatomyositis
eczema
epidermolysis bullosa acquisita

herpes gestationis
mucocutaneous candidiasis
pemphigus
pustulosis palmoplantaris
scleroderma
Sweet's syndrome
systemic lupus erythematosus
vitiligo

# Tinea versicolor

burn (severe case)
Cushing's disease
diabetes mellitus
herpes gestationis
hyperhidrosis
ichthyosis
immunosuppression

malnutrition
oral contraceptive pills
post-adrenalectomy
pregnancy
steroid treatment (systemic)
striae

# Toxic epidermal necrolysis

AIDS
Aspergillosis
Crohn's disease

Drugs:
Alkaseltzer
Allopurinol
Amiodarone
Antibiotics(esp. penicillin and tetracyclines)
Anticonvulsants
Antipyrine
Barbiturates
Brompheniramine
Chlorpromazine
Dapsone
Ethambutol
Fansidar
Fenoprofen
Gold
Griseofulvin
Ipecac
Isoniazid
NSAIDs(esp. phenylbutazone)

Pentamidine
Phenolphthalein
Quinine
Streptomycin
Sulfonamides
Tolbutamide
Trimethoprim

Escherichia Coli (septicemia)
graft versus host disease*
Herpes simplex
Measles Virus
Varicella-Zoster Virus
Idopathic
internal carcinoma (leukemia, lymphoma)
systemic lupus erythematosus
Vaccinations
BCG
Diphtheria toxiod
Measles
Poliomyelitis
Tetanus antitoxin

# Unilateral nevoid telangiectasia

chronic liver disease associated with alcoholism
high estrogen

pregnancy

# Urticarial vasculitis

chronic liver disease associated with alcoholism
high estrogen
pregnancy
relapsing polychondritis
unilateral nevoid telangiectasia

Sjögren's syndrome
systemic lupus erythematosus*
viral infections (especially with Epstein–Barr and
hepatitis B)

# Vitiligo

Addison's disease
alopecia areata
atrophic gastritis
candidiasis (chronic mucocutaneous)
chloroquine
clofazimine
dermatitis herpetiformis
diabetes mellitus (insulin dependent)
Down's syndrome

halo nevus
hyperthyroidism (including Grave's disease)
hypothyroidism (including Hashimoto's
thyroiditis)
malignant melanoma
pernicious anemia
polyglandular autoimmune syndromes (types I,
II, III)
uveitis

# Xanthoma & lipid association

eruptive-increased chylomicron
plane-increased cholestrol
tendinous-increased LDL

tuberous-increased chylomicron & VLDL
xanthelasma-50% of people have normal lipid

# SECTION TWO

## Body systems and skin disorders

The skin is the most visible and easily-accessible organ of the body. It is important diagnostically, opening a window to the diseases affecting the internal organs. Recognition of the dermatologic manifestation of systemic diseases is important for practically all practicing clinicians.

This section reviews different pathologic states of body systems as they relate to skin manifestations. '=' denotes the association

# Auditory

albinism (AD, AR)
Cockayne's syndrome
congenital syphilis
ectodermal dysplasia
KID syndrome (keratitis, ichthyosis, deafness)

knuckle pads, leukonychia, and deafness
   syndrome
pili torti
Refsum's syndrome
relapsing polychondritis
Waardenburg's syndrome
xeroderma pigmentosum

# Bone

**Infectious**
early congenital syphilis (periostitis*,
   metaphyseal changes, osteitis, pathologic
   fractures)
late congenital syphilis and late (acquired)
   syphilis (periostitis (which results in Saber
   shins, frontal bossing, Higoumenakis' Sign
   (swelling of sternoclavicular joint)),
   gummatous osteitis, osteomyelitis)
osteomyelitis (sinus tract and, uncommonly,
   squamous cell carcinoma)
secondary syphilis (periostitis*, osteomyelitis,
   osteitis)

**Medicinal**
retinoids (hyperostoses or osteophyte
   formation)
steroids (aseptic necrosis of bone,
   osteoporosis)
vinyl chloride (acro-osteolysis (most commonly
   of the thumb))

**Metabolic**
metastatic calcinosis cutis (in presence of
   increased calcium or phosphorus)

**Idiopathic**
acne conglobata (erosive and proliferative
   arthritis of the skeleton, indistinguishable
   from the changes noted in seronegative
   spondyloarthropathy)
acne fulminans (lytic bone lesions consistent
   with osteomyelitis, most commonly on the
   clavicles)
hypophosphatasia (shallow depression to deep
   pits of skin, defective osteogenesis,
   rickets-like bony changes (alkaline
   phosphatase deficiency in liver, bone and
   kidney))
dermatomyositis (ectopic and dystrophic
   calcification in 40–70% of children;
   'popcorn-like' findings on X-ray)
multicentric reticulohistiocytosis (destructive
   lesions of periosteum and bone; most
   commonly affect interphalangeal joints of
   hands; 'accordion hand' is noted in the end
   stage)

pachydermoperiostosis (periostitis, painful subperiosteal new bone formation)

POEMS syndrome (polyneuropathy, organomegaly (liver, spleen, lymph nodes), endocrinopathy (amenorrhea, gynecomastia, impotence), M-protein, skin changes (angiomas, hyperpigmentation, hypertrichosis, induration), sclerotic bony changes)

psoriasis (atlantoaxial subluxation, erosion and fusion of sternomandibular joints, erosions and spurs of calcaneus)

Reiter's disease (arthritis, very similar to the psoriatic type, but more commonly lower extremities (knees, toes, heels) are involved, and there is increased frequency of sacroilitis)

sarcoidosis (hands most commonly affected; common changes include acrosclerosis, cysts, latticework or honeycomb pattern; osteoporosis of nasal bones in lupus pernio)

scleroderma (dermal and subcutaneous calcification are most characteristic; other changes include flexion derformities; resorption of digital tufts, demineralization and generalized osteoporisis)

## Neoplastic

enchondroma (may clinically present as paronychia in the distal phalanx)

histiocytosis X (painful lytic lesions; exophthalmos results from orbital bony lesions)

mastocytosis (generalized osteoporosis and osteosclerosis (possibly secondary to heparin, histamine and other substances released from mast cells)

subungual exostosis (often underlying cause of pincer nails)

## Congenital

alkapotonuria (ochronosis) (AR, slate blue or black skin and skeletal pigmentation, generalized osteopenia)

Buschke–Ollendorff syndrome (AD, osteopoikilosis (focal areas of bony sclerosis), elastomas (dermatofibrosis lenticularis disseminata))

chondrodysplasia punctata (atrophic skin lesions, ichthyosis, punctate (calcification)

stippling in epiphyseal regions in the first year of life)

Conrad–Hunermann syndrome ('classic') (AD, asymmetric shortening of the extremities, vertebral and paravertebral stippling, calcification of larynx and trachea)

non-rhizomelic lethal subtype of Conrad–Hunermann syndrome (AR, more coarse and more profound laryngeal and tracheal calcifications)

XD condrodysplasia punctata (hexadactyly is unique and diagnostic)

AR rhizomelic type (absent laryngeal and tracheal calcifications, symmetric shortening of the upper extremities)

Cobb's syndrome (associated intraspinal angioma with an overlying nevus flammeus or angiokeratoma circumscriptum)

ectodermal dysplasias (odontodysplasia is characteristic in most varieties)

Ehlers–Danlos syndrome (characteristic molluscoid pseudo-tumors develop over pressure points; subcutaneous masses (spheroids) form secondary to hematomas or fat herniation)

Gardner's syndrome (AD, epidermoid and desmoid cysts, fibromas, lipomas, intestinal polyposis, osteomas and dental abnormalities)

Goltz syndrome (focal, dermal, hypoplasia) (XD, linear bands of dermal hypoplasia following lines of Blaschko; in 80%, bony defects are associated (most commonly abnormalities of hands and feet); characteristic *osteopathia striata* (fine, opaque, parallel, vertical bands in the metaphysis of long bones)

hypomelanosis of Ito (AD, asymmetry of face or arms, leg length discrepancy, kyphoscoliosis; streaks or whorls of hypopigmentation along the lines of Blaschko)

incontinentia pigmenti (XD, whorl-like hyperpigmentation, characteristic marked hypodentia ('pegged teeth'), microcephaly, occult spina bifida)

Jaffe–Campanacci syndrome (hyperpigmented macules; multiple non-ossifying fibromas)

Klippel–Trenaunay syndrome (angio-osteohypertrophy) (port-wine stains, varicose veins, soft tissue and bony hypertrophy; characteristic elongation of bones on X-rays) linear nevus sebaceous syndrome (seizure, eye abnormalities and mental retardation; 65% with skeletal abnormalities)

lipoid proteinosis (AR, characteristic *intracranial calcifications* (bilateral 'bean-shaped' calcification of hippocampus is pathognomonic))

Maffucci's syndrome (multiple bilateral asymmetric enchondromas (mostly of metacarpal and phalangeal bones); capillary and cavernous hemangiomas and lymphangiomas)

McCune–Allbright syndrome (polyostotic fibrous dysplasia) (hyperpigmented macules; characteristic discrete cyst-like bony changes which appear moth-eaten or mottled; pathologic fractures occur commonly)

nail–patella syndrome (hereditary osteo-onychodysostosis) (AD, nail dystrophies; absent or hypoplastic patella and elbow; pathognomonic finding (seen in 80% of patients) is bilaterally symmetrical osseous horns that arise from posterior aspect of iliac wings)

Neurofibromatosis (AD, 40% of patients have bone abnormalities; most commonly kyphoscoliosis; 0.5–1% have congenital pseudoarthroses (but neurofibromatosis accounts for 50% of cases of patients with congenital pseudoarthrosis))

nevoid basal cell carcinoma syndrome (odontogenic cysts of jaw (75% of patients); characteristic lamellar calcification of falx cerebri, tentorium or the peteroclinoid ligaments (80% of patients))

Parkes–Weber syndrome (Klippel–Trenaunay syndrome plus arteriovenous fistulas)

proteus syndrome (epidermal nevi, subcutaneous masses; asymmetry and bony hypertrophy of the extremities)

pseudoxanthoma elasticum (AR, involves skin, eyes and blood vessels; X-ray reveals soft tissue and vascular calcifications)

Rothmund–Thomson syndrome (congenital poikiloderma, bony hypoplasia and bony defects)

spina bifida occulata (sacral lipomas, dermal sinuses, deep dimples, hairy tufts, aplasia cutis, and dermoid cysts)

Sturge–Weber syndrome (port-wine stain and ipsilateral meningeal angiomatosis; pathognomonic opaque, double-contoured ('railroad track') sinusoidal lines that follow the convolutions of the brain and which represent calcium deposits, seen on X-ray)

trichorhinophalangeal syndrome (AD, triad of fine sparse hair, pear-shaped nose with elongated philtrum, and stubby fingers; commonly, cone-shaped epiphysis noted on X-ray of phalanx)

tuberous sclerosis (AD, intracranial calcifications (commonly in children), sclerosis of skull bones (commonly in adults))

## BONE PAIN

histiocytosis X
mastocytosis
metastatic malignant melanoma

# Cardiovascular

## CARDIOVASCULAR DISORDERS AND SKIN DISEASES AND SYNDROMES

coarctation of aorta = Turner's syndrome – pterygium colli (redundant skin on sides of neck)

constrictive pericarditis, tricuspid valvular disease = jaundice

hypertension = pseudoxanthoma elasticum, neurofibromatosis

increased risk of coronary artery disease = earlobe crease, familial hyperlipidemia, Kawasaki's disease, Werner's syndrome, xanthomatosis

mitral valve prolapse = Ehlers–Danlos syndrome, Marfan's syndrome

myocarditis, arrhythmias, cardiac failure, thromboembolism = Chagas' disease (American trypanosomiasis)

post-bypass surgery = dermatitis along saphenous vein graft scar

post-myocardial infarction = shoulder–hand syndrome

pulmonic stenosis/obstructive cardiomyopathy = Moynahan's syndrome

subacute bacterial endocarditis = clubbing, Janeway lesions, Osler's node (5%), petechiae (50%), purpura, subungual splinter hemorrhages

## NAIL CHANGES AND CARDIOVASCULAR DISORDERS

aortic regurgitation = Quincke's pulsations (flushing of nailbeds synchronous with heartbeat)

cyanotic heart disease = clubbing

heart failure = reddish lunulae

ischemia = nail dystrophy

vasculitis = periungual infarcts, splinter hemorrhages

## SKIN DISEASES AND CARDIOVASCULAR DISORDERS

amyloidosis = cardiomegaly, conduction abnormalities, congestive heart failure, orthostatic hypotension

Behçet's syndrome = pericarditis

carcinoid syndrome = fibrotic plaques of the pulmonic and tricuspid valves, right-sided heart failure, tricuspid insufficiency and/or pulmonic stenosis

cutis laxa = aortic dilatation/rupture, cor pulmonale

Degos' disease = pericardial effusion, pericarditis

dermatomyositis = conduction abnormalities, congestive heart failure, non-specific EKG changes, myocarditis, pericarditis

Ehlers–Danlos syndrome = aortic/pulmonary artery dilatation, mitral/tricuspid valve prolapse

exfoliative erythroderma = high output heart failure

Fabry's disease = cardiomyopathy, coronary artery disease, hypertension, valvular dysfunction

hemochromatosis = restrictive cardiomyopathy, supraventricular arrhythmias with or without congestive heart failure

**Infectious**
*Fungal*
    pericarditis = histoplasmosis
*Bacterial*
    endocarditis = gonococcal, meningococcal, staphylococcal, streptococcal
myocarditis = diphtheria

*Parasitic*
   myocarditis = toxoplasmosis,
   trypanosomiasis
*Spirochetal*
   arrhythmias, myocarditis = Lyme disease
*Viral*
   myocarditis = coxsackie B. cytomegalovirus,
   infectious mononucleosis, rubella, varicella
Kawasaki's disease = arrhythmias, coronary
   artery aneurysm, myocardial infarction,
   myocarditis, ventricular hypertrophy
LAMB (NAME) syndrome = atrial myxoma
LEOPARD syndrome = EKG abnormalities
lipoid proteinosis = arrhythmia, conduction
   abnormalities
lymphomatoid granulomatosis = pulmonary
   vasculitis
Marfan's syndrome = ascending aortic
   aneurysm*, mitral valve prolapse*
multicentric reticulohistiocytosis = congestive
   heart failure, coronary artery disease
neurofibromatosis = coarctation of aorta,
   hypertension with pheochromocytoma
periarteritis nodosa = coronary artery disease,
   hypertension

progeria = atherosclerosis, coronary artery
   disease
pseudoxanthoma elasticum = aortic aneurysm,
   atherosclerosis hypertension
relapsing polychondritis = aortic insufficiency or
   aneurysm
Reiter's syndrome = aortic insufficiency,
   conduction abnormalities, pericarditis
rheumatic fever = pericarditis, valvular disease
rheumatoid arthritis = pericarditis
sarcoidosis = conduction abnormalities,
   congestive heart failure
scleroderma = conduction abnormalities, cor
   pulmonale, hypertension, pericarditis
systemic lupus erythematosus:
   adult = coronary arteritis, hypertension,
   pericarditis
   neonatal = congenital heart block
tuberous sclerosis = congestive heart failure,
   rhabdomyoma
vasculitis = coronary heart disease
Werner's syndrome = coronary atherosclerosis

# Endocrine

## ADRENAL

### Hypercortisolism
acanthosis nigricans
acne[+]
atrophic and friable skin
decreased vascular tone (cutis marmorata)
prone to dermatophytosis and tinea versicolor
hirsutism (mild)[+]
hyperpigmentation
hypertrichosis
increased vascular fragility (ecchymosis,
   petechiae)
central obesity (buffalo hump, moon facies)
plethora[+]
poor wound healing
striae
telangiectasia

### Hypocortisolism
hyperpigmentation
loss of body hair[+] (axilla)
mucocutaneous candidiasis
vitiligo

### Adrenal insufficiency
histoplasmosis
paracoccidiodomycosis
tuberculosis

## PANCREAS

### Diabetes mellitus
*Autonomic neuropathy*
atrophy
decreased sweating in lower extremities
edema

erythema
increased sweating in face

*Diabetic foot*
cellulitis
deep infections
fissuring
neuropathic ulcers (mal perforans)

*Infections*
candidiasis (pruritus vulvae, recurrent
    balanoprosthitis leading to phimosis)
carbunculosis
dermatophytosis
erysipelas
erythrasma
malignant external otisis (*Pseudomonas*)
nonclostridial gas gangrene
phycomycetes

*Macroangiopathy*
atrophy
coldness of toes
hair loss
mottling on dependence
nail dystrophy
pallor on elevation

*Microangiopathy*
blush or telangiectasias of proximal nail fold
erysipelas-like erythema (legs and feet)
wet gangrene of foot

*Nails*
acute and chronic paronychia
Beau's line
leukonychia
onychauxis (thickening, darkening, and surface
    irregularities)
onychocryptosis (ingrown toenails)
onychogryposis
onycholysis
onychomadesis
onychomycosis
pterygium
pterygium inversum unguis
Rosenau's depressions
splinter hemorrhages
telangiectasia (proximal nail fold)
yellow nail

*Sensory neuropathy*
aching
burning

numbness
tingling

*Miscellaneous*
diabetic bullae
diabetic dermopathy (shin spots, M > F, seen in
    50% of patients)
disseminated granuloma annulare
necrobiosis lipoidica diabeticorum (F : M 3 : 1)
scleredema of diabetes mellitus (scleredema
    adultorum; M : F 4 : 1)
waxy skin and stiff joints (diabetic digital
    sclerosis)
xanthomatosis
yellow skin (face, palms and soles)

*Other conditions associated with increased
incidence of diabetes mellitus*
acromegaly
Cushing's syndrome
flushed face
lipoatrophy
lipohypertrophy
oral changes (angular stomatitis, periodontal
    disease)
peripheral edema
pigmented purpura
pruritus (generalized)

*Skin diseases associated with increased incidence of
diabetes mellitus*
cutaneous perforating disease of diabetes
    mellitus and renal failure (Kyrle's disease)
dermatitis herpetiformis
Kaposi's sarcoma
lichen planus
lipoid proteinosis (AR)
scleroderma
vitiligo
Werner's syndrome (AR)

*Other possible associations with diabetes mellitus*
alopecia
cutaneous porphyrias (porphyria cutanea
    tarda[+])
Degos' disease
Dupuytren's contractures
hemochromatosis
intracutaneous fat herniation
lipodystrophies
pseudoxanthoma elasticum
psoriasis
pustulosis palmaris et plantaris
scalp pruritus

## PARATHYROID

### Increase
Darier's disease
ichtyosis linearis circumflexa
ichtyosis vulgaris
lamellar ichtyosis
nonbullous congenital ichthyosiform
    erythroderma
pityriasis rubra pilaris
pruritus
subcutaneous calcification

### Decrease
*Hair*
alopecia areata
coarse, sparse, patchy alopecia

*Nail*
brittle
opaque
transverse ridges

*Skin*
dry
eczematous dermatitis
exfoliative dermatitis
hyperkeratotic
maculopapular eruption
puffy
scaly

Primary hypoparathyroidism associated with
    chronic mucocutaneous candidiasis

## PITUITARY

### Excess growth hormone
acanthosis nigricans
coarsening of facial features
cutis verticis gyrata
dermal thickening[#]
excessive eccrine and apocrine sweating
    (offensive body odor and greasy skin)
fibromas (20–30%)
furrowing
hyperpigmentation (40%)
hypertrichosis[+] (50%)
macroglossia
soft tissue swelling of hands and feet
thick and hard nails

### Panhypopituitarism
decreased sebaceous secretion and decreased
    sweating
expressionless facies
fine wrinkling around eyes and mouth
increased sensitivity to sunlight
loss of body hair
pallor and yellow tinge of skin
xerosis

## SEX HORMONES

### Androgen excess
acne
hyperpigmentation of areolae/axillae/external
    genitalia/nipples/perineum
precocious puberty with virilization in
    preadolescent children
thickened and coarsened skin
virilization in adult female

### Estrogen excess
amelioration of acne
hair loss
gynecomastia (in male)
melasma
precocious puberty (in female)
testicular atrophy
vaginal candidiasis

## THYROID

### Hyperthyroidism
**Hair**
alopecia areata
diffuse alopecia
fine, soft and rapid growth

*Nail*
clubbing with thyroid acropachy
koilonychia
onycholysis
Plummer's nail

*Skin*
fine, moist, smooth, soft, velvety, warm[#]
    dermatographism[+]
elephantitis nostras
erythema (palmar)
exophthalmos (in Grave's disease only)
facial flushing

hyperhidrosis
hyperpigmentation (diffuse or patchy)
palmar erythema
pretibial myxedema (only in Grave's disease, 5% of patients)
pruritus (generalized)
red elbow
telangiectasis
urticaria (chronic)
vitiligo (only in Grave's disease, 7% of patients)
urticaria

### Hypothyroidism
*Hair*
brittle, coarse, decreased body hair, dull
increase percentage of telogen hair, dry
loss of outer third of eyebrows[+]
patchy alopecia and diffuse thinning of scalp hair
slow growth (in beard, genitals and scalp)

*Nail*
brittle
onycholysis (rare)
slow growth

striated
thin

*Skin*
carotenemia
coarse
cold
dry
easy bruisability
edematous
fine wrinkling
hyperkeratosis (palmoplantar)
ichthyosis
macroglossia
myxedema[++]
pale
poor wound healing
puffy
yellowish tint (palms, soles and nasolabial folds)

*Congenital hypothyroidism*
acral swelling
periorbital puffiness
thick lips
yellow discoloration of skin

# Gastrointestinal

## ABDOMINAL PAIN AND SKIN

Degos' disease
Fabry's disease
Henoch–Schönlein purpura
herpes zoster
porphyrin disorders (hereditary coproporphyria, variegate porphyria)

## CHRONIC LIVER DISEASE

abdominal vein dilation
body hair loss
gynecomastia
jaundice
palmar erythema

peripheral edema
pigmentary changes
purpura
spider angioma

## DYSPHAGIA AND SKIN

### Bullous disorders
bullous pemphigoid
dermatitis herpetiformis
dystrophic epidermolysis bullosa
pemphigus vulgaris

### Carcinoma of esophagus
arsenic ingestion

celiac disease
dermatitis herpetiformis
Plummer–Vinson syndrome
tylosis

**collagen vascular disease**
dermatomyositis
systemic sclerosis

**Other**
acanthosis nigricans
Behçet's syndrome
Darier's disease
lichen planus
Stevens–Johnson syndrome

## GASTROINTESTINAL BLEED AND SKIN

### INFLAMMATORY DISEASES
Crohn's disease
Henoch-Schonlein purpura
Polyarteritis nodsa
Ulcerative colitis

**Inherited connective tissue defects**
Ehlers–Danlos syndrome type IV
pseudoxanthoma elasticum

### INHERITED POLYPOSIS SYNDROMES
Cowden's syndrome (multiple hamartoma
    syndrome)
Gardner's syndrome
Peutz-Jeghers syndrome

**Vascular abnormalities**
blue rubber bleb nevus syndrome
Kaposi's sarcoma
leukocytoclastic vasculitis
malignant atrophic papulosis (Degos' disease)
Osler–Weber–Rendu syndrome

## INFLAMMATORY BOWEL DISEASE AND SKIN

annular erythema

aphthous ulcers
bowel-associated dermatosis–arthritis
    syndrome
clubbing of fingernails
cutaneous Crohn's disease
epidermolysis bullosa acquisita
eruptions at colostomy and ileostomy sites
erythema nodosum
erythema multiforme
fissure
fistulae
granulomas
lichen planus
malnutrition
metastatic Crohn's disease
mucous membrane lesions
pyoderma gangrenosum
urticaria
vasculitis (vascular thrombosis)
vitiligo

## LIVER DISEASE AND SKIN

**Nail**
brittleness
clubbing
flat nails
striations
watch-glass deformity
white bands
white nails

**Skin**
amyloidosis (primary) (hepatosplenomegaly,
    purpura, skin infiltration)
biliary cirrhosis (clubbing, pruritus,
    scleroderma, xanthomas)
chronic active hepatitis (allergic capillaritis,
    clubbing, lupus-like eruptions, splinter
    hemorrhage)
erythropoietic protoporphyria
    (erythematous/purpuric plaques, gallstones,
    hepatic necrosis)
Gaucher's disease (hepatosplenomegaly, skin
    pigmentation)
Gianotti–Crosti syndrome (hepatitis, papular
    acrodermatitis)
graft versus host disease (erythematous
    eruption, hepatitis, lichen planus-like
    eruption, scleroderma-like eruption)
hemochromatosis (skin pigmentation)

hepatitis B infection (urticarial eruption)
hyperlipidemia (abdominal pain, eruptive
xanthomas, hepatosplenomegaly)
mastocytosis (hepatomegaly, nodular and
plaque eruption)

### Other
chloasma hepaticum (perioral/periorbital)
corkscrew scleral vessels
decreased growth of facial hair in males
Dupuytren's contracture
guttae hypomelanosis (patchy depigmentation)
gynecomastia
jaundice
loss of axillary/forearm/pubic hair
melanosis
palmar erythema
spider nevus
striae distensae
swelling of parotid gland
telangiectatic changes

## MALABSORPTION AND SKIN

### Non-specific changes
acquired ichthyosis
decreased elasticity of skin
eczematous and psoriasiform eruptions
hair and nail abnormalities
hyperpigmentation
intestinal bypass syndrome
thinning of skin

### Specific nutritional deficiency
celiac disease
dermatitis herpetiformis
polyarteritis and other vasculitides
systemic sclerosis
folate-, iron-, zinc-poor hair growth
hypoalbuminemia (transverse white bands on
nails)
iron – koilonychia
zinc – acrodermatitis enteropathica

## PANCREATIC DISEASE AND SKIN

acute pancreatitis and blood extravasation
(Cullen's and Turner's signs)
chronic pancreatitis and fat necrosis with
painful subcutaneous nodules
diabetes mellitus
fibrocystic disease and sodium loss in sweat
glucagonoma
hemochromatosis
pancreatic carcinoma and migratory superficial
thrombophlebitis

## PRIMARY BILIARY CIRRHOSIS AND SKIN

hyperpigmentation (in butterfly configuration)
jaundice
pruritus
xanthomas

## POLYPOSIS AND SKIN

Canada–Cronkhite syndrome
Cowden's disease (AD)
Gardner's syndrome (AD)
Muir–Torre syndrome (AD)
neurofibromatosis (AD)
Peutz–Jeghers syndrome

## OTHER

### Diarrhea
carcinoid syndrome
dermatitis herpetiformis (rare)
mastocytosis

### Jaundice
cholangitis
hepatitis
leptospirosis
pancreatitis
Q fever
yellow fever

**Peptic ulcer disease**
telangiectasia macularis eruptiva perstans

**Pyloric atresia**
junctional epidermolysis bullosa

# Hematologic

## ANEMIA

dermatitis herpetiformis
erythroderma
psoriasis
toxic epidermal necrolysis

## ANEMIA (hypochromic signs)

glossitis
koilonychia
pallor

## ANEMIA OF IRON DEFICIENCY

pruritus

## ANEMIA OF SICKLE CELL DISEASE

hemosiderosis and melanosis of legs
leg ulcers (75% of patients)

## COLD AGGLUTININS

Usually in the elderly

acrocyanosis
gangrene
Raynaud's phenomenon

## EOSINOPHILIA

**Vascular**
allergic granulomatosis
angioedema
periarteritis nodosa
systemic mastocytosis
urticaria
vasculitis

**Infectious**
*Fungal*
    chronic mucocutaneous candidiasis
    coccidiomycosis
*Bacterial*
    scarlet fever
    leprosy
*Parasitic*
    parasitic infections
    scabies
    schistosomiasis
*Spirochetal*
    secondary syphilis
*Viral*
    erythema infectiosum

**Traumatic**
insect bite

**Allergic**
atopic dermatitis
exfoliative dermatitis
graft versus host disease

**Medicinal**
drug hypersensitivity reactions

**Idiopathic**

*Bullous disorders*

    bullous pemphigoid

    dermatitis herpetiformis

    herpes gestationis

    pemphigus

*Collagen vascular disease*

    eosinophilic fasciitis

    rheumatoid arthritis

*Other*

    angiolymphoid hyperplasia with eosinophilia

    eosinophilia myalgia syndrome

    eosinophilic cellulitis (Well's syndrome)

    eosinophilic granuloma

    eosinophilic pustular folliculitis

    erythema nodosum

    erythema toxicum neonatorum

    hypereosinophilic syndrome

    granuloma faciale

    sarcoidosis

**Neoplastic**

angioimmunoblastic lymphadenopathy

lymphomatoid papulosis

mycosis fungoides

Waldenstrom's macroglobulinemia

**Congenital**

incontinentia pigmenti (XD, first stage, erythema and bullae)

## HODGKIN'S DISEASE

**Non-specific**

exfoliative dermatitis

hyperpigmentation/melanoderma (pale mucous membranes, but involves nipples)

prurigo-like papules

pruritis (25%; can be localized or generalized)

urticaria

**Specific**

relatively uncommon:

nodules

plaques

tumors

ulcerative lesions as a result of direct tumor invasion

## LEUKEMIA (acute), ERYTHEMATOUS PAPULES AND NODULES

Most frequent oral changes include gingival hyperplasia and hemorrhage, petechiae, ulceration, and loosening of teeth

bacterial or fungal sepsis

drug eruption

leukemia cutis

neutrophilic eccrine hidradenitis

Sweet's syndrome

## LEUKOCYTOSIS IN ABSENCE OF INFECTION

erythema multiforme

erythroderma*

pustular miliaria

pustular psoriasis

## LEUKOPENIA

anaphylactic shock

chickenpox

leishmaniasis

measles

rickettsialpox

Rocky Mountain spotted fever

rubella

systemic lupus erythematosus

## MULTIPLE MYELOMA

**Specific**

plasmacytoma (if metastatic to skin, poor prognostic sign)

**Non-specific**

alopecia

amyloidosis

angioedema

cold urticaria

drug eruptions

generalized anhidrosis

ichthyosiform or desquamative dermatitis

petechiae
planar xanthoma
pruritic dermatitis
purpura
pyoderma gangrenosum
Raynaud's phenomenon
scleroderma-like lesions
skin infections

## NEUTROPHILIA

Sweet's syndrome
Von Zambusch pustular psoriasis

## PARAPROTEINEMIA

amyloidosis
angioedema
angioimmunoblastic lymphadenopathy

edema
generalized plane xanthoma, eruptive
    xanthoma, tuberous xanthoma
macroglossia
myeloma (plasmacytoma)
necrobiotic xanthogranuloma
purpura
pyoderma gangrenosum
Raynaud's phenomenon
scleroderma
Sneddon–Wilkinson disease

## THROMBOCYTOPENIA

Kasabach–Merritt syndrome
Letterer–Siwe disease
lupus erythematosus
strawberry angiomas (especially if rapidly
    enlarging)
Wiskott–Aldrich syndrome

# Joints

## ACUTE ARTHRITIS, FEVER AND RASH

acute rheumatic fever
chronic gonococcemia
erythema multiforme
Henoch–Shönlein purpura
rat-bite fever (*Streptobacillus moniliformis*)
subacute bacterial endocarditis

## ACUTE ARTHRITIS AND SKIN ERUPTION

acute dermatomyositis
acute rheumatic fever
acute rheumatoid arthritis
gonococcal arthritis
gout
Henoch–Schönlein purpura
hepatitis

infectious mononucleosis
juvenile rheumatoid arthritis
Kawasaki's disease
psoriatic arthritis
Reiter's syndrome
serum sickness
systemic lupus erythematosus
subacute bacterial endocarditis

## ARTHRALGIA AND SKIN DISEASE

Behçet's syndrome
bowel bypass syndrome
dermatomyositis
erythema elevatum diutinum
gout
mastocytosis
multicentric reticulohistiocytosis
psoriasis
Reiter's disease

rheumatoid arthritis
scleroderma
systemic lupus erythematosus

## PSORIATIC ARTHRITIS

anklosing (psoriatic) spondylitis (5%)
arthritis mutilans (5%)
asymmetric oligoarthritis (few joints of fingers
　　and toes, 70%)
classical psoriatic arthritis (primarily distal
　　interphalangeal joints, 5%)
symmetrical polyarthritis (clinically similar to
　　rheumatoid arthritis, 15%)

## RHEUMATOID ARTHRITIS

### Skin changes in rheumatoid arthritis
Subcutaneous nodules
*Vascular changes*
erythema multiforme
erythema nodosum
leg ulcers
leukocytoclastic vasculitis
necrotizing venulitis
periungual telangiectasia
segmental hyalinizing vasculitis
splinter hemorrhages (most common)
systemic arteritis (infarcts and gangrene of
　　digits, skin ulcers, systemic vasculitis)
urticaria

*Other skin changes*
atrophy

hyperpigmentation
localized hyperhidrosis
palmar erythema
purpura
skin transparency
yellow nail syndrome
yellow skin

### Disorders associated with rheumatoid arthritis
*Bullous disorders*
bullous pemphigoid
cicatricial pemphigoid
dermatitis herpetiformis
epidermolysis bullosa acquisita
pemphigus foliaceus/vulgaris

*Collagen vascular diseases*
overlap syndrome with dermatomyositis
scleroderma
systemic lupus erythematosus

*Other*
alopecia areata
amyloidosis
erythema elevatum diutinum
erythromelalgia
Felty's syndrome (granulocytopenia,
　　rheumatoid arthritis, splenomegaly)
Mondor's disease
pyoderma gangrenosum
Raynaud's phenomenon
Sjögren's syndrome
subcorneal pustular dermatosis
vitiligo

# Ophthalmic

## ANGIOMAS, GLAUCOMA, RETINAL HYALINE BODIES, TUMORS

(Any, some or all)

neurofibromatosis (AD)

Sturge–Weber syndrome
tuberous sclerosis (AD)
Von Hippel–Lindau disease

## BLEPHARITIS, CONJUNCTIVITIS, KERATITIS, UVEITIS

(Any, some or all, otherwise indicated in parentheses)

**Vascular**
periarteritis nodosa
Wegener's granulomatosis

**Infectious**
*Fungal*
    candidiasis
    dermatophytosis
    histoplasmosis
*Bacterial*
    Chlamydia trachomatis
    lepromatous leprosy
    lymphogranuloma venereum
    staphylococcal
*Infestation*
    lice
*Parasitic*
    toxoplasmosis
*Spirochetal*
    syphilis
*Viral*
    herpes simplex
    herpes zoster
    measles
    molluscum contagiosum
    rubella
    smallpox

**Traumatic**
tobacco–alcohol amblyopia (loss of central vision)

**Allergic**
atopic dermatitis
seborrheic dermatitis

**Medicinal**
accutane

chloroquine (retinopathy)
psoralen
steroids (glaucoma)

**Metabolic**
acrodermatitis
diabetes mellitus
niacin excess (reversible loss of central vision)
vitamin A deficiency
vitamin A toxicity (papilledema)
vitamin C deficiency (orbital hemorrhage and proptosis)

**Idiopathic**
*Bullous disorders*
    dermatitis herpetiformis
epidermolysis bullosa (acquired and dystrophic)
cicatricial pemphigoid
hydroa vacciniforme
pemphigus foliaceous
porphyria
Stevens–Johnson syndrome
toxic epidermal necrolysis
*Collagen vascular disease*
    dermatomyositis
rheumatoid arthritis (Sjögren's syndrome)
scleroderma
systemic lupus erythematosus
*Other*
    Behçet's syndrome
graft versus host disease (dry eye syndrome)
lichen planus
pityriasis rubra pilaris
psoriasis
relapsing polychondritis
rosacea
sarcoidosis
Vogt–Koyanagi–Harada syndrome

**Neoplastic**
leukemic/lymphomatous infiltrate
necrobiotic xanthogranuloma

**Hematologic**
hemolytic anemia (hemorrhage)
sickle cell disease (angioid streaks)

173

**Congenital**
albinism (AD, AR)
ataxia telangiectasia (conjunctival telangiectasis, AR)
Down's syndrome
epidermolysis bullosa
ichthyosis
Marfan's syndrome (AD, lens discoloration)
pseudoxanthoma elasticum (AD, AR, angioid streaks)
xeroderma pigmentosum (AR)

## CATARACTS

**Infectious**
syphilis
tuberculosis

**Allergic**
atopic dermatitis

**Medicinal**
chlorpromazine
psoralen
steroids

**Metabolic**
diabetes mellitus
hypoparathyroidism

**Idiopathic**
Behçet's syndrome
pemphigus foliaceus

rheumatoid arthritis
sarcoidosis
scleroderma
Vogt–Koyanag–Harada syndrome

**Congenital**
Down's syndrome
Cockayne's syndrome
dyskeratosis congenita (XR)
Fabry's disease
ectodermal dysplasia
ichthyosis
incontinentia pigmenti
Refsum's disease
Rothmund–Thomson syndrome (AR)
Werner's syndrome (AR)
Wilson's disease (AR)

## INFECTIONS INVOLVING EYE AND SKIN

herpes simplex
herpes zoster
gonorrhea
molluscum contagiosum
tuberculosis
vaccinia
varicella

## OCULAR SCARRING

cicatricial pemphigoid
dystrophic forms of inherited epidermolysis bullosa
epidermolysis bullosa acquisita

# Other

## SARCOIDOSIS

cataracts
glaucoma
papilloedema (but not pingvecula)
uveitis

## SJÖGREN'S SYNDROME

Associated with HLA-B8 and HLA-DW2, and thus occasionally seen with dermatitis herpetiformis in the same patient

alopecia (patchy)

decreased sweating*
hyper- or hypopigmentation
keratoconjunctivitis sicca
nasal dryness and crusting
pruritus*
Raynaud's phenomenon
thrombotic thrombocytopenic purpura

vaginal dryness and dyspareunia
vasculitis
   cryoglobulinemia
   hypergammaglobulinemic purpura
xerosis*
xerostomia

# Pulmonary

Associated pulmonary disorders are noted in brackets

## Vascular

allergic granulomatosis (Churg–Strauss
   syndrome)
polyarteritis nodosa (rare)
Wegener's granulomatosis

## Infectious

*Fungal*
   blastomycosis
   coccidiomycosis
   histoplasmosis
*Bacterial*
   tuberculosis
*Parasitic*
   cutaneous larva migrans [transient
   pulmonary infiltrate]

## Traumatic

fat embolism syndrome [triad of cerebral
   dysfunction, petechiae, respiratory
   insufficiency after long bone fracture]

## Allergic

atopic dermatitis [asthma (and hay fever)]

## Metabolic

cystic fibrosis [(progressive lung disease with
   chronic bronchitis, emphysema and cor
   pulmonale), excessive skin wrinkling (when
   palms and soles immersed in water)]

## Idiopathic

amyloidosis
lipoid proteinosis
lymphomatoid granulomatosis
multicentric reticulohistiocytosis
progressive systemic sclerosis
relapsing polychondritis
rheumatoid arthritis
sarcoidosis
Sweet's syndrome (rare)
systemic lupus erythematosus
yellow nail syndrome [pleural effusions]

## Congenital

Osler–Weber–Rendu syndrome [pulmonary
   arteriovenous fistulas]

# Renal

## END STAGE RENAL DISEASE

benign nodular calcification
calciphylaxis
ecchymosis
elastosis
half & half nails
hyperpigmentation
ichtyosis (acquired)
pallor
perforating disorders
poor skin trugor
porphyria cutanea tarda
pruritus
sallow yellow cast
pseudoporphyria
uremic frost
xerosis

## RENAL DISEASE AND SKIN AND MULTISYSTEM DISEASE

alkaptonuria = nephrolithiasis, nephropathy
amyloidosis = nephrotic syndrome, renal failure
blastomycosis = diffuse glomerulonephritis
Fabry's disease (angiokeratoma corporis diffusum) = uremia
furuncle = perinephric abscess
gout = nephritis secondary to tophi deposits in the interstitial tissue
Henoch–Schönlein purpura = acute glomerulonephritis
herpes zoster/varicella = hemorrhagic cystitis
impetigo contagiosa = acute poststreptococcal glomerulonephritis
lipodystrophy (partial) = glomerulonephritis
nail–patella syndrome = chronic glomerulonephritis, dysplastic kidney

Osler–Weber–Rendu syndrome = renovascular abnormalities
polyarteritis nodosa = acute glomerulitis
pseudoxanthoma elasticum = hypertension, kidney stones
sarcoidosis = nephrocalcinosis
syphilis = nephrotic syndrome
systemic lupus erythematosus = nephritis, renal failure
tuberous sclerosis = angiomyolipomas of kidney, (hamartomas that replace kidney)
Von Hippel–Lindau disease = hypernephroma, polycystic kidney disease
Von Recklinghausen's disease (neurofibromatosis) = renal artery stenosis, renal tumors
Wegener's granulomatosis = focal necrotizing glomerulonephritis

### Other
calcium deposits (calciphylaxis)
diabetes mellitus
dysproteinemias
familial mediterranean fever
scleroderma
sickle cell anemia
xanthomas

## DIALYSIS-RELATED SKIN DISEASE

Kyrle's disease (more in Blacks)
porphyria cutanea tarda (pseudo-porphyria cutanea tarda)
pruritus* (up to 80%)
purpura
self-limited bullous dermatosis
splinter hemorrhages

gingival friability
ulcerative stomatitis
uremic glossitis
xerostomia

Cushing's syndrome (secondary to steroid
   administration)
increased incidence of infections, especially viral
   (chronic erosive ulcerative herpes simplex,
   verrucae), and Norwegian scabies

Kaposi's sarcoma
squamous cell carcinoma

cutaneous calcification
diffuse hyperpigmentation
half-and-half nail
pruritus
scattered ecchymosis and petechiae
sparse body hair
uremic frost
xerosis
yellow cast (retained carotene, urochromes,
   etc.)

# Teeth changes

actinomycosis = dental abscess
Apert's syndrome (acrocephalosyndacyly) =
   retarded dental eruption and malocclusion
dyskeratosis congenita (XD) = most commonly
   edentulous, extensive caries, wide
   separation, crowding, malformation
ectodermal dysplasis = 'peg tooth' and hypo- or
   adontia
Ehlers–Danlos syndrome type VIII (AD) –
   periodontitis, complete loss of permanant
   teeth by 2nd or 3rd decade of life
epulis fissuratum = inflammatory fibrous
   hyperplasia associated with ill-fitting
   dentures
erythropoietic porphyria = erythrodontia
focal dermal hypoplasia (Goltz's syndrome, XR)
   = abnormal number and form of teeth
Gardner's syndrome (AD) = supernumary
   unerupted teeth, dentigerous cysts and
   odontomas

histiocytosis X = tooth mobility, premature
   tooth loss
incontinentia pigmenti = delayed dentition,
   pegged or conical crowns, malformation and
   missing teeth
junctional epidermolysis bullosa = cobblestone
   appearance, enamel pits
late congenital syphilis = Hutchinsons's teeth
   (malformation of central upper incisors)
oculodentodigital dysplasia (AD) = enamel
   hypoplasia
Papillon–Lefevre syndrome (AR) = premature
   destruction of periodontal ligament results
   in loss of the deciduous and permanent
   teeth
Sjögren–Larsson syndrome (AR) = dental
   enamel dysplasia, serrated teeth

# Voice changes

In most instances, hoarseness is the usual
finding, unless otherwise indicated

**Infectious**
candidiasis
epidemic typhus (dysphonia secondary to
cranial nerve paralysis)
histoplasmosis
papillomas (involving the larynx)
secondary syphilis

**Metabolic**
hypothyroidism

**Idiopathic**
amyloidosis (tongue infiltration may result in
difficulty or hoarseness)
angioedema (difficulty speaking)
dermatomyositis (dysphonia)
Epidermolysis bullosa simplex (Dowling-Meara)
erythema multiforme
Junctional epidermolysis bullosa (Herlitz
variant)
pemphigus vulgaris
relapsing polychondritis
sarcoidosis
systemic lupus erythematosus

**Neoplastic**
eruptive keratoacanthoma

**congenital**
Cornelia de Lange syndrome (low pitched,
feeble, growling cry)
Farber's syndrome
lipoid proteinosis
pachyonychia congenita

## PAIN-PRODUCING DISEASES WHICH MAY VOLUNTARILY INHIBIT SPEAKING

aphthous stomatitis
Behçet's syndrome
cicatricial pemphigoid
hand–foot–mouth disease
infectious pharyngitis
lichen planus
primary herpetic gingivostomatitis

# SECTION THREE

## Diseases and their features

This section is divided into several subsections.
Each subsection highlights the characteristic findings
of different categories of the disease process

# Contact dermatitis

ALLERGENS THAT CROSS-REACT WITH OTHER ALLERGENS

## Balsam of Peru cross-reacts with:

benzoin
benzyl alcohol
benzyl benzoate
cinnamon
clove
colophony
eugenol
'oriental' tiger balm
propolis (bee glue)
tincture of benzoin
vanilla
peel of citrus fruits

*Bacitracin* co-reacts with:
neomycin (thus avoid Baciguent, Bacitin, Polysporin ointment)

*Benzocaine* cross-reacts with:
aniline dyes
hair dyes
oral hypoglycemic agents
other benzoate ester anesthetics (cocaine, procaine, tetracaine)
paraminobenzoic acid (PABA)
paraminosalicylic acid
*p*-phenylenediamine
procainamide
sulfonamides

*Colophony (rosin)* cross-reacts with:
balsam of Peru
pine resin
spruce resin
turpentine
wood tar

*D&C Yellow No 11* (a quinoline dye) cross-reacts with:
(quinoline compounds) chloroquine, ethoxyquin, vioform

*Epoxy resin* (bisphenol A) cross-reacts with:
ethylenedeiamine
diethylstilbestrol

*Ethylenediamine* cross-reacts with:
aminophylline
antihistamine (ethylenediamine type, Atarax, Meclizine, Piperazine, Phenergan, Vistral) capsules/creams/tablets
epoxy resin
Lanolin alcohol (wool wax alcohol)
Eucerin

Mycolog (Kenacomb) cream
Vasocon A (but not with EDTA)

*Foods that cross-react with latex:*

*Avocado*
*Banana*
*Celery*
*Chestnut*
*Fig*
*Papaya*
*Passion fruit*
*Peach*

*Formaldehyde* cross-reacts with:
Quaternium 15

*Neomycin* cross-reacts with:
[coreacts with Bacitracin]
gentamicin [COREACTS WITH BACITRACIN]
kanamycin
streptomycin
tobramycin

*Paraphenylenediamine* cross-reacts with:
aniline and azo dyes
diuretics (thiazides)
hydroquinone
local anesthetics (ester type;benzocaine,
  procaine)
PABA esters
*para*-aminosalicylic acid
resorcin green
sulfonamides
sulfonoureas

*Poison Ivy (Rhus* group) cross-reacts with:
cashew-nut shell oil
ginkgo fruit pulp
Japanese lacquer tree
mango rind
marking-nut tree of India
*Rhus* (oak, sumac, oleoresin,
  pentadecylclatechol, urushiol)

*Psoralen* cross-reacts with:
lime

*Quatrenium 15* cross-reacts with:
formaldehyde

*Quinoline mix* cross-reacts with:
iodoquinol (diodoquin), Vioform

*Slfonamides* cross-react with:
hydrochlorothiazide

*Thimerosal (merthiolate)* cross-reacts with:
ammoniated mercury
mercuric chloride
mercurochrome
mercurous chloride
metallic mercury
mercury sulfide
phenylmercuric salts

*Turpentine* cross-reacts with:
balsam of Peru
benzoin
chrysanthemum
colophony
pine
pyrethrum and ragweed oleoresin
spruce
skin of citrus fruits

*Vanilla* cross-reacts with:
balsam of Peru

benzoin
benzoic acid
cinnamon
clove colophony (rosin)

## FORMALDEHYDE-RELEASING PRESERVATIVES

2-bromo-2-nitroprpane-1,3-diol (Bronopol)
diazolidinyl urea (Germall II)
1,2-dibromo-2,4-dicyanobutane (one
  constituent of Euxyl K400)
DMD Hydantoin
imidazolidinyl urea (Germall 115)
quaternium-15 (Dowicil 200)

## DETECTION OF CONTACT DERMATITIS

**chromium**
diphenylcarbazide test

**cobalt**
2-nitroso-1-naphthol-4-sulfonic acid test

**formaldehyde**
chromotropic acid test

**group A (hydrocortisone type) corticosteroid**
Tixocotol-21-pivalate

**nickel**
dimethylglyoxime test (a red precipitate
  indicates positive reaction)

**PLANT dermatitis**
sesquiterpene lactone mix

**rubber allergy**
thiuram mix

## MOST COMMON ALLERGEN/SENSITIZER

### antihistamines (topical)

balsam of Peru
cosmetics
ethylaminobenzoate (benzocaine)
ethylenediamine hydrochloride
merbromin (mercurochrome)
mercaptobenzothiazole
neomycin
nickel
perfumes
poison ivy, oak, and sumac
potassium dichromate
thimerosal (merthiolate)

### In airborne allergic contact dermatitis
burning of poison ivy
compositae (ragweed, chrysanthemum) (may lead to photosensitivity in about 50% of patients, and has been associated with persistent light reaction)
pollen
ragweed

### In allergic cement dermatitis
dichromate (rarely cobalt and nickel)

### In allergic cheilitis
carrots
coffee
menthol
orange peel

### In allergic contact dermatitis to plants
oleoresin fraction

### In antibiotic-induced allergic contact dermatitis
neomycin
penicillin
streptomycin

### In contact leukoderma (vitiligo)
butylcatechol
para-tertiary butylphenol
phenolic detergents

### In contact urticaria
ammonium persulfate
bacitracin
benzoic acid
benzoyl peroxide
cinnamic acid
cinnamic aldehyde
diethyltoluamide (DET)
dimethyl sulfoxide (DMSO)
latex
raw meat and sea food
sorbic acid
trafuril (an ester of nicotinic acid)

May also be caused by metals such as nickel, rhodium, and platinum salts

### In cook's fingers
Diallyldisulfide (in garlic–onion)

### In cosmetics
fragrance
Quaternium 15
lanolin and derivatives

### In dentists (in US)
acrylic monomers

### In diaper dermatitis
ammonia (only occurs with alkaline urine, in reality not a sensitizer, but an irritant)

### in eye preparations
thimerosol

### In eyelid dermatitis
facial cosmetics
nail polish (toluene sulfonamide/formaldehyde resin)

### In florist
chrysanthemum

### In fragrance
cinnamic aldehyde
cinnamic alcohol

### In general (overall)
nickel

### In hair bleach
ammonium persulfate

### In hairdressers
acrylates (in nail cosmetics)
*Para*-phenylenediamine (from use of permanent and semi-permanent hair dyes)
nickel
glyceryl monothioglycolate (in permanent wave solution)

(Other allergens include formaldehyde, hair dyes, perfumes, rubber gloves)

### In hydrocortisone cream (over-the-counter preparations)
preservatives in the vehicle (parabens, Quaternium-15)

### In industrial sensitizer
chromates (found in cement, leather, bleaches, detergents, glue, matches, shaving cream and lotion)
industry (foundry, printing, pulp, welding)

### In leather dermatitis
chromates

### In lemon and orange peel
limonene (a terpene, which may cross-react with bergamot and turpentine)

### In metal dermatitis
chromium (most commonly seen in males; commonest source is cement in building industry)
nickel (the most common cause; in general, females > > males)

### In mycolog cream
ethylenediamine

### In nail polish (laquers)
toluene sulfonamide/formaldehyde resin

### In nose piece of eyeglass frame
resorcinoimonobenzoate (a UV light absorber)

### In permanent waving solution (acid or heat perms)
glycerol thioglycolate

### In photoallergic dermatitis
musk ambrette
p-aminobenzoic acid

### In phytophotodermatitis (which is a phototoxic reaction to UVA)
psoralens in celery, parsley, and wild parsnip

### In plastic (synthetic resin) dermatitis
acrylic nails and (uncured acrylic) dentures
epoxy and formaldehyde resin glues and cements
nail lacquer (toluene sulfonamide/formaldehyde resin)

### In Poison Ivy (Japanese Lacquer Tree, Oak, Sumac)
catechols (a component of the oleoresin (urushiol) of the sap of *Rhus* plants)

### In preservative
formaldehyde-releasing Quaternium-15
least allergenic is paraban mix

**In preservative Kathon CG**
methylchloroisothiazolinone

**In Shaving Preparations**
fragrances (especially musk ambrette)

**In Shoe Dermatitis**
mercaptobenzothiazole and tetraethylthiuram
potassium dichromate
*Para*-tertiary butylphenol formaldehyde resin

**In Sunscreens**
PABA

**In surfactant in shampoo**
cocamidopropyl betaine

**In Textile Dye Dermatitis**
azo dyes

**In Toothpastes**
cinnamic aldehyde and alcohol

**In Weed Dermatitis**
sesquiterpene lactones

**In Women**
nickel

PRINCIPAL SENSITIZER

**In Desert Heliotrope**
hydroquinone

**In Ophthalmic Lens Solutions**
benzalkonium chloride and merthiolate

**In Paper Dermatitis**
*Duplicating paper*
*azo dyes*
  *hydroquinone*

*Paper towel*
  *Formaldehyde resin*
  *Toilet paper*
  *Fragrance*
  *Typewriter paper*
  *Colophony (rosin)*

**In Ragweed, Chrysanthemum, Pyrethrum, sagebush**
sesquiterpene lactones

**In Rosein (Colophony)**
abietic acid

**In Rubber**
accelerators (carbamates,
    mercaptobenzothiazoles, thiurams)
antioxidants (*para*-phenylenediamine, phenols)

Most commonly seen with gloves

**In Shoe Dermatitis**
*Dyes*
azo dyes
  *Leather*
  formaldehyde and potassium dichromate
    (tanning agents)
    *Rubber, rubber cement*
  carbamates (accelerator)
  mercaptobenzothiazole (accelerator)
  monobenzyl ether of hydroquinone
    (antioxidant)
  *para-tertiary* butylphenol-formaldehyde resin
    tetraethylthiuram (accelerator)
  *Shoe eyelets*
  nickel
Most sensitive to allergens: eyelids, face
Most resistant to allergens: palms and soles,
    scalp, mucous membranes

**In tulips**
tuliposidea

## SYSTEMIC CONTACT DERMATITIS

Seen when a sensitive individual ingests the sensitizer. Topical sensitizers are followed by the relevant systemic sensitizers.

### Azo dyes, benzocaine, PABA, para-phenylenediamine, silvadene
azo dyes
oral hypoglycemic agents
p-aminosalicylic acid
procaine
procainamide
saccharin
sulfonamides

### Chloral hydrate
chloral hydrate

### Cobalt
vitamin $B_{12}$

### Diphenhydramine
diphenhydramine
doxylamine
dramamine

### Ethylenediamine and tripelennamine
aminophylline
ethylenediamine antihistamines (Phenergan)

### Formaldehyde
mandelamine
methenamine

### Fragrance
cinnamon

### Hydrazine
hydralazine
isoniazid
Nardil

### Iodine
potassium iodide

### Mercurials
calomel
mercurial diuretics

### Neomycin
neomycin

### Penicillin
penicillin

### Phenothiazines
phenothiazine antihistamines
phenothiazines

### Quinine
quinine
quinidine

### Resorcinol
throat trochees containing resorcin

### Streptomycin
streptomycin

### Thiamine
thiamine

### Thiurams
alcohol
Antabuse

## TATTOO SENSITIZERS

### Black tattoo
carbon

### Blue tattoo
cobalt aluminate

**Brown tattoo**
ferric sulfate

**Green tattoo**
chromium or chromic oxide

**Red tattoo**
cadmium yellow (phototoxic reactions)
mercury sulfide (red cinnabar)

**Violet tattoo**
manganese

**white tattoo**
Titanium or Zinc oxide

**Yellow tattoo**
cadmium yellow (phototoxic reactions)

IN TURPENTINE

oxidation product of the terpane δ-3-carene

IN TRANSIENT
NON-ALLERGIC
URTICARIA OF THE LIPS

sorbic acid (contained in salad dressings)

MISCELLANEOUS

Airborne-irritant reactions compared to airborne-allergen reactions are more common, but are more difficult to demonstrate. Most cases of contact dermatitis from airborne substances are caused by agents in the form of solid particles. A common site of contact dermatitis from airborne substances is the upper eyelid. A characteristic site of involvement with airborne substances in women (but not in men) is the legs. Airborne pyrethroids may cause paresthesia.

Allergic contact stomatitis may mimic the oral changes seen in a vitamin deficiency, and results in a burning sensation, loss of taste, and numbness.

Antabuse or Alcohol ingestion can flare dermatitis due to thiurams (e.g. rubber-glove dermatitis).

Azo dyes in pharmaceuticals may produce asthma, fixed drug eruption, purpura and urticaria.

Balsam of Peru is a marker of fragrance sensitivity and is positive in 50% of cases of perfume allergy.

Black dermographism is a physical process in which substances in cosmetics (e.g. carbon, pumice, zinc oxide) that are harder than gold, nickel, or silver, remove fine metallic particles from jewelry and other metallic objects by friction. A thin metallic powder is deposited on the skin and causes a black discoloration. Only stainless steel and chromium are harder than other agents in cosmetics, and thus produce no black dermographism.

Dermal contact dermatitis: In an allergic contact dermatitis, most commonly with neomycin, nickel or ragweed, edema and erythema may occur without the usual eczematous skin changes. Pathologically, these eruptions will show a dense perivascular lymphocytic infiltrate without any epidermal changes.

Early mycosis fungoides and Sézary syndrome are clinical and pathological mimickers of chronic contact dermatitis.

Fiberglass dermatitis is usually an irritant type of contact dermatitis. This eruption is more common in individuals with fair skin and blue eyes. The eruption may consist of folliculitis, linear erosions, petechiae, telangiectasia and urticaria, and can be mistaken for scabies.

Formaldehyde is detected by chromotropic acid. It is released by Bronopol (in Eucerin cream and lotion), imidazolidinyl urea (Germal 115), methenamine (Dr. Scholl's Foot

Magic®, Dehydral, Mandelamine), and Quaternium-15.

Nickel is released by boiling water and detergents, and permanent wave solutions (used by hairdressers).

Para-tertiary-butylphenol formaldehyde *resin* can induce allergic contact dermatitis; it may also cause skin depigmentation, and may occasionally cross-react with formaldehyde.

Phototoxic reactions are primarily in the UVA range, and usually occur on the first exposure and resemble sunburn. They are due to non-immunologic mechanisms. Most common causes are psoralens and tar.

Solvents produce dry fissured dermatitis; they may also produce chemical lymphangitis and peripheral neuropathy.

Soluble' and 'Synthetic' *industrial fluids* may produce eczematous eruptions (primarily irritant type). The insoluble industrial fluids, 'Neat' oils, may produce oil acne, carcinomas, and keratoses.

Thiurams are used in insecticides and fungicides and are often on lawns and garden plants.

Vitamin B$_{12}$ (cyanocobalamin) injection or oral use can cause flare-ups in cobalt-sensitive patients.

# Diseases and etiology

In this subsection, infectious diseases are alphabetically listed followed by their cause

**Acquired cold urticaria** = associated with
Epstein–Barr virus
**Actinomycosis**
*Actinomyces israeli* (anaerobic, gram-positive)
**Adult T cell Leukemia**–*lymphoma*
*HTLV-1*
**Anthrax**
*Bacillus anthracis*
**Aphthae, minor**
– *Streptococcus sanguis* strain 2A
– Viral
**Aspergillosis**
*Aspergillus flavus* (most common cause of primary cutaneous aspergillosis)
*A. fumigatus* (most common cause of disseminated aspergillosis)
**Bacillary angiomatosis**
*Bartonella henselae*
*Bartonella quintana*
**Bartonellosis**
*Bartonella bacilliformis*

**Bejel (endemic syphilis)**
*Treponema pallidum*
**Black Piedra**
Piedra hortai
**Blastomycosis**
Blastomyces dermatitidis
**Blistering distal dactylitis**
Group A β-hemolytic streptococci
**Boston exanthem**
echovirus 16
**Botryomycosis (actinophytosis)**
*Staphylococcus aureus*\*
also seen with streptococci, *Escherichia coli*, proteus, and *Pseudomonas*
**Bullous impetigo**
staphylococci
phage 71
coagulase positive
**Burkett's lymphoma**
Epstein-Barr Virus

**Cat-scratch disease**
*Bartonella henselae*, (*Afipia felis* in minority of cases)

**Cellulitis**
*Hemophilus influenzae* (especially in children)
*Staphylococcus aureus*
*Streptococcus pyogenes**

**Chancroid**
*Hemophilus ducreyi*

**Chromoblastomycosis**
*Cladosporium carrionii*
*Fonsecaea compacta*
*Fonsecaea pedrosoi*
*Phillophora verrucosae*

**Coccidioidomycosis**
*Coccidioides immitis*

**Cryoglobulinemia**
hepatitis B infection (in 75% of cases)

**Cryptococcosis**
*Cryptococcus neoformans*

**Cutaneous larve migrans**
*Ancylostoma braziliense*

**Cutaneous larva currens**
*Strongyloides stercoralis*

**Cutaneous T-cell Lymphoma**
Human T Lymphocytic Virus (HTLV, in some patients)

**Cysticercosis**
*Taenia solium* (pork tapeworm)

**Degos' disease**
paramyxovirus-like particles noted in endothelial cells and fibroblasts, on electron microscopy

**Dermatomyositis/polymyositis**
picornavirus proteins

**Diphtheria**
*Corynebacterium diphtheriae*

**Ecthyma**
β-hemolytic streptococci

**Ecthyma contagiosum (orf)**
orf virus

**Ecthyma gangrenosum**
*Pseudomonas aeruginosa* (most commonly)

**Erysipelas**
*β-hemolytic Group A streptococci*

**Erysipeloid**
*Erysipelothrix (Rhusionathrix) insidiosa*

**Erythema infectiosum (fifth disease)**
parvovirus B19

**Erythema multiforme**
Herpes Simplex Virus

**Erythrasma**
*Corynebacterium minutissimum*

**Filariasis**
*Brugia malayi* or *timori*
*Wuchereria bancrofti*

**Fournier's gangrene**
Group A streptococci, or a mixed infection with anaerobes and enteric bacilli

**Gianoti–Crosti Syndrome**
papular acrodermatitis of childhood
coxsackie virus
cytomegalovirus
Epstein–Barr Virus*
Hepatitis B Virus*
parainfluenza virus

**Glanders**
*Pseudomonas mallei*

**Gonococcemia**
*Neisseria gonorrhoeae*

**Gram negative folliculitis**
*Enterobacter*
*Klebsiella*
*Proteus* (from deep cystic lesions)

**Granuloma annulare**
– viral, associated with Epstein–Barr virus and HIV

**Granuloma inguinale**
*Calymmatobacterium (Donovania) granulomatis*

**Hand–foot–mouth disease**
coxsackievirus A 5, 9, 10

**Hairy cell leukemia**
HTLV-II

**Hairy leukoplakia**
Epstein–Barr virus

**Herpangina**
coxsackievirus A 1–10 (picornavirus group)

**Histoplasmosis**
*Histoplasma capsulatum*

**Impetigo contagiosum**
Group A streptococci

**Impetigo of Bockhart**
*Staphylococcus aureus*

**Infectious mononucleosis**
Epstein–Barr virus

**Kaposi Sarcoma**
Human Herpes Virus 8

**Kawasaki disease**
–staphylococcal superantigen

**Leishmaniasis**
American (mucocutaneous): *Leishmaniasis braziliensis*
cutaneous (oriental sore): *L. tropica*
systemic (kala-azar): *L. donovani*

**Leprosy**
*Mycobacterium leprae*

**Leptospirosis**
pretibial fever (anicteric leptospirosis:
*Leptospira autumalis* (spirochete)
Weil's disease (icteric leptospirosis):
*Leptospira interrogans*
**Lichen planus**
hepatitis C (associated)
**Lyme disease**
*Borrelia burgdorferi*
**Lymphogranuloma venereum**
*Chlamydia trachomatis*
**Measles**
paramyxovirus
**Meleney's gangrene (progressive
bacterial synergistic gangrene)**
microaerophilic non-hemolytic
streptococcus *(Peptostreptococcus)*
**Melioidosis**
*Pseudomonas pseudomallei*
**Milker's nodule**
paravaccinia virua
**Mycetoma (Madura foot)**
about 20 different organisms; *Nocardia
brasiliensis* is the most common, but
*Pseudallescheria boydii* in the USA
**Mycosis fungoides**
HTLV-I
**Necrotizing fasciitis**
Bacteroides
β-hemolytic streptococci
enterococci
*Pseudomonas*
staphylococci
**Nocardiosis**
*Nocardia asteroids* (Gram-positive and
acid-fast, most common in N. America)
**Oral hairy leukoplakia**
Epstein-Barr Virus
**Orf**
parapoxvirus
**Paracoccidioidomycosis (South American
blastomycosis)**
*Paracoccidioides brasiliensis*
**Paronychia**
fungal
gram-negative bacteria
herpes
*Staphylococcus aureus*\*
streptococci
**Pinta**
Treponema carateum
**Pinworm (enterobiasis)**
*Enterobius vermicularis*

**Pitted keratolysis**
*Corynebacterium*
*Dermatophillus congolensis*
*Micrococcus sedentarius*
**Pityriasis rosea**
Herpes Simplex virus-7 (associated)
**Plague**
*Yersinia pestis*
**Psittacosis**
*Chlamydia psittaci*
**Purpura fulminans**
Group A streptococci
**Pyomyositis**
*Staphylococcus aureus*
**Q Fever**
*Rickettsia burnetti*
**Rat-bite fever**
*Spirillum moniliformis* (in the USA)
*Spirillum minor*
**Reiter's syndrome**
campylobacter
*Chlamydia trachomatis*
– Shigella
– Yersinia
*Ureaplasma urealyticum*
**Relapsing fever (tick fever)**
*Borrelia recurrentis*
*B. duttonii*
**Rhinoscleroma**
*Klebsiella rhinoscleromatis*
**Rickettsialpox**
*Rickettsia akari*
**Rocky Mountain spotted fever**
*Rickettsia rickettsii*
**Roseola infantum (exanthem subitium)**
human herpes virus 6 & 7
**Rubella**
togavirus
**Scarlet fever**
Group A streptococci
**Sporotrichosis**
*Sporothrix schenckii*
**Squamous cell Ca of foreskin**
*Mycobacterium smegmatis*
**Staphylococcal scalded skin syndrome**
*Staphylococcus aureus* II
phage 71
**Syphilis**
*Treponema pallidum*
**Systemic sclerosis**
retroviral P30 proteins
**Tinea (pityriasis) versicolor**
*Pityrosporum ovale (obiculare)*

**Toxic shock syndrome**
*Staphylococcus aureus*
**Trench fever**
*Rickettsia quintana*
**Trichinosis**
*Trichinella spiralis*
**Trichomycosis axillaris**
*Corynebacterium tenuis*
**Trypanosomiasis**
African: *Trypanosoma gambiense, T. rhodesiense*
American (Chagas' disease): *T. cruzi*
**Tuberculosis**
Bacillus–Calmette–Guerin
*Mycobacterium bovis*
*Mycobacterium tuberculosis*
**Tularemia**
*Francisella tularenesis*
**Typhus**
endemic typhus: *Rickettsia typhi*
epidemic typhus (and Brill's disease): *Rickettsia prowazekii*
scrub typhus: *Ricketssia tsutsugamushi*
**Tyzzer's disease**
*Bacillus piliformis* (occurs in patients infected with HIV)
**Varicella-zoster**
Herpes Virus 3
**Warts**
human papillomavirus (HPV):
bowenoid papulosis: HPV-16, 18, 31, 33, 51
butcher's wart: HPV-7
cervical & vaginal atypias: HPV-16, 18, 31, 33, 51

condyloma acuminata: HPV-(6, 11,low cancer risk) (16, 18, 31,33,51 high cancer risk)
epidermal cysts: 60
epidermodysplasia verruciformis: HPV-3,5*, 8, 9, 10, 12, 14, 15, 17, 19–26, 38, 47, 50
focal epithelial hyperplasia: HPV-13*, 32
genital warts in children: HPV-2, 6, 11
keatoacanthoma: HPV-9, 16, 19, 25, 37
laryngeal carcinoma: HPV-30
oral leukoplakia: HPV-11,16
periungal squamous cell ca: HPV-16
pigmented wart: 65
squamous cell carcinoma in renal allograft recipients: HPV-5/8
squamous cell ca of penis: HPV16
verruca plana (flat wart): HPV-3,10,28,49
verruca vulgaris: HPV-2,4, 7
verruca vulgaris (filiform): HPV-2
verruca vulgaris (palmoplantar, deep, hyperkeratotic): HPV-1
verruca vulgaris (palmoplantar, mosaic type): HPV-2, 4
verrucous carcinoma (Buschke-Loewenstein tumor): HPV6,11
Vincent's angina: 'fusospirochetal complex' (*Bacteroides fusiformis* in associated with *Borrelia vincentii* and other organisms)
**White piedra**
*Trichosporon beigelii*
**Yaws**
*Treponema pertenue*

# Etiology and diseases

In this subsection diseases are listed according to their etiology

**Actinomycosis**
*Acrinomyces israelii* (*anaerobic, gram-positive)

**Anthrax**
*Bacillus anthracis*
**Bacillary angiomatosis**
*Bartonella henselae*
*Rochalimaea quintana*

**Bartonellosis (Oroya fever)**
*Bartonella bacilliformis*
**Blistering distal dactylitis**
Group A β-hemolytic streptococci
**Botryomycosis** (actinophytosis)
*Staphylococcus aureus*
**Bullous impetigo**
staphylococci
phage 71
coagulase positive
**Cat-scratch disease**
bartonella henselae
**Cellulitis**
*Hemophilus influenzae* (especially in children)
*Staphylococcus aureus*
*Streptococcus pyogenes**
**Chancroid**
*Hemophilus ducreyi*
**Diphtheria**
*Corynebacterium diphtheriae*
**Ecthyma**
β-hemolytic streptococci
**Ecthyma gangrenosum**
*Pseudomonas aeruginosa*
**Erysipelas**
β-hemolytic Group A streptococci
**Erysipeloid**
*Erysipelothrix (Rhusionathrix) insidiosa*
**Erythrasma**
*Corynebacterium minutissimum*
**Fournier's gangrene**
Group A streptococci, or a mixed infection
with anaerobes and enteric bacilli
**Glanders**
*Pseudomonas mallei*
**Gonococcemia**
*Neisseria gonorrhoeae*
**Granuloma inguinale**
*Calymmatobacterium (Donovania) granulomatis*
**Impetigo contagiosum**
*Group A streptococci*
**Impetigo of Bockhart**
*Staphylococcus aureus*
**Leprosy**
*Mycobacterium leprae*
**Leptospirosis**
pretibial fever (anicteric leptospirosis):
*Leptospira autumalis* (spirochete)
Weill's disease (icteric leptospirosis):
*Leptospira Interrogans*
**Lyme disease**
*Borrelia burgdorferi*

**Lymphogranuloma venereum**
*Chlamydia trochamatis*
**Meleney's gangrene (progressive
bacterial synergistic gangrene)**
Microaerophilic non-hemolytic
streptococcus (*Peptostreptococcus*)
**Melioidosis**
*Pseudomonas pseudomallei*
**Mycetoma (Madura foot)**
about 20 different organisms; *Nocardia
brasiliensis* is the most common, but
*Pseudallescheria boydii* in the USA
**Necrotizing fasciitis**
Bacteroides
β-hemolytic streptococci
enterococci
Pseudomonas
staphylococci
**Nocardiosis**
*Nocardia asteroides* (gram-positive and
acid-fast, most common in N. America)
*N. brasiliensis*
**Psittacosis**
*Chlamydia psittaci*
**Pitted keratolysis**
*Corynebacterium*
*Dermatophillus congolensis*
*Micrococcus sedentarius*
**Plague**
*Yersinia pestis*
**Purpura fulminans**
Group A streptococci
**Pyomyositis**
*Staphylococcus aureus*
**Q Fever**
*Rickettsia burnetti*
**Rat-bite fever**
*Spirillum moniliformis* (in the USA)
*Spirillum minor*
**Relapsing fever (tick fever)**
*Borrelia recurrentis*
*B. duttonii*
**Rhinoscleroma**
*Klebsiella rhinoscleromatis*
**Rickettsialpox**
*Ricketssia akari*
**Rocky Mountain spotted fever**
*Rickettsia rickettsii*
**Roseola (exanthum subitum)**
*Herpes virus 6 & 7*
**Scarlet fever**
Group A streptococci

**Staphylococcal scalded skin syndrome**
  *Staphylococcus aureus II*
  phage 71
**Syphilis**
  *Treponema pallidum*
**Toxic shock syndrome**
  *Staphylococcus aureus*
**Trench fever**
  *Rickettsia quintana*
**Trichomycosis axillaris**
  *Corynebacterium tenuis*
**Tuberculosis**
  Bacillus–Calmette–Guerin
  *Mycobacterium bovis*
  *Mycobacterium tuberculosis*
**Tularemia**
  *Francisella tularenesis*
**Typhus**
  endemic typhus: *Rickettsia typhi*
  epidemic typhus: *Rickettsia prowazekii*
  scrub typhus: *Rickettsia tsutsugamushi*

FUNGAL INFECTIONS

**Aspergillosis**
  *Aspergillus flavus* (most common cause of
  primary cutaneous aspergillosis)
  *A. fumigatus* (most common cause of
  disseminated aspergillosis)
  *A. niger*
**Black piedra**
  *Piedra hortai*
**Blastomycosis**
  *Blastomyces dermatitidis*
**Candidiasis**
  *Candidia albicans*
  *C. krusei*
  *C. tropicalis*
**Chromoblastomycosis (chromomycosis)**
  *Fonsecaea pedrosoi*
**Coccidioidomycosis**
  *Coccidioides immitis*
**Cryptococcosis**
  *Cryptococcus neoformans*
**Histoplasmosis**
  *Histoplasma capsulatum*
  African histoplasmosis: *H. duboisis*)
**Lobomycosis**
  *Loboa loboi*
**Paracoccidioidomycosis (South American
  blastomycosis)**
  *Paracoccidioides brasiliensis*

**Phycomycosis (mucormycosis)**
  *Mucor* and *Rhizopus* species of fungi
**Sporotrichosis**
  *Sporothrix schenckii*
**Tinea (pityriasis) versicolor**
  *Pityrosporum ovale (obiculare)*
**White piedra**
  *Trichosporon beigelli*

PARASITIC INFECTIONS

**Cutaneous larva migrans**
  *Ancylostoma braziliense*
**Cysticercosis**
  *Taenia solium* (pork tapeworm)
**Leishmaniasis**
  American (mucocutaneous): *Leishmania
  braziliensis*
  Cutaneous (oriental sore): *L. tropica*
  Systemic (Kala-Azar): *L. donovani*
**Pinworm (enterobiasis)**
  *Enterobius vermicularis*
**Trichinosis**
  *Trichinella spiralis*
**Trypanosomiasis**
  African: *Trypanosoma gambiense, T.
  rhodesiense*
  American (Chagas' disease): *T. cruzi*

VIRAL INFECTIONS

**Boston exanthem**
  echovirus 16
**Dermatomyositis/polymyositis**
  picornavirus proteins
**Ecthyma contagiosum (orf)**
  orf virus (parapoxvirus)
**Erythema infectiosum (fifth disease)**
  parvovirus B19
**Hand–foot–mouth disease**
  coxsackivirus A 5, 9, 10
**Hairy leukoplakia**
  Epstein–Barr virus
**Herpangina**
  coxsackievirus A1–10

**Herpes viruses (HSV):**
Cytomegalovirus- HSV5
Erythema multiforme-HSV1&2
Exanthum subitum (roseola)-HSV6

**Epstein–Barr virus**
Burkett's lymphoma
Infectious mononucleosis
Large cell lymphomas
Nasopharangeal carcinoma
Oral hairy leukoplakia

Kaposi-Sarcoma- HSV8 (associated)
Pityriasis Rosea-HSV-7
Varicell-Zoster-HSV3

**Infectious mononucleosis**
Epstein–Barr virus

**Measles**
paramyxovirus
**Orf**
parapoxvirus
**Roseola infantum (exanthem subitium)**
human herpesvirus 6
**Rubella**
togavirus
**Systemic sclerosis**
retroviral P30 proteins
**Wart viruses**
(see Diseases and Etiology for details)

# Diseases and immune deficiency

This subsection lists a number of diseases in which an immunological deficiency has been detected

**Ataxia telangiectasia**
defective T-cell response to some antigens
**Burton's disease**
lack of all immunoglobulins and antibodies
**Chediak–Higashi syndrome**
defective granulocytes
**Defective granulocyte function**
C3 deficiency
**Di George syndrome (congenital thymic aplasia)**
absent T cells
neonatal tetany (most frequent presenting sign)
**Hereditary angioneurotic edema**
C1 esterase deficiency
**Job's syndrome**
various defects of granulocyte function

**Leiner's disease**
C5 deficiency (decreased opsonic activity)
**Lupus erythematosus**
C2 deficiency
**Nezelof syndrome**
deficienct T-cell response
**Partial lipodystrophy**
type II hypercatabolism of C3 (C3 deficiency)
**Recurrent *Neisseria* infections**
C6, C7, C8 deficiencies
**Severe combined immunodeficiency**
decreased C1q, very low immunoglobulins
**Wiskott–Aldrich syndrome**
defective T- and B-cell responses (due to defective antigen recognition)

# Diseases and their incubation periods

This subsection is a compilation of infectious diseases and their usual incubation periods.
If known, the average incubation period is given in parentheses

**Bartonellosis**
19–30 days

**Bejel (primary)**
3–5 weeks

**Blastomycosis**
about 45 days

**Brucellosis**
6–9 months (5–21 days)

**Cat-Scratch disease**
2–4 days

**Chancroid**
12 hours to 5 days

**Chickenpox (varicella)**
9–21 days (14 days)

**Coccidioidmycosis**
1–4 weeks

**Condyloma accuminata**
3 weeks to 8 months (3 months)

**Coxsackievirus**
A-5: 5–7 days
A-9: 2–12 days

**Cutaneous atypical mycobacteria
infection (swimming pool granuloma)**
few weeks to few months
A-10 (hand, foot, and mouth disease):
    3–5 days
B-5: 4–7 days

**Duke's disease (fourth disease)**
9–20 days

**Echovirus**
2: 3–6 days
4 and 9: 5–8 days
16: 3–8 days

**Erythema infectiosum (fifth disease)**
7–28 days (16 days)

**Gonorrhea**
1–14 days (3–5 days)

**Granuloma inguinale**
8–90 days

**Hepatitis A**
15–50 days

**Hepatitis C**
4–12 weeks

**Herpangina**
2–9 days (3–5 days)

**Herpes simplex (facial–oral)**
5–10 days

**Herpes simplex (genital)**
3–14 days (5 days)

**Herpes simplex virus type I**
3–5 days

**Herpesvirus simiae infection**
2–3 days

**Herpes zoster**
unknown

**Histoplasmosis**
7–14 days

**Infectious mononucleosis**
Few days to several weeks

**Leishmaniasis (cutaneous)**
2–4 weeks to 3 months

**Leprosy**
several months to 2–3 years

**Leptospirosis**
8–15 days

**Lyme disease**
1–36 days (9 days)

**Lymphogranuloma venereum**
3–30 days (7 days)

**Measles (rubeola)**
10 days

**Molluscum contagiosum**
2 weeks to 2 months

**Monkeypox**
7–24 days

**Orf (ecthyma contagiosum)**
3–6 days

**Pinta**
  primary: 1–2 weeks
  secondary: 5 months to 1 year
**Plague**
  1–6 days
**Psittacosis**
  1–2 weeks
**Sporotrichosis**
  3 days to 12 weeks (3 weeks)
**Rat-bite fever**
  1–6 days
**Reovirus 2**
  3–6 days
**Rocky Mountain spotted fever**
  5–7 days
**Roseola infantum (exanthem subitum)**
  5–15 days
**Rubella (German measles)**
  14–21 days (18 days)
**Scabies**
  2–6 weeks (onset of symptoms)
**Scarlet fever**
  2–5 days (1–7 days)

**Smallpox (variola)**
  12–30 days
**Streptobacillus moniliformis**
  1–10 days
**Syphilis**
  neurosyphilis: 5–35 years
  primary chancre: 3–90 days (3 weeks)
  secondary: 1–3 months (6–8 weeks)
**Tinea capitis**
  2–4 days
**Tuberculosis**
  *Mycobacterium ulcerans:* 3 months
  primary inoculation: 2–4 weeks
**Tularemia**
  2–10 days
**Wart**
  1–12 months (2–3 months)
**Yaws**
  primary: 3–5 weeks
  secondary: 2–6 months
  latent: months to years

# Diseases and their vectors

This subsection is an alphabetical listing of diseases and their known vectors

**Anthrax**
  sheep
**African trypanosomiasis**
  tsetse fly
**American trypanosomiasis**
  deer fly, kissing bug (reduviid bug, assassin bug)
**Arboviruses**
  mosquitoes, ticks
**Babesiosis**
  hard ticks
**Bacillary angiomatosis**
  cats
**Bartonellosis (Carrion's disease)**
  sandfly
**Boutonneuse fever**
  rabbit flea

**Dengue**
  *Aedes aegypti* mosquito
**Ehrlichiosis**
  hard ticks
**Erythema chronica migran**
  ticks
**Filariasis**
  mosquitoes
**Glanders**
  horses
**Leishmaniasis (kala-azar)**
  sandfly
**Loaiasis**
  horse fly, mango fly (*Chrysops*)
**Lyme disease**
  *Ixodis dammini, I. pacificus* and *I. ricinus* (in Europe)

**Murine typhus**
rat flea feces
**Onchocerciasis**
black fly (genus *Simulidae*)
**Orf**
sheep
**Plague**
rat flea (*Xenopsylla cheopis* and *X. braziliensis*), squirrel flea (*Diamanus montanus*)
**Q fever**
(inhalation of dried) tick feces
**Relapsing fever**
louse, tick
**Rickettsialpox**
rodent mite (*Allodumanyssus sanguineus*)
**Rocky Mountain spotted fever**
hard-wood tick (*Ixodidae* group; *Dermacentor andersoni* in western USA, *D. variabilis* (dog tick) in eastern USA

**Scrub typhus**
mites(chiggers)
**Seabather's eruption**
*Linuche unguiculata* (sea lice)
**Swimmer's itch**
*avian schistosomes*
**Trench fever**
louse
**Tularemia**
deerfly, mosquito, squirrel flea (*Diamanus montanus*), tick*
**Typhus**
endemic typhus: rat flea (*Xenopsylla cheopis* and *X. braziliensis*)
epidemic typhus: body louse (*Pediculus species*)
scrub typhus: Trombiculid red mite

# Vectors and their diseases

**Avian schistosomes**
swimmer's itch
**Black fly** = *Pemphigus foliaceaus (Fogo selvagum)*
*Black fly, buffalo gnat, turkey gnat*
onchocerciasis
**Deer fly, greenheads, horse fly, mango fly**
loa loa
*Dermacentor variabilis (dog tick)*
human granulocytic ehrlichiosis
*Ixodes scapularies (deer tick)*
human granulocytic ehrlichiosis
**Mite**
murine typhus, plague, Q fever, rickettsialpox, scrub typhus
**Mosquito**
dengue, filariasis (by *Clulex fatigans*), malaria, yellow fever

*Pediculus corporis*
epidemic typhus, louse-borne relapsing fever, trench fever
**Sandfly**
bartonellosis, leishmaniasis
**Tick**
Colorado tick fever, lyme disease, plague, Rocky Mountain spotted fever, relapsing fever, tularemia, western equine encephalitis
*Triatoma* species
Chagas' disease
**Tsetse fly, (house fly, stable fly)**
African trypanosomiasis

# Diseases transmitted through animals

**Anthrax**
cattle
**Cat-scratch disease**
cats*, chickens, dogs, monkeys
**Cowpox**
cows
**Cysticercosis cutis**
pork tapeworm
**Glanders**
donkeys, horses, mules
**Hepatitis B**
bed bugs
**Herpesvirus simiae infection**
monkeys
**Human cowpox**
cats and rodents

**Leptospirosis**
dogs (USA), rats (most of the world)
**Milker's nodule**
cows
**Orf (Ecthyma contagiosum)**
goats, sheep
**Rat-bite fever**
rats
**Rickettsialpox**
house mice
**Trichinosis**
bears, pigs
**Tularemia**
rodents (rabbits)
**Vibro vulnificus**
raw oysters and other seafood

# Diseases with pentad features

In this subsection five major characteristic findings of different diseases are cited

**Allergic granulomatosis (Churg–Strauss syndrome)**
1   Asthma
2   Debilitation and fever
3   Hypereosinophilia
4   Multisystemic vasculitis
5   Papules and macules on extremities and scalp
*Bloom's syndrome*
1   Cafe-au-lait spots
2   Cheilitis
3   Congenital facial telangiectatic erythema
4   Photosensitivity
5   Stunted growth (dwarfism; AR)

**Chediak–Higashi syndrome (AR)**
1   Azurophilic leukocytic inclusions
2   Early death (before age 20; recurrent pyogenic sinopulmonary infections, especially with *Staphylococcus aureus*)
3   Hematologic and neurologic abnormalities
4   Partial oculocutaneous albinism (tyrosinase-positive)
5   Photophobia
**CREST syndrome**
1   Calcinosis
2   Raynaud's phenomenon
3   Esophageal immotility
4   Sclerodactyly

5 Telangiectasia

## Cronkhite–Canada syndrome

1 Alopecia
2 Generalized gastrointestinal polyposis
3 Malabsorption
4 Onychodystrophy
5 Skin pigmentation

## DeSanctis–Cacchione syndrome

1 Dwarfism
2 Gonadal hypoplasia
3 Mental deficiency
4 Microcephaly
5 Xeroderma pigmentosum

## Felty's syndrome

1 Granulocytopenia
2 Leg ulcers
3 Rheumatoid arthritis
4 Skin nodules and pigmentation
5 Splenomegaly

## Glucagonoma

1 Distinctive skin rash (migratory necrolytic erythema)
2 Glossitis
3 Glucose intolerance
4 Islet cell carcinoma of pancreas (secreting glucagon)
5 Normocytic normochromic anemia

## Focal dermal hypoplasia (Goltz syndrome) (XD)

1 Colobomata of eyes or microphthalmia
2 Hypoplasia of hair, nails and teeth, linear areas of hypoplasia (striae distensae), periorofacial papillomatosis
3 Large ulcers (due to congenital abscence of skin)
4 'Lobster-claw' deformity (lack of digit)
5 Soft yellow nodules (herniation of fat through an underdeveloped dermis), linear or cribiform reddish–tan atrophic patches in conjunction with fat herniation (mostly on axillae, buttocks, thighs)

## Hartnup disease

1 Constant aminoaciduria
2 Intermittent cerebellar ataxia
3 Pellagra-like dermatitis following sun exposure
4 Photosensitivity
5 Psychiatric manifestations

## Henoch–Schönlein purpura

1 Abdominal pain and gastrointestinal bleeding
2 Arthralgia
3 Hematuria
4 Immune deposits (IgA and C3 around cutaneous vessels)
5 Intermittent purpura

## Hurler's syndrome

(AR, $\alpha$-L-iduronidase deficiency; most common mucopolysaccharidoses)

1 Chondrodystrophy, hepatosplenomegaly; high association of cardiac and respiratory failure
2 Dwarfism, macrocephaly with frontal bulging, short neck
3 Hypertrichosis
4 Protuberant tongue and very coarse facial features
5 Saddle-nose deformity

## Marfan's syndrome (AD)

1 Cardiovascular abnormalities (ascending aortic aneurysm, mitral valve prolapse)
2 Dental abnormalities
3 Ocular abnormalities (ectopia lentis)
4 Skeletal abnormalities (loose-jointedness, tallness, etc.)
5 Striae distensae

## Pachyonychia congenita

1 Follicular keratosis (especially of elbows and knees), and blistering
2 Keratitis and cataracts
3 Leukokeratosis of the mucous membranes (oral white sponge nevus)
4 Nails excessively thickened
5 Palmar and plantar hyperkeratosis (subungual hyperkeratosis) and hyperhidrosis

(Other features: AD, corneal dyskeratosis, focal or diffuse grayish-white, striate or spotted opacities on buccal mucosa, lips, and lateral tongue. Natal teeth and dental abnormalities. Partial, diffuse alopecia)

## POEMS syndrome

1 Polyneuropathy
2 Organomegaly (heart, kidneys, spleen)
3 Endocrinopathy
4 M Protein

5  Skin changes (angiomas, clubbed nails, hyperpigmentation, hypertrichosis, leukonychia, sweating, thickening)

**Richner–Hanhart syndrome (tyrosinemia II) (AR)**
1  Deficiency of hepatic tyrosine aminotransferase
2  Bradyphalangia
3  Hyperkeratotic and erosive lesions of palms and soles (keratoderma)
4  Keratitis (corneal ulcers)
5  Mental retardation

**Sweet's syndrome (acute febrile neutrophilic dermatosis)**
1  Arthritis and iritis
2  Association with malignancy (especially acute myeloid leukemia) or *Yersinia* infection
3  Fever
4  Leukocytosis (neutrophilia)
5  Skin eruption (painful, tender, rapidly extending erythematous plaques, one-third of which are studded with pustules; on face, neck and extremities)

# Diseases with tetrad features

**Alezzandrini's syndrome**
1  Deafness (may or may not be present)
2  Ipsilateral poliosis
3  Ipsilateral vitiligo on the face
4  Unilateral degenerative retinitis

**Apert's syndrome**
1  Craniosynostosis
2  Cutaneous and ocular hypopigmentation
3  Midface malformation, symmetric syndactyly
4  Severe acneiform eruption, seborrhea

**Ataxia telangiectasia (AR)**
1  Cerebellar ataxia
2  Choreic and athetoid movements and pseudopalsy of the eyes
3  Oculocutaneous telangiectasia
4  Sinopulmonary infections

**Blue rubber-bleb nevus (AD)**
1  Association with intestinal hemangiomas
2  Blue to purple rubbery nodules
3  Pressure will express blood, leaving an empty wrinkled sac
4  Spontaneously painful and tender to palpation

**Dyskeratosis congenital**
1  Leukoplakia of buccal mucosa
2  Nail dystrophy
3  Ocular manifestations, including cataracts

4  Skin tan–gray, mottled hyper- or hypopigmented macule or reticulated patches, atrophy and telangiectasia (poikiloderma vasculare atrophicans)
(Other features: XR; diffuse alopecia; esophageal/lacrimal duct/urethra may be stenotic; hyperhidrosis and hyperkeratosis of palms and soles; increased incidence of squamous cell carcinoma of cervix/esophagus/mouth/skin/rectum/vagina; multiple dental caries and early loss of teeth; subnormal intelligence (50%))

**Hyperimmunoglobulin E syndrome**
1  Defective neutrophil chemotaxis
2  Extreme elevation of serum IgE (10–100 × normal)
3  Peripheral blood eosinophilia and personal or family history of atopy
4  Recurrent skiun infections (*Staphylococcus* usually, but also *Streptococcus*)

**Job's syndrome**
1  Chronic, recurrent *Staphylococcus* (cold abscesses)
2  Hyperextensible joints
3  Red hair
4  Women with major features of hyperimmunoglobulin E syndrome

**Leiner's disease (erythroderma desquamativum)**
1 Intractable, severe diarrhea
2 Marked wasting and dystrophy
3 Recurrent local and systemic infections (C5 deficiency)
4 Seborrheic dermatitis

**Pachydermoperiostosis**
seen in males only
(AD, may result in pulmonary disease, acquired form associated with lung carcinoma)
1 Furrowed thickening of the skin of the face and scalp (leonine facies), cutis verticis gyrata
2 Hypertrophic osteoarthropathy, hyperplasia of forearms and legs

3 Increased sebaceous activity
4 Palmoplantar keratoderma

**Russel–Silver syndrome (AD)**
1 Blue sclera
2 Café-au-lait spots
3 Short immature bones
4 Triangular facies

**Tuberous sclerosis**
1 Angiofibromas (adenoma sebaceum, seen in 94% of patients over age 4)
2 Ash-leaf macules (in about 85%), shagreen patch, subungual fibromas
3 Epilepsy
4 Mental retardation

# Diseases with triad features

**Acrodermatitis enteropathica**
(Classically appears at the time of weaning from breast to cow's milk; AD)
1 Alopecia
2 Dermatitis
3 Diarrhea

**Adiposis dolorosa (Dercum's disease)**
1 Obese, menopausal women
2 Symmetric, tender, multiple lipomas
3 Weakness and psychiatric diseases

**Albright's hereditary osteodystrophy**
1 Pseudohypoparathyroidism and pseudopseudohypoparathyroidism, tetany
2 Short stature, short metacarpals, short metatarsals
3 Short broad nails, soft tissue calcification, cataracts, mental retardation, defective teeth

**Albright's syndrome**
1 Fibroud dysplasia of long bones
2 Large pigmented macules (cafe-au-lait spots, usually unilateral and stop abruptly in midline)
3 Sexual precocity

**Bazex syndrome (AD)**

1 Basal cell carcinomas (small and multiple, on face, arising in adolescence or early adulthood)
2 Follicular atrophoderma (widened follicular openings like 'ice-pick marks', especially on the extremities)
3 Localized anhidrosis or generalized hypohidrosis and congenital hypotrichosis on the scalp and body

**Behçet's syndrome**
1 Recurrent genital aphthous ulcers (almost 100%)
2 Recurrent oral aphthous ulcers
3 Uveitis or retinal vasculitis

Other features: pathergy; erythema nodosum; papulopustular or acniform lesions; thrombophelbitis. HLA-B5 associated with ocular disease, predominantly; HLA-B27 associated with seronegative arthritis, predominantly.

**Cobb syndrome**
1 Angiokeratoma circumscriptum, or
2 Nevus flammeus
3 Angioma in spinal cord within a segment or two of the involved dermatome

**Diffuse neonatal hemangiomatosis**

201

1 cutaneous hemangiomas
2 congestive heart failure
3 hepatomegaly

**Disseminated candidiasis**
1 Diffuse muscle tenderness
2 Fever
3 Papular rash

**Ectodermal dysplasia**
Anhidrotic ectodermal dysplasia
(XR, characteristic facies: prominent frontal
bosses and a depressed nasal bridge; may
also have nail dystrophy
1 Hypodontia or anodontia
2 Hypohidrosis or anhidrosis
3 Hypotrichosis

**Hidrotic ectodermal dysplasia**
(AD, primarily a disorder of keratinization; may
also have dental abnormalities)
1 Hair defects (sparse, hypotrichosis)
2 Nail dystrophy
3 Palmoplantar keratoderma

**Fat embolism syndrome**
1 Cerebral dysfunction
2 Petechiae
3 Respiratory insufficiency

**Favre–Racouchot syndrome (nodular
elastoidosis)**
1 Follicular cysts
2 Giant comedones
3 Yellow, furrowed skin with large folds

**Grinspan's syndrome**
1 Diabetes mellitus
2 Hypertension
3 Oral lichen planus

**Hand–Schüller–Christian disease**
1 Defects in membranous bones (especially
cranium)
2 Diabetes insipidus
3 Exophthalmos

**Hemochromatosis (bronze diabetes)**
1 Diabetes mellitus
2 Gray to brown skin and mucous membrane
hyperpigmentation
3 Hepatomegaly (often cirrhosis, heart
disease and hypogonadism)

**Klippel–Trenaunay–Weber syndrome**
1 Arteriovenous aneurysm and cutaneous
telangiectasia
2 Hemangiomas
3 Overgrowth of bone and soft tissue of an
extremity or portion of trunk

**Kwashiorkor**
1 Depigmentation of hair (flag sign) and of
skin
2 Edema (hypoalbuminemia)
3 Retarded growth

**Lyme disease (if in the endemic area)**
1 Cranial neuritis
2 Meningitis
3 Radiculoneuritis

**Melkerson–Rosenthal syndrome**
1 Recurrent (intermittent) facial paralysis
(usually unilateral) or paresis
2 Recurrent soft, non-pitting edema of lips or
face
3 Scrotal (plicated) tongue

**Papillon–LeFèvre syndrome**
1 Ectopic calcification in choroid plexus and
tentorium
2 Palmoplantar hyperkeratosis
3 Periodontosis

**Pellagra (niacin or tryptophan deficiency)**
1 Dementia
2 Dermatitis (fiery-red, symmetrical eruption
on the face, neck (Casal's necklace),
wrists, and dorsum of hands; painful
fissures and ulcerations of the mucous
membrane
3 Diarrhea

**Plummer–Vinson syndrome (sideropenic
dysphagia)**
(Primarily in middle-aged women)

1 Atrophic changes of the oral mucosa
2 Chronic dysphagia (an absolute
requirement for diagnosis)
3 Hypochromic anemia (iron deficiency)

**Poikiloderma**
1 Atrophy
2 Dyschromia (hyper- and/or
hypopigmentation)
3 Telangiectasia

**Prolidase deficiency (AR)**
1 Chronic otitis media, sinusitis, chronic
recurrent by ulceration
2 Papulopustular dermatitis, diffuse
telangiectasia
3 Reticulocytosis, splenomegaly

**Reiter's syndrome**
1 Arthritis ( 90%, most disabling, persistent
feature)

2   Conjunctivitis
3   Non-gonococcal urethritis, circinate balanitis, keratoderma blenorrhagica

**Severe combined immunodeficiency**
1   Intractable diarrhea
2   Moniliasis of oropharynx and skin
3   Pneumonia

**Sézary syndrome**
1   Generalized erythroderma with intense pruritus
2   Peripheral lymphadenopathy
3   Presence of Sézary cells in the cellular infiltrate of skin and in the peripheral blood

**Thrombotic thrombocytopenic purpura**
1   Hemolytic anemia
2   Neurologic manifestations
3   Thrombocytopenic purpura

**Toxic vinyl chloride disease**
(An occupational hazard in the manufacture of polyvinyl chloride)

1   Lytic bone lesions
2   Raynaud's phenomenon

3   Scleroderma

**Wegener's granulomatosis**
1   Extensive necrotizing vasculitis of arteries and veins (almost always lungs)
2   Focal necrotizing glomerulitis
3   Necrotizing granulomatous lesions in upper and lower respiratory tract

**Wiskott–Aldrich syndrome**
1   Chronic eczematous dermatitis resembling atopic dermatitis
2   Increased susceptibility to recurrent infections in male infants (pyodermas, otitis media)
3   Thrombocytopenic purpura (intrinsic platelet abnormality), hepatosplenomegaly

**Yellow-nail syndrome**
1   Lymphedema
2   Pleural effusions
3   Yellow nails, dystrophic shape, absent cuticles, slow growth, transverse ridging, *Pseudomonas* infection

# Features of fungal infections

In this subsection fungal diseases are classified according to various criteria, highlighting major characteristic features, colony appearance and microscopic findings

## DERMATOPHYTES BY BODY REGION

### Tinea barbe
Trichophyton verrucosum*, *T. mentagrophytes, Microsporum canis* (less common); almost always caused by zoophilic fungus. Coarse hair is uniquely susceptible. Infection is usually unilateral.

### Tinea capitis
*Microsporum audouinii*, *M. canis*, *Trichophyton mentagrophytes*, *T. tonsurans** (most common)

### Tinea corporis (tinea circinata)
*Microsporum canis, Trichophyton mentagrophytes, T. rubrum*, (these three are the most common), T. tonsurans, T. verrucosum*
*Verrucous epidermophyton* is a variety of tinea corporis, caused by *Epidermophyton floccosum*; verrucous-like lesions occur on the head, neck and buttocks.

### Tinea cruris
*Epidermophyton floccosum*, *Trichophyton rubrum*, *T. mentagrophyes*; almost exclusively seen in men.

### Tinea faciale

Usually *Trichophyton* species, occasionally *Microsporum canis*; scaly plaques with or without active borders, atrophy, photoexacerbation and telangiectasia may mimic lupus erythematosus.

### Tinea pedis

Scaly: *Trichyphyton rubrum*\* (60%), *Epidermophyton floccosum* (total 10%)
Vesicular: *T. mentagrophytes* var. *interdigitale* (25%), *E. floccosum* (total 10%)

### Tinea unguium

*Trichophyton rubrum*\*, *T. mentagrophytes var interdigitale E. floccosum*

## DERMATOPHYTES BY ECOLOGY

(Partial listing)

### Anthropophilic Fungi

Primarily infect humans
*Epidermophyton floccosum*
*Microsporum audouinii, M. ferrugineum*
*Trichophyton concentricum, T. gourvilli, T. meninii, T. mentagrophytes, T. rubrum, T. schoenleinii, T. soudanense, T. tonsurans*\*, *T. violaceum, T. yaoundei*

### Geophilic Fungi

Primarily live in soil. Colonies generally have a granular texture. Characteristically show hair perforation *in vitro*.

*Microsporum cookei, M. fulvum, M. gypseum* (most common geophilic infection isolated in humans), *M. nanum, M. vanberuseghemii*
*Trichophyton ajelloi, T. terrestre*

### Zoophilic Fungi

Primarily infect animals

*Microsporum canis, M. distortum (M. canis* var. *distortum), M. equinum, M. gallinae, M. nanum*
*Trichophytan mentahrophytes, T. verrucosum*

## DERMATOPHYTES BY SCALP HAIR INVASION IN VIVO

### Ectothrix Infection Of Hair

A sheath formed around the hair shaft by a mosaic of round arthrospores. In infections with *Microsporum* species, hairs tend to break off a few millimeters above the scalp and give the appearance of dots.

*Microsporum audouinii, M. canis, M. ferrugineum, M. fulvum, M. gypseum, Trichophyton menginii, T. mentagrophytes, T. rubrum, T. verrucosum*

### Endothrix Infections Of Hair

A mosaic pattern of round arthrospores are found within the hair shaft. Hairs tend to break off at the surface of the scalp.
*Trichophyton gourvilli, T. schoenleinii, T. soudanense, T. tonsurans*\*, *T. violaceum, T. yaoundei*
('Black dot ringworm', so called because the infected hair follicle resembles a black dot, is most commonly seen with *T. tonsurans* and *T. violaceum*)

### Favus

A severe, chronic form of tinea capitis, infections of glabrous skin and/or nails, in which characteristic yellowish cup-shaped crusts (scutula) form within the hair follicle and eventually lead to scarring alopecia. Scutula may cause a characteristic 'mousy' odor. Athroconidia and air spaces (vacuolation) are seen microscopically in a linear arrangement within the hair shaft, from degenerating hyphae on the hair preparation.

*Microsporum gypseum, Trichophyton schoenleinii* (most common cause), *T. violaceum*

## ONYCHOMYCOSIS

### Distal Subungual Onychomycosis

Most common; invades stratum corneum

### Proximal Subungual Onychomycosis
Least common; invades stratum corneum. Most common fungus is *Trichophyton rubrum*

### Proximal white Onchomycosis
A combination of proximal subungual onchomycosis and white subungual onchomycosis. Caused by *Trichophyton rubrum, & Trichophyton megninis, and seen in patients with AIDS*

### White Subungual Onychomycosis
Most rare form. Most common fungus is *Trichophyton mentagrophytes*; invades dorsal surface of nail plate; also *Aspergillus, Cephalosporium* and *Fusarium oxysporum*; fingernails are not affected.

### Candida onychomycosis
Invades nail plate via the hyponychial epithelium; seen in patients with chronic mucocutaneous candidiasis

## SUPERFICIAL MYCOSIS

These are *non-invasive* (but are capable of causing invasive disease, especially in an immunocompromised host), do not destroy the hair shaft, and do not evoke a significant host response.

### Piedra
Asymptomatic fungal infection of hair shaft. Cured by shaving the infected hair.

### Black Piedra
Macroscopic colony appearance: small, black–green, velvety colony with a raised center
Microscopic appearance: chlamydospore-like, dark, septate hyphae
Special features: caused by *Piedra hortae*; *pigmented* (dark brown), firmly attached concretions ('stones') on the hair shaft

### White Piedra
Macroscopic colony appearance: white–cream (pale yellow), yeast-like, with a heaped center; radial folds
Microscopic appearance: septate hyphae that fragment into arthroconidia
Special features: caused by *Trichosporon (Cutaneum) Beigelii*; white, soft nodules that are easily separated from the hair shaft

### Pityriasis (tinea) versicolor
Caused by *Malassezia furfur (Pityrosporum ovale, P. obiculare)*. Potassium hydroxide preparation is diagnostic, showing 'spaghetti and meatball' appearance. Requires *lipids* for growth.

### Tinea Nigra Palmaris
Also known as superficial phaeohyphomycosis. Caused by *Exophiala (Cladosporium or Phaeonnellomyces) werneckii*. A brownish-black, non-scaly macule/patch on the palms. Most common in tropical and subtropical areas. (Griseofulvin is not an effective treatment). Potassium hydroxide preparation demonstrates *hyaline to pigmented hyphae* and *yeast cells*.
Macroscopic colony appearance: early yeast phase; later mold phase; pigmented; black, moist, heaped-up colony
Microscopic appearance: hyaline to pigmented hyphae and yeast cells on potassium hydroxide preparation

## DIMORPHIC FUNGI

These demonstrate yeast-like structures in tissue when cultured at 37°C, and show hyphae when grown at 25°C:
*Blastomyces dermatitidis*
    *Coccidioides immitis*
*Histoplasma capsulatum*
*Paracoccidioides brasiliensis*
*Sporothrix schenckii*

# Laboratory characteristics of fungal infections

Conidia are smooth-walled, large, clavate or club shaped.

E. floccosum

Macroscopic colony appearance: khaki to olive-green; reverse yellow (mustard yellow) to tan; flat with elevated center; folded center and radial grooves

Microscopic appearance: macroconidia only (*no microconidia*); smooth walls (not warty); multi-celled – 'clavate' or club-shaped

Characteristic macroconidia have rough (spiny or echinulate) walls; they may be spindle-shaped and thick

M. audouinii

Macroscopic colony appearance: buff (tanish white) to grayish; *'mouse fur'* (velvety) texture; reverse is salmon-colored (best seen on potato dextrose agar)

Microscopic appearance: unique pectinate (comblike); septate hyphae; terminal chlamydospores

Special features: does not grow on polished rice (as opposed to *M. canis*); does not perforate hair *in vitro*; ectothrix hair invasion; fluorescent tinea capitis

M. canis

Macroscopic colony appearance: whitish with yellowish periphery; reverse is yellow to brown; periphery is fuzzy, hairy, has 'cotton tufts' texture (color and texture reminder of a tabby cat)

Microscopic appearance: macroconidia are spindle-shaped with knob-like ends

Special features: grows on polished rice; ectothrix hair invasion and fluorescence

M. cookei

Macroscopic colony appearance: granular colony with deep grape-red pigment under the surface; reverse is purple–red

Microscopic appearance: thick-walled echinulate macroconidia

Special features: rare cause of human infection

M. ferrugineum

Macroscopic colony appearance: rust colored

Microscopic appearance: bamboo hyphae

Special features: causes infection similar to *M. audouinii*; fluorescent; *in vivo* hair invasion; mostly in Asia and Africa

M. gallinae

Macroscopic colony appearance: lateral diffusion of pinkish pigment far beyond the extent of the gross colony

Special features: causes infection in chickens

M. gypseum

Macroscopic colony appearance: tan to cinnamon–buff color with white edge; reverse is yellow; texture is granular or suede-like

Microscopic appearance: numerous symmetrical cucumber-like macroconidia

Special features: ectothrix; may or may not fluoresce; perforates hair *in vitro*

M. nanum

Microscopic colony appearance: looks like pig shells

Special features: cause of pig ringworm; ectothrix; no fluorescence

M. vanbreuseghemi

Microscopic colony appearance: long, tapered conidia

Microconidia are often diagnostic. They are thin and smooth-walled, often one-celled.

T. mentagrophytes

Macroscopic colony appearance: buff to white color; may have red non-diffusing pigment under the surface

Microscopic appearance: coiled or spiral hyphae; 'grape-like' arrangement of microconidia

Special features: no fluorescence; positive hair perforation test (as opposed to *T. rubrum*); urease test positive in 5–7 days (as opposed to *T. rubrum*)

*T. rubrum*

Macroscopic colony appearance: white to cream; reverse port-wine or blood-red

Microscopic appearance: diagnostic tear-drop or peg-shaped (pencil-shaped) microconidia occur in lateral distribution, off the side of the hyphae

Special features: ectothrix and endothrix hair infection; negative hair perforation *in vitro*; non-fluorescent; urease negative in 5–7 days; causes a moccasin type of *T. pedis* (dry and scaly soles); produces pigment on corn meal agar

*T. schoenleinii*

Macroscopic colony appearance: irregular, heaped-up and folded with a glabrous, waxy surface; yellowish white to brown in color

Microscopic appearance: antler-like (favic chandeliers) hyphae

Special features: blue–white hair fluorescence; causes favus

*T. tonsurans*

Macroscopic colony appearance: flat, powdery to suede-like surface; reverse is reddish-brown

Microscopic appearance: many teardrop or balloon form microconidia

Special features: partial thiamine requirement for growth endothrix

*T. verrucosum*

Macroscopic colony appearance: glabrous white, heaped; reverse is yellowish

Microscopic appearance: rat-tail macroconidia; chain of chlamydospores; sparse mycelium

Special features: thiamine requirement and partial requirement for inositol; may mimic bacterial furunculosis

## CANDIDIASIS

*Candida albicans*

Macroscopic colony appearance: moist, pasty, smooth, cream to white

Microscopic appearance: yeast cells are short, ovoid; pseudo-hyphae

Special features: negative urea test; can grow on media containing cycloheximide (e.g. dermatophyte test medium or mycosel®)

## DERMATOMYCOSIS

Infection of skin or nail by a non-dermatophyte mold that produces a 'tinea-like' eruption

*Hendersonela toruloidea*

Macroscopic colony appearance: light colored colony that darkens, developing grey or greenish hues; texture is cottony to velvety

Microscopic appearance: non-pigmented hyphae on potassium hydroxide; similar to dermatophytes

Special features: grows poorly on cyclohexidine-containing media; produces 'tinea' manum, 'tinea' pedis and onychomycosis; occurs in endemic areas

*Scytalidium hyalinum*

Macroscopic colony appearance: light-colored, cottony mold

Microscopic appearance: non-pigmented hyphae on potassium hydroxide

Special features: thought to be an albino variant of *Hendersonela toruloidea*

## MISCELLANEOUS

### Ascending Lymphangitis Spread

Most characteristically seen with sporotrichosis and atypical acid-fast bacteria. (Also seen with blastomycosis, coccidiomycosis, histoplasmosis and nocardiosis)

### Aspergillosis

Produces characteristic necrotizing suppurative inflammation, blood vessel invasion and thrombosis. The most important predisposing factor is metabolic acidosis (especially in diabetic ketoacidosis).

### Asteroid Bodies

Spores with radiating fingers of eosinophilic material found in sporotrichosis

**'Boxcar' chlamydospores**
Characteristic of coccidiomycosis

**Chromoblastomycosis**
Potassium hydroxide shows 'sclerotic bodies' or 'copper pennies'

**Dematiaceous Fungi**
Molds that have brown, septate hyphae in tissue

**Dermatophytids**
A generalized or localized skin reaction to the fungal antigen

erythema annulare centrifugum
erysipelas-like
erythema nodosum
follicular papules
urticaria
vesicular id of hands and feet

**Disseminated Candidiasis**
Suggested by a triad of erythematous skin lesions, fever, and myalgia, in a patient with sepsis who is not responding to antibiotic therapy. Predisposing factors include:

broad spectrum antibiotics
corticosteroid therapy
hyperglycemia
intravenous catheters
neutropenia (most common)

Candidiasis is the most common and aspergillosis is the second most common cause of systemic fungal infection in immunocompromised patients.

**Distinguished hyphael structures**
Bamboo hyphae: *Microsporum ferrugineum*
Pectinate hyphae: *Microsporum audoinii*
Racquet hyphae: *Trichophyton schoenleinii*
Tangled hyphae: *Trichophyton violaceum*

**Fluorescence under Wood's light**
Fluorescence thought to be produced by Pteridines

Blue–white fluorescence seen with *Trichophyton schoenleinii*
Bright green (yellow–green) fluorescence seen with *Microsporum audouinii, M. canis, M. distortum, M. ferrugeneum*, and *M. gypseum*
Yellowish fluorecence seen with tinea versicolor

**Hair perforation in vitro**
Geophilic dermatophytes
*Microsporum canis*
*Trichophyton mentagrophytes*
*T. tonsurans* var. *sulphureum*

**Kerion**
In tinea capitis, usually seen with zoophilic species and occasionally with geophilic species. It is the host's cellular immune response (delayed type hypersensitivity, a 'localized-id reaction') to infection with a dermatophyte. It consists of an inflammatory, boggy mass studded with broken hairs, and oozing purulent material from the follicular orifices. Most frequently caused by *Microsporum canis* and *Trichophyton mentagrophytes*

**Loboa Loboi**
The organism found in keloidal blastomycosis

**Majocchi's granuloma**
A deep pustular type of tinea corporis (circinata) which resembles a carbuncle or a kerion; seen on glabrous skin, most commonly on the shins or wrists. A perifollicular granuloma; it is an annular, boggy, circumscribed, crusty, raised granuloma in which the hair follicles are distended with viscid purulent material.

*Trichophyton mentagrophytes**
*T. rubrum**
*T. tonsurans*
*T. violaceum*

**Mucormycosis**
Produces characteristic necrotizing suppurative inflammation, blood vessel invasion and

thrombosis (seen with aspergillosis, as well). The most important predisposing factor is metabolic acidosis (especially in diabetic ketoacidosis)

### Myospherulosis
Thought to represent an alteration in red blood cells, usually produced by petrolatum or lanolin, with an accompanying foreign body response

### Slow-growing Colonies
*Trichophyton concentricum*
*T. schoenleinii*
*T. soudanense*
*T. verrucosum*

*T. violaceum*
*T. yaounde*

### Special Nutritional Requirements
Histidine: *Trichophyton megninii*
Inositol and thiamine: *T. verrucosum*
Niacin: *T. equinum*
Thiamine: *T. concentricum, T. tonsurans, T. verrucosum, T. violaceum*

### Tinea Imbricata
*Trichophyton concentricum*; autosomal recessive inheritance for susceptibility to this infection; endemic in Pacific Islands; produces concentric rings in an infected area; there may be generalized pruritus

# Immunologic and other diagnostic tests

## NORMAL COMPLEMENT FUNCTION

C1q: binds antibody
C3a: activation of mast cells and basophils; mast cell degranulation
C3b: opsonization, phagocytosis
C4a: activation of mast cells and basophils
C5a: chemotactic factor (eosinophils, monocytes, neutrophils)
C5b, 6, 7, 8, 9 (membrane attack complex): membrane damage; cell lysis
C5, 6, 7: neutrophil chemotaxis
C5b: basophil chemotaxis

## LABORATORY TESTS

### Acrodermatitis enteropathica
zinc deficiency
### Acrodynia
mercury (blood, urine)
C1 esterase inhibitor deficiency; decreased C4
### Angioedema

ANA PATTERNS:
Centomere- CREST, Raynaud's phenomenon
Homogenous- systemic lupus erythematosus (drug induced)
Mitochondrial-primary biliary cirrhosis
Nucleolar- scleroderma
Particulate- mixed connective tissue disease, systemic lupus erythematosus
Peripheral- systemic lupus erythematosus
Rim- systemic lupus erythematosus
Speckled- mixed connective tissue disease (high titers), scleroderma (low titers)

ANA POSITIVE:
Allergic encephalitis
Auto immune liver disease
Autoimmune thyroiditis
dermatomyositis
Mixed Connective tissue disease
Polymyositis
Sjogren's syndrome
Systemic lupus erythematosus

ANTIGENS & DISEASES
Alpha 6 beta 4: junctional epidermolysis bullosa with pyloric atresia

Desmoglein-1: pemphigous foliaceous
Desmoglein-3: pemphigus vulgaris
Desmoplakin: paraneoplastic pemphigus
Ladinin: linear IgA
Laminin-5: generalized atrophic benign
   epidermolysis bullosa (laminin-5 & bullos
   pemphigoid antigen2), junctional
   epidermolysis bullosa letalis (Herlitz's
   disease)

**Ataxia telangiectasia**
α-fetoprotein and carinoembryonic antigen
   (CEA) levels increased
**Atopic dermatitis**
increased IgE
**Bloom's syndrome**
cultured blood leukocytes
**Bullous erythematosus**
autoantibody to type VII collagen
**Carcinoid syndrome**
increased serotonin
**C2 deficiency**
anti-Ro (SS-A)
**Carcinoid syndrome**
increased urinary 5-hydroxyindoleactic acid
**Chediak–Higashi syndrome**
neutrophil morphology, giant, abnormal
   lyosomal granules

*CHOLESTROL ESTERS (lipids) DOUBLY
   REFRACTILE:*
**Dermatofibroma**
**Erythema elevatum diutinum**
**Fabry's disease**
**Had-Schuller-Christian disease**
**Juvenile xanthogranuloma**
**Other** *(amyloid stained with Congo red, silica,
   starch granules, suture material, urate crystals
   of gout, wooden splinters)*
**Xanthelasma (of hyperlipoproteinemia)**
**Xanthoma (plane or tuberous)**

**Chronic granulomatous disease**
neutrophil chemiluminescence
**Cyclic neutropenia**
decreased neutrophils
**Dermatitis herpetiforms**
endomysial antibodies
**Dermatomyositis/polymyositis**
ANA (50–75%), Anti-Jo-1 antibodies associated
   with fibrosing alveolitis; antibodies to
   endomysium, gliadin, reticulin; IgA2 deposits,
   mainly

***Drug-induced lupus erythematosus***
ANA (100%), anti-histone antibody
***Epidermolysis bullosa acquisita***
autoantibody to type VII collagen
***Epidermolysis bullosa (junctional type)***
19-DEJ-1 (antibody to
   hemidesmosome-anchoring filament, AA3)
***Epidermolysis bullosa simplex***
antibodies to bullous pemphigoid antigen
***Fabry's disease***
decreased serum alpha galactosidase
***Fogo selvagem***
increased serum thymosin alpha
***Gianotti–Crosti syndrome***
elevated hepatic enzymes, vital titers
***Hereditary angioedema***
low serum C4 level (choice screening test); low
   or normal C1 inhibitor level
***Herlitz junctional epidermolysis bullosa***
GB3 antibodies
***Herpes gestationis***
HG factor

HYPERCALCEMIA (OR CALCIFICATION):
Albright's hereditary osteodystrophy
Osteoma cutis
Primary hyperparathyroidism
Subcutaneous fat necrosis of the newborn

IMMUNOFLUORESCENCE PATTERNS:
BULLOUS PEMPHIGOID- Linear band of IgG
CICTRICIAL PEMPHIGOID- linear band of IgG
CHRONIC BULLOUS DISEASE OF
   CHILDHOOD- linear band of IgA
DERMATITIS HERPETIFORMIS- granular
   deposits of IgA
HERPES GESTATIONIS- linear band of C3 only
***Job's syndrome***
IgE levels increased
***LEOPARD syndrome***
electrocardiogram
***Linear IgA bullous disease (A subset only)***
autoantibodies to type VII collagen only
***Mastocytosis***
increased 24 h urine histamine
***Mixed connective tissue disease***
anti-histone antibody, anti-nRNP at high titers,
   extractable nuclear antigen (ENA), speckled
   pattern ANA (100%)
***MORPHEA (GENERALIZED)***
**Anti-histone antibodies**
***Necrolytic migratory erythema***

marked rise in glucagon, and decreased amino acid concentrations

**Neonatal lupus erythematosus**
anti-Ro (SS-A)

**Partial lipodystrophy**
serum C3 levels

**Papular dermatitis of pregnancy**
marked elevation of 24 h urinary chorionic gonadotropin

**Pemphigus vulgaris**
glycocalyx antibodies

**Phenylketonuria**
increased blood levels of phenylalanine. A few drops of ferric chloride added to the urine, turns it green (because of phenylpyruvic acid)

**Polymyositis**
anti-Jo-1 and anti-Mi-2, anti-RNA synthetase autoantibodies

**Polymyositis/scleroderma/systemic lupus erythematosus overlap syndrome**
KU antibodies, Anti-U1RNP

**Porphyria cutanea tarda**
under Wood's lamp, pinkish red fluorescence; (addition of a few drops of hydrochloric acid or acetic acid to the urine intensifies the fluorescence)

**Primary biliary cirrhosis**
anti-mitochondrial antibodies

**Recessive dystrophic epidermolysis bullosa**
KF-1 antibodies

**Rheumatoid arthritis**
ANA (40–60%), rheumatoid factor (90%)

**Sarcoidosis**
angiotensin-converting enzyme serum levels increased in 60% of patients; helpful to monitor diseased activity; increased serum calcium levels; Kveim test is positive in 80% of acute cases; CXR (hilar adenopathy, 70%)

**Scleroderma**
CREST syndrome
anticentromere antibody (considered a marker for this; implies good prognosis); speckled nuclear pattern ANA

**Diffuse scleroderma**
ANA (94%), SC1-70 antibodies (implies poor prognosis)

**Linear scleroderma**
antibodies to single-stranded DNA; rapid progression and telangiectasia; anti-fibrillarin antibody

**Localized scleroderma**
eosinophilia – active disease
elevated IgG – contractures

positive ANA – prolonged disease course
single-stranded DNA antibodies – diffuse skin disease
increased serum intercellular adhesion molecules

**Scleroderma with myositis**
Pm-SCL particle

**Sjögren's syndrome**
ANA (80%); anti-La (SS-B)*; anti-Ro (SS-A)

**Subacute cutaneous lupus erythematosus**
anti-Ro (SS-A)

**Sweat color**
chromhidrosis: blue-black
ochronosis: brown
occupational exposure to copper: blue
rifampin: red

**Sweet's syndrome**
antibodies to neutrophil cytoplasmic antibodies

**Systemic lupus erythematosus**
*ANA*
(95–100% of patients, useful for screening); may also be posisive in autoimmune thyroid disease, chronic infection, malignancy; also in 5% of healthy people, and even more in healthy people above the age of 55
*Antibody to double-stranded DNA*
active nephritis; positive in 50–70% of systemic lupus erythematosus patients
*Antibody to ribosomal antibody*
lupus psychosis
*Antibody to single-stranded DNA*
suggestive of systemic disease in patients with cutaneous LE; also seen in patients with rheumatoid arthritis
*C3, C4, CH$_{50}$ decrease*
useful for follow up of treatment
*Fluorescent ANA*
almost diagnostic of systemic lupus erythematosus at a titer of 1 : 160 or higher, with a peripheral staining pattern
*Lupus band test*
  *For diagnosis*
involved and uninvolved sun-exposed skin (negative in DLE, positive in 80% of untreated systemic lupus erythematosus patients)
  *For prognosis*
uninvolved sun-protected skin (positive in 50% of patients with systemic lupus erythematosus, and in 83% of patients with diffuse renal disease)
Sm antibodies (prognostic value; occur in 25% of patients, indicative of significant

renal involvement); 83% of patients with anti-Sm antibodies have systemic lupus erythematosus (most specific autoantibody for SLE)

*ANA fluorescence patterns*

*Homogeneous pattern*

systemic lupus erythematosus and any connective tissue disease

*Nucleolar pattern*

Raynaud's phenomenon, scleroderma, (rare in mixed connective tissue disease and uncommon in systemic lupus erythematosus)

*Particulate pattern*

mixed connective tissue disease; scleroderma; systemic lupus erythematosus

*Peripheral pattern*

active systemic lupus erythematosus (very specific); commonly positive in systemic lupus erythematosus with nephritis

*Speckled pattern*

CREST/scleroderma, Raynaud's phenomenon

*Acute cutaneous lupus erythematosus*

ANA

anti-ds DNA

anti-sm

low complement

lupus band test (98% in involved skin; 70% in uninvolved skin)

*Subacute cutaneous lupus erythematosus*

ANA

anti Ro/SSA, anti La/SSB

HLA-DR3

lupus band test (50% in involved skin; 30% in uninvolved skin)

**Systemic scleroderma**

anti-DNA topoisomerase I autoantibody

**Vasculitis**

anti-Ro (SS-A)

**Wegener's granulomatosis**

antineutrophil cytoplasmic antibody (also seen in primary sclerosing cholangitis & in ulcerative colitis)

**Wiskott–Aldrich syndrome**

deficiency of sialoproticn (CD43) on the surface of lymphocytes and platelets

**Xeroderma pigmentosum**

recovery rate of DNA synthesis after ultraviolet light exposure

*False-positive FTA-ABS test*

addition to drug

alcoholic cirrhosis

collagen vascular diseases (mixed connective tissue disease, rheumatoid arthritis, scleroderma, systemic lupus erythematosus)

herpes simplex virus (genital)

pregnancy

*False-positive Kveim test*

brucellosis

Crohn's disease

tuberculosis

*False-positive VDRL test*

*Acute (< 6 months)*

atypical pneumonia

chickenpox

drug addiction

infectious mononucleosis

malaria

measles

pregnancy

smallpox vaccination

systemic lupus erythematosus (drug-induced)

*Chronic (> 6 months)*

cirrhosis of liver

collagen vascular diseases (mixed connective tissue disease, rheumatoid arthritis, scleroderma, systemic lupus erythematosus)

drug addiction

familial

Hashimoto's thyroiditis

leprosy

lymphoma

metastatic disease of the liver

myeloma

sarcoidosis

Sjögren's syndrome

*HLA related diseases*

*HLA-B8 and HLA Dw2*

celiac disease

chronic active hepatitis

juvenile onset diabetes mellitus

myasthenia gravis

Sjögren's disease

systemic lupus erythematosus

*HLA-DR3*

Addison's disease

chronic active hepatitis

Grave's disease

myasthenia gravis

Sjögren's disease

systemic lupus erythematosus

# Nail changes in skin diseases

## ALOPECIA AREATA

pitting

## DARIER'S DISEASE

distal V-shaped notch
red, longitudinal subungual streaks
wedge-shaped subungual hyperkeratosis
white, longitudinal subungual streaks

## LICHEN PLANUS

longitudinal grooves and ridges of the nail plate
(onychorrhexis)
nail atrophy

onycholysis
onychomadesis
pterygium formation*
subungual hyperkeratosis
subungual hyperpigmentation
thinning of nail plate

## PSORIASIS

brownish macule ('oil drop' or yellowing –
defect in nailbed)
onychodystrophy
onycholysis – nail bed defect
pitting – defective keratinization of proximal
nail fold
subungual hyperkeratosis

# Some diseases and syndromes highlighted

Some main features of different groups of diseases or syndromes

## GROUP ONE

Four *autosomally dominant* inherited syndromes
where different associated *malignant*
diseases may occur

### Cowden's Disease (Multiple Hamartoma Syndrome)
AD
adenoid facies; high arched palate
acromelanosis, cafe-au-lait spots, fibrocystic
breast disease (53–60% of females),

hemangiomas, lipomas, neuromas, palmar
pits, thyroid adenoma and/or goiter (59%)
increased risk of carcinoma of breast (30–50%)
and thyroid (12%), and also of the
gastrointestinal tract
multiple tricholemmomas (83%) (when closely
set, may give cobblestone appearance)
papillomatosis of oral mucosa (83%)
Cowden's fibromas
one third of patients have polyposis (most
commonly in the rectosigmoid)

## Gardner's syndrome

AD, the most common hereditary polyposis syndrome

epidermoid cysts (50–100%), fibromas, desmoids, osteomatosis of mandible and maxilla (75%)

intestinal polyposis with malignant transformation

lifetime risk of colonic cancer is 100%

pigmented lesions of ocular fundus (90%)

Turcot's syndrome – association of familial polyposis syndrome with neoplasm of the central nervous system

## Muir–Torre syndrome

AD

sebaceous adenoma (most common and most specific), carcinoma, epithelioma, hyperplasia; skin tumors; keratoacanthoma

gastrointestinal cancers (especially colon), larynx or endometrial carcinoma

## Multiple Mucosal Neuroma syndrome (Sipple's syndrome)

AD

conjunctival, nasal, oral, upper gastrointestinal neuromas

medullary thyroid carcinoma, pheochromocytoma

'blueberry' lips, marfanoid features, joint laxity, arachnodactyly

## GROUP TWO

*Diagnostic criteria*

## Cat-scratch disease

Three of four criteria needed for diagnosis:
1  cat contact
2  failure to show other causes
3  positive skin test
4  regional adenopathy

## Infectious Mononucleosis

Generalized adenopathy is a hallmark; 50% of patients have upper eyelid swelling

## Kawasaki's Disease

Five of six criteria needed for diagnosis:
1  conjunctival injection (uveitis in 70% of patients)
2  changes of lips and oral cavity (swollen red tongue)
3  fever for at least 5 days
4  lymph node enlargement (usually confined to the neck nodes)
5  polymorphous exanthem of the skin
6  swelling, peeling, redness of palms and soles

## Lupus erythematosus Diagnostic Criteria

Four or more of 11 criteria needed serially or simultaneously:
1  ANA positive
2  discoid eruption
3  hematologic – hemolytic anemia, leukopenia, lymphopenia, thrombocytopenia
4  immunologic – anti-Sm antibody, anti-DNA antibody, false positive serologic test for syphilis, positive LE-cell prep
5  joint involvement – non-erosive arthritis involving two or more peripheral joints
6  malar eruption
7  neurologic – psychosis, seizure
8  oral ulcers
9  photosensitivity
10  renal – persistent proteinuria greater than 0.5 g/d, cellular casts
11  serositis – pericarditis, pleurisy

## Neurofibromatosis

*In adults*

six or more cafe-au-lait spots > 1.5 cm in diameter

*In children*

five or more cafe-au-lait spots > 0.5 cm in diameter

axillary freckling (Crowe's sign) is pathognomonic

Lisch nodules (hamartomatous lesions of the iris) seen in 94% of patients after age 6

## Tuberous sclerosis

Diagnostic triad

1   angiofibroma
2   mental deficiency
3   seizure

*Pathognomonic skin lesions*
hypopigmented macules (70–90%; early marker)
periungual, subungual, and gingival fibromas
shagreen's patches (21–83%, between the ages
   of 2 and 5)
tooth pits (1–2 mm enamel defects); > 5 is
   pathognomonic
*Other findings*
increased cafe-au-lait spots
increased incidence in patients with partial
   albinism
sclerotic calcification in brain

GROUP THREE

*Ehlers–Danlos syndrome*

**Type I**
AD
easy bruisability
marked skin fragility and poor wound healing
skin and joint hyperextensibility

**Type II**
AD
digits, joints, hypermobile

**Type III**
AD
large-joint hypermobility

**Type IV**
(arterial type)
AD and AR
decreased type III collagen synthesis
fragile very bruisable skin
arterial rupture
perforation of intestines

**Type V**
XR
lysyl oxidase deficiency
hernias

mitral and tricuspid valve prolapse
dwarfism

**Type VI**
(ocular type)
AR
*lysyl hydroxylase deficiency*
joint and skin hypermobility
kyphoscoliosis
retinal detachment
intraocular bleeding

**Type VII**
AR
procollagen aminoprotease deficiency
dwarfism
joint hypermobility
hip dislocation

**Type VIII**
(periodontal type)
   AD
significant skin fragility
severe periodontitis

**Type IX**
XR, X-linked cutis laxa
*lysyl oxidase deficiency*
copper metabolism abnormal
bladder diverticula
hernias
joint laxity
hyperextensible skin

**Type X**
(fibronectin type)
AR
fibronectin abnormality
striae
easy bruisability (platelet aggregation defect)

**Type XI**
AD
skin normal
joint dislocation and laxity

*Epidermolysis Bullosa*

### Epidermolysis Bullosa Simplex

Bullae are intraepidermal, primarily basilar, except that in the superficialis type, they are subcorneal.

*Localized epidermolysis bullosa simplex*
1   Epidermolysis bullosa simplex of hands and feet (Weber–Cockayne, AD); onset in infancy to early childhood
2   Epidermolysis bullosa simplex with anodontia/hypodontia (Kallin syndrome, AR); mostly on hands and/or feet; thickened or curved nails; childhood alopecia with brittle hair

*Generalized epidermolysis bullosa simplex*
1   Epidermolysis bullosa simplex, herpetiformis (AD); onset at birth; grouping of blisters; generalized, esophageal involvement
2   Epidermolysis bullosa simplex, Koebner variant
3   Epidermolysis bullosa simplex Mendes da Costa variant (XR)
4   Epidermolysis bullosa simplex Ogna variant (AD); characteristic mechanical fragility; onychogryposis
5   Epidermolysis bullosa simplex superficialis (AD)
6   Epidermolysis bullosa simplex with mottled pigmentation with or without keratoderma (AD)
7   Epidermolysis bullosa simplex with or without associated neuromuscular disease (epidermolysis bullosa simplex letalis, AR); onset at birth or early infancy; scarring alopecia; congenital myasthenia gravis

### Epidermolysis Bullosa Junctional

Bullae are intralamina lucida

*Localized junctional epidermolysis bullosa*
1   Junctional epidermolysis bullosa acral (minimus, AR)
2   Junctional epidermolysis bullosa inversa (AR)
3   Junctional epidermolysis bullosa localized, other
4   Junctional epidermolysis bullosa progressiva (neurotropica) variant (AR)

*Generalized junctional epidermolysis bullosa*
1   Junctional epidermolysis bullosa cicatricial (AR); characteristic acral muscular deformities
2   Junctional epidermolysis bullosa gravis (Herlitz) variant (AR); characteristic exuberant granulation tissue
3   Junctional epidermolysis bullosa mitis variant (non-Herlitz variant, generalized atrophic benign epidermolysis bullosa, AR)

### Dystrophic Epidermolysis Bullosa

Bullae are sub-lamina densa

*Localized dystrophic epidermolysis bullosa*
1   Dystrophic epidermolysis bullosa acral (minimus)
2   Dystrophic epidermolysis bullosa centripetal
3   Dystrophic epidermolysis bullosa inversa
4   Dystrophic epidermolysis bullosa localized, other
5   Dystrophic epidermolysis bullosa pretibial

*Generalized dystrophic epidermolysis bullosa*
*Autosomal dominant*
1   Dystrophic epidermolysis bullosa albopapuloidea (Pasini variant); milia, scarring and atrophy are commonly present
2   Dystrophic epidermolysis bullosa hyperplasique (Cockayne–Touraine variant); milia, scarring and atrophy are commonly present
3   Transient bullous dermolysis of the newborn
*Autosomal recessive*
most frequently reported epidermolysis bullosa complicated by squamous cell ca.

1 Recessive dystrophic epidermolysis bullosa, gravis, (Hallopeau–Siemens variant); milia, scarring and atrophy are commonly present

2 Recessive dystrophic epidermolysis bullosa mitis

## GROUP FIVE

### Histiocytic syndromes

### Histiocytosis X

Proliferation of Langerhans cells. On electronmicroscopy, Birbeck granules are noted.

*Eosinophilic granuloma (chronic localized Histiocytosis X)*
Least severe, most common form; occurs in children more than six years old and in young adults; usually confined to bone; has a tendency to spontaneous healing

*Hand–Schüller–Christian disease (chronic disseminated histiocytosis X)*
Triad of (1) diabetes insipidus, (2) exophthalmus, (3) multiple bone defects, especially cranium; moderate severity, occasional fatal outcome; occurs before age 30, most commonly between two and six years; may involve lymph nodes, liver, spleen, lungs, and may result in chronic otitis media from mastoid involvement

*Letterer–Siwe disease (generalized histiocytosis X)*
Most severe, malignant, poor prognosis. Present at birth or before age two. Anemia; fever; hepatosplenomegaly; lymphadenopathy; bone lesions (good prognosis); thrombocytopenia (poor prognosis); skin eruption in 80–100% of cases; reddish-orange papules with crust in seborrheic distribution, and a petechial component which may resemble Darier's disease

### Non-Histiocytosis X
*Benign*
*With lipidization*

1 Generalized xanthelasma (plane xanthoma); 50% of cases associated with lymphoproliferative disorders, multiple myeloma, and paraproteinemia. On electronmicroscopy birbeck granules and dense bodies noted

2 Juvenile xanthogranuloma; onset before age 1; 30% present at birth; may occasionally have systemic involvement. On electronmicroscopy, myeloid bodies and fat droplets noted

3 Necrobiotic xanthogranuloma; inflammatory xanthomatous nodules and plaques that ulcerate and heal with scarring, especially occurring in the periorbital areas. Associated with lymphoproliferative disorders, multiple myeloma, and paraproteinemia (100% of cases). On electronmicroscopy, laminated bodies noted

4 Papular xanthoma

5 Xanthoma disseminatum; as a rule involves the mucous membranes; onset in adulthood; 50% have mild diabetes insipidus. On electronmicroscopy, myeloid bodies and fat droplets noted

*Without lipidization*

1 Benign cephalic histiocytosis; on electronmicroscopy, comma-shaped, worm-like bodies (20%) and coated vesicles (100%) noted

2 Congenital self-healing reticulohistiocytosis; on electronmicroscopy, laminated and dense bodies noted; present in perinatal period or at birth

3 Familial derm–chondro–corneal dystrophy (Francois syndrome)

4 Familial histiocytic dermatoarthritis

5 Generalized eruptive histiocytoma

6 Multicentric reticulohistiocytosis; on electronmicroscopy, numerous lysozomes and pleomorphic cytoplasmic inclusions; characteristically, histiocytes accumulate in skin and bones; symmetrical distal arthritis in two thirds of cases

7 Nodular non-X histiocytosis

8  Progressive nodular histiocytosis; on electronmicroscopy, pleomorphic cytoplasmic inclusions noted

*Malignant*
Lethal in a few months. Severe pancytopenia, and extensive invasion of reticuloendothelial organs (e.g. bone marrow, spleen)
1  Erytherophagocytic syndrome with lymphoma
2  Malignant fibrous histiocytoma
3  Malignant histiocytosis
4  Monocytic leukemia

*Pseudo-malignant*
1  Atypical fibroxanthoma
2  Cytophagic panniculitis
3  Familial erythrophagocytic lymphohistiocytosis
4  Regressing atypical histiocytosis; multiple fungating, ulcerative papules and nodules
5  Sinus histiocytosis with massive lymphadenopathy; on electronmicroscopy, cluster of comma-shaped bodies noted
6  Viral associated hemophagocytic syndrome

## GROUP SIX

### Ichthyosis, Major Types
*Epidermolytic hyperkeratosis (bullous congenital ichthyosiform erythroderma)*
AD
incidence 1/300 000
onset at birth
*Clinical*
coarse, verrucous grayish-brown scales, especially in flexures; bullae (especially in infancy and childhood)
normal-appearing skin in middle of hyperkeratotic area
unpleasant odor; frequent skin infections
prenatal diagnosis possible
*Pathological*
large, coarse keratohyalin granules; vacuolization of granular layer

*Ichthyosis vulgaris*
AD
incidence 1/300

onset in childhood
*Clinical*
fine scales; primarily extensor areas; flexures spared; palmoplantar hyperkeratosis; lateral aspect of legs with fish-like scales; associated with atopy and keratosis pilaris
*Pathological*
hyperkeratosis; decreased to absent granular layer

*Lamella ichthyosis*
AR
incidence 1/300 000
onset at birth
*Clinical*
large, thick scales; may be verrucous, especially around joints; universal involvement; fissured and hyperkeratotic palms and soles; nails with grooves and ridges; mucous membrane and lips spared
often born encased in collodion membrane
*ectropion*\*, no sweating, thus hyperpyrexia
frequent skin infections
*Pathological*
hyperkeratosis; thickened granular layer

*X-Linked Ichthyosis*
XR
incidence 1/6000
onset at birth or infancy
*Clinical*
large, yellow–brown–black scales, thus dirty appearance; commonly involves lateral face and neck; variable involvement of flexures; palms and soles are spared
corneal opacities, steroid sulfatase (arylsulfatase C) deficiency
prenatal diagnosis possible
*Pathological*
hyperkeratosis; normal granular layer

### Ichthyosis, Minor Types

*CHILD syndrome (congenital hemidysplasia with ichthyosiform erythroderma and limb defects)*
XD
onset at birth to few weeks of infancy
unilateral scaling; erythroderma
congenital hemidysplasia; ipsilateral hypoplasia of bones and brain

*Conradi's disease*
AR
onset at birth to infancy
whorl-like scaling; heals with atrophy
bilateral cataracts; dwarfism; shortenings of
    humerus and femur; high arched palate

*Erythrokeratodermia variabilis*
AD
onset few months to three years
two kinds of lesion: symmetrical and sharply
    marginated patches of erythema;
    yellow-brown hyperkeratotic plaques of
    erythema

*Harlequin fetus*
AR
onset at birth
rigid skin; thick plaques of stratum corneum;
    armor-like skin split by deep fissures
absent or rudimentary ear; eclabium; ectropion

*Ichthyosis linearis circumflexa*
inheritance –
onset at birth to infancy
polycyclic lesion with a migratory
    hyperkeratotic margin; peripheral
    double-edged scale
–atopy
trichorrhexis invaginata (Netherton's
    syndrome)

*KID syndrome (congenital ichthyosiform syndrome
with deafness and keratitis)*
inheritance –
onset in infancy
verrucoid plaques, extensive congenital
    ichthyosiform eruption
hypotrichosis
nail dystrophy
neurosensory deafness
partial anhidrosis
vascularization of cornea (vascularizing
    keratitis)

*Refsum's disease*
AR
onset in childhood
deficiency of α-phyanic acid α-hydroxylase
resembles ichthyosis vulgaris
cataracts and night blindness
motor and sensory deafness
polyneuritis

improvement with dietary restriction of
    phytanic acid; chlorophyll-free diet

*Rud's syndrome*
–AR
onset in infancy
similar to lamellar ichthyosis
mental deficiency; seizures; short stature;
    hypogonadism

*Sjögren–Larsson syndrome*
AR
onset at birth
similar to a mild form of lamellar ichthyosis
mental deficiency
macular degeneration of retina
spastic paralysis

*Trichothiodystrophy (Tay's or BIDS syndrome
(Brittle hair, Intellectual impairment, Decreased
fertility, Short stature)*
AR
onset at birth
sparse, brittle hair; skin red and scaly;
    keratoderma of palms and soles
decreased fertility; intellectual impairment;
    short stature
IBIDS = Ichthyosis + BIDS
PIBIDS = Photosensitivity + IBIDS
SIBIDS = Osteosclerosis + IBIDS

## GROUP SEVEN

*Keratodermas*

### Acquired Keratoderma
Arsenical keratosis
Calluses, corns
Disorders associated with palmoplantar
    keratoderma
cancer-associated paraneoplastic syndromes
contact dermatitis
dermatophyte infections
eczematous dermatitis
epidermal nevus
lichen planus
pityriasis rubra pilaris
psoriasis
Reiter's syndrome
syphilis
tuberculosis

verruca

yaws

Focal acral hyperkeratosis

Almost exclusively seen in black female patients; papules on the medial and lateral aspect of hands and feet, clinically identical to acrokeratoelastoidosis

Glucan-induced keratoderma in AIDS

Keratoderma climacterium

Hyperkeratosis of plams and soles (especially the heels and areas of trauma), starting at about the time of the menopause; fissuring is a common feature

Keratoelastoidosis marginalis (degenerative collagenous plaques of the hands)

occurs in older white men with a history of excessive sun exposure and manual labor

Keratosis punctata of palmar creases

most common in Blacks, primarily in the creases of the palms or fingers; strong association with personal family history of *atopy*

Porokeratosis plantaris discreta

well-defined, rubbery papule, in non-weight-bearing areas, with a 4 : 1 female preponderance

*Porokeratotic eccrine ostial and dermal duct nevus*

---

### Inherited Keratoderma

*Autosomal dominant*

Acrokeratoelastoidosis of Costa

AD; most common in women; firm, round papules on the dorsa of hands, knuckles, and lateral aspect of palms and soles

Greither disease (progressive palmoplantar keratoderma)

AD; similar to Unna–Thost disease; onset in infancy or pre-school years; however, keratoderma progresses to non-palmoplantar areas by the time of puberty

Hereditary palmoplantar keratoderma (Unna–Thost disease)

AD; frequent associated hyperhidrosis, knuckle pads, ocasional deafness

Howell–Evans syndrome

AD; familial keratoderma associated with carcinoma of the esophagus

Keratosis palmaris plantaris nummularis

AD; onset in childhood; nummular plaques which become painful are noted in pressure areas

Keratosis punctata palmaris et plantaris

AD; firm, discrete papules on palms and soles; association with intestinal (especially colonic) carcinoma, hyperhidrosis, and oral leukoplakia

Mutilating keratoderma of Vohwinkel

AD; diffuse honeycomb palmoplantar hyperkeratosis, associated with 'starfish' hyperkeratosis on backs of hands and feet, linear keratoses of elbows and knees, and pseudoainhum (annular constriction) of the digits; also associated with a high frequency of hearing loss and scarring alopecia

Porokeratosis palmaris plantaris et disseminata

AD; onset in late teens; punctate hyperkeratotic plug with a raised margin and depressed center

Punctate keratoderma

AD; onset after puberty; pits with keratinous plug

Striate keratoderma

AD; onset in adolescence; linear lesions, radiating distally along the palmar surface of the fingers; blisters may form; associated with corneal opacities and papillomatous lesions of the buccal mucosa

*Autosomal recessive*

Mal de Meleda

AR; seen in people living in the island of Meleda; onset in infancy; associated with hyperhidrosis, bromhidrosis, physical and mental retardation; nail changes are common

Papillon–Lefevre

AR; onset in preschool years; keratoderma palmaris et plantaris with periodontopathia (destruction of the supporting tissues of both primary and secondary dentition, resulting in tooth loss); calcification of falx and tentorium; nail dystrophy and mental retardation also seen

Tyrosinemia II (Richner–Hanhart syndrome)

painful blisters, erosions, and crusts of palms and soles; onset in infancy; associated with corneal dystrophy, hyperhidrosis, keratitis, mental retardation, bradyphalangia, oligophrenia, and deficiency of hepatic tyrosine aminotransferase

Other inherited disorders associated with palmoplantar keratoderma

basal cell nevus syndrome

Darier's disease

dyskeratosis congenita
hidrotic ectodermal dysplasia
ichthyosis vulgaris
lamellar ichthyosis
non-bullous congenital ichthyosiform
    erythroderma
pachyonychia congenita
Unknown inheritance *(Olmsted's syndrome)*
congenital, symmetrical, sharply marginated,
    mutilating keratoderma

## Mastocytosis

### Generalized Mastocytosis
*Diffuse cutaneous mastocytosis*
Almost always starts in early infancy with
    generalized red–brown infiltrated lesions
    which urticate on stroking. If bullae are the
    predominant lesions, the term *bullous
    mastocytosis* is used. If there is generalized
    erythroderma, where the skin has a
    leather-grain appearance, the term
    *erythrodermic mastocytosis* is applied
The entire skin may be thickened, doughy or
    boggy and at times lichenified. The
    infiltration with mast cells produces a
    peculiar orange color
Visceral lesions are common, but usually
    improve with time

*Generalized cutaneous mastocytosis (urticaria
pigmentosa)*
Most common, dozens to hundreds of brown
    lesions that urticate on stoking. Usually
    begins during the first week of life

*Telangiectasia macularis eruptiva perstans*
Usually in adults, an extensive eruption of
    brownish-red macules with fine
    telangiectasias, and little or no urtication on
    stroking

### Localized Mastocytoma
Almost exclusively in infants, often a solitary
    lesion which urticates on stroking, and
    sometimes forms a bulla; commonly occurs
    on the dorsum of the hand near the wrist.
    Most involute spontaneously by age 10

### Malignant Mastocytosis
Rare development of mast-cell leukemia; more
    commonly develops in adults

### Systemic Mastocytosis
Mast-cell proliferation may involve almost any
    organ but most commonly it involves blood,
    bone, the gastrointestinal tract, liver, lymph
    nodes, and spleen; most commonly occurs
    in adults; most skin lesions are of the
    nodular type
Symptoms of systemic involvement may include
    flushing, headache, intense pruritus,
    gastrointestinal symptoms, hypotension,
    abnormalities of blood clotting, syncope, and
    tachycardia
Increased level of urinary telemethylimidazole
    acetic acid is diagnostic

## Perforating disorders

### Major Types
*Elastosis perforans serpiginosa*
Not very common; M : F ratio is 4 : 1; usually
    presents in the third decade of life
Skin-colored to erythematous keratotic papules
    (0.2–0.5 cm) usually in a symmetrical circular
    or serpiginous pattern, and usually confined
    to one anatomic site (most commonly nape
    and sides of the neck, face, and the upper
    extremities)
Lesions last from 6 months to 5 years and then
    spontaneously resolve, leaving a superficial
    scar; Koebner phenomenon is usually
    present
Most commonly associated with Down's
    syndrome, Ehlers–Danlos syndrome,
    Marfan's syndrome, osteogenesis imperfecta
    and pseudoxanthoma elasticum; similar
    lesions noted in patients being treated with
    penicillamine
Abnormal elastic fibers are extruded through
    the epidermis

*Kyrle's disease (hyperkeratotis follicularis et
parafollicularis in cuteum penetrans)*
A rare disorder with an average age of onset of
    30; most of the patients are diabetic; it

occurs anywhere, especially palms and soles and mucosa (most commonly on the extensor surface of the extremities)

Follicular or extrafollicular, flesh-colored to grayish pinhead-shaped papules which progress to dome-shaped papules with a central keratotic plug; papules may coalesce into verrucous plaques

*Perforating disorder of renal disease (uremic follicular hyperkeratosis)*

A relatively common disorder in dialysis patients, and more commonly seen in Blacks; most frequently, lesions develop within a few months after renal dialysis; almost all patients have chronic renal failure and most have diabetic nephropathy and retinopathy

Many hyperpigmented umbilicated papules (0.2–1 cm) with a central plug, mainly on the extensor aspect of extremities (especially knees and elbows); intense pruritus and Koebner phenomenon are common; spontaneous resolution may occur, leaving atrophic scars

*Perforating folliculitis (uremic follicular hyperkeratosis)*

The most common perforating disorder. It is more frequent in uremic patients. The follicular infundibulum is disrupted and perforated

Erythematous follicular (a constant feature, not so with Kyrle's disease) papules (0.2–0.8 cm) with a central keratinous plug, commonly occurring on hair-bearing extremities and buttocks

*Reactive perforating collagenosis*

Rare; may show autosomal recessive inheritance; typically occurs in infancy and childhood. The acquired adult form is often associated with chronic renal failure and diabetes mellitus. The disease is less active during the summer; Koebner phenomenon is present

Centrally umbilicated papules (0.51 cm) with erosions, commonly occur in exposed areas; it resolves in 6–10 weeks, leaving a small scar

Precipitated by superficial trauma; altered collagen is extruded by transepidermal elimination

**Minor Types**

Calcinosis cutis

Chondrodermatitis nodularis helicis

Lichen planus

Necrobiosis lipoidica diabeticorum

*Perforating granuloma annulare*

Mostly in children, and on sun-exposed extremities. Flesh-colored papules with central umbilication and crust. Lesions worsen in the summer and improve in the winter. Most lesions spontaneously resolve over several weeks, leaving punctate hyperpigmented scars. No Koebner phenomenon

*Perforating pseudoxanthoma elasticum*

Periumbilical hyperpigmented atrophic patches or plaques in middle-aged, multiparous women; commonly associated with hypertension and obesity

Perforating rheumatoid nodules

## GROUP TEN

*Porokeratosis*

*Disseminated superficial actinic porokeratosis*

AD; M : F 1 : 3; most common type; may have hundreds of lesions. Generalized, bilateral, symmetrical, sun-exposed, mostly extremities, size of 0.5–1 cm surrounded by a narrow, slightly raised, hyperkeratotic ridge without any distinct furrow. Onset in third and fourth decades; not seen in Blacks (so far)

*Linear porokeratosis*

Inheritance –; M : F ratio 1 : 1; rare; few to many lesions; unilateral, linear, clinically similar to Mibelli type; resembles linear verrucous epidermal nevus. Lichenoid plaques; small annular and hyperkeratotic plaques with central atrophy and a characteristic peripheral ridge. Onset from birth to adulthood

*Porokeratosis of Mibelli*
AD; M : F ratio 2–3 : I; rare; only a few lesions. Localized, usually unilateral, brownish, keratotic papule may gradually enlarge (peripheral extension) into an annular, irregular plaque with a smooth atrophic center and prominent hyperkeratotic, thread-like, furrowed (diagnostic) border; ranges in size from < I cm to > 20 cm
onset in childhood

*Porokeratosis palmaris, plantaris, et disseminata*
AD; M : F ratio 2 : I; rare; hundreds of lesions present; generalized, sun-exposed and non-sun-exposed. First start in palms and soles and spread to involve trunk and extremities symmetrically; lesions uniform and well demarcated with a distinct peripheral ridge. Onset in adolescence to adulthood
cv. *punctate porokeratosis*: numerous punctate, I–2 mm seed-like keratotic plugs limited to the palms and soles

## GROUP ELEVEN

Porphyrias
Abbreviations used:
ALA = δ-aminolevulinic acid
COPRO = coproporphyrin
ISOCOPRO = isocoproporphyrin
PBG = porphobilinogen
PROTO = protoporphyrin
URO = uroporphyrin

## Erythropoietic

*Erythropoietic coproporphyria*
Very rare

*Erythropoietic porphyria (Gunther's disease)*
AR; onset in infancy to first decade; marked photosensitivity. Increase URO and COPRO in red blood cells and urine, and only COPRO in stool. Erythrodentia
Uroporphyrinogen III cosynthetase deficiency

*Erythropoietic protoporphyria*
AD; onset in early childhood; 'aged knuckles', increased PROTO in feces, plasma, and red blood cells. Deficiency of ferrochelatase (heme synthetase)

## Hepatic

*Acute intermittent porphyria*
AD; onset ages 10–40; more common in Scandinavia (Swedish porphyria); attacks often precipitated by drugs and consist of neurologic–visceral symptoms. During and between attacks, urinary ALA and PBG increased
Uroporphyrinogen I synthetase deficiency

*Hereditary (idiopathic) coproporphyria*
AD; onset at any age; rare; during and between attacks, urinary and fecal COPRO III highly elevated
Coproporphyrinogen oxidase deficiency

*Porphyria cutanea tarda*
Acquired or hereditary (–AD); onset in third to fourth decade; increased urinary URO, increase ISOCOPRO in urine and feces
Uroporphyrinogen decarboxylase deficiency

*Variegate porphyria*
AD; common in South Africa (South African porphyria, protocoporporphyria hereditaria); onset 15–30 years old. During acute attack, urinary ALA and PBG increased (normal between attacks); PROTO, COPRO, and X-porphyrin are increased in feces
Protoporphyrinogen oxidase deficiency

## Erythropoietic/Hepatic

*Hepatoerythropoietic (hepatoerythrocytic) porphyria*
Onset before age 2; very rare; increased urinary URO (I–III) and 7-carboxyl porphyrin III. Increased PROTO in red blood cells; increased COPRO, ISOCOPRO, and URO in feces
Uroporphyrinogen decarboxylase deficiency

# SECTION FOUR

## Common Drug-Related Diseases (DRUG ERUPTIONS)

General classification of drug eruptions:

Erythema multiforme
Erythema nodosum
Exacerbation of pre-existing dermatological disease
Fixed drug eruption
Lichenoid drug eruption
Miscellaneous drug eruption
Morbilliform drug eruption (most common)
Pigmentary alteration
Photosensitivity drug eruptions
Toxic epidermal necrolysis (most serious)
Urticarial drug eruptions (second most common)
Vasculitis (palpable purpura)

# General eruptions associated with or caused by medications

| Typical drug eruptions | Rate of occurrence |
|---|---|
| Anaphylaxix | 1.5% |
| Angioedmea/urticaria | 26% |
| Erythema multiforme | 5% |
| Exanthematous (maculopapular or morbilliform) | 46% |
| Exfoliative dermatitis | 4% |
| Fixed drug eruption | 10% |
| Photosensitivity | 3% |
| Stevens–Johnson syndorme | 4% |
| Toxic epidermal necrolysis | 1% |

In this subsection, skin diseases are alphabetically listed with the associated/causative medication(s)

**Acanthosis nigricans**
diethylstilbestrol
glucocorticoids
niacinamide
nicotinic acid
oral contraceptive pills
**Acrodynia**
mercury
**Alopecia**
allopurinol
anticoagulants
antithyroid drugs
β-blockers
chemotheraoy (alkylating agents, antimetabolites, cyclophosphamide, methotrexate)
colchicine
dilantin
heavy metals
hypocholesteremic agents
levodopa
non-steroidal anti-inflammatory drugs
oral contraceptive pills
quinacrine
testosterone (in females)
thallium
trimethadione
vitamin A derivatives
**Acneiform (pustular) eruption**
actinomycin D

cyanocobalamin
dilantin
ethambutol
haldol
halogens
hormones (ACTH, androgens*, corticosteroids*, oral contraceptive pills)
isoniazid
lithium
phenobarbital
tar preparations
trimethadione
vitamin B$_{12}$
**Anetoderma-like eruption**
penicillamine
**Basal cell carcinoma, Bowen's disease*, squamous cell carcinoma**
arsenic
**Black hairy tongue**
methyldopa
penicillin
tetracycline

**Bullous drug eruptions**

**Bullous fixed drug eruption:**
Mefenamic acid
paclitaxel
paracetamol(acetaminophen)
phenylbutaone

piroxicam
sulfonamides
vinburnine

**Bullous lichen planus:**
radiocontrast dye

**Bullous pemphigoid:**
chloroquine
furosemide
penicillamine
penicillins

**Cicatricial pemphigoid:**
Indomethacin
Oral pracotolol
Penicillamine
Topical pilocarpine

**Epidermolysis bullosa acquisita:**
Furosemide
Penicillamine
Sulfonamides

**Erythema multiforme:**
benzothiazides
furosemide
nonsteroidal anti-inflammatory drugs
penicillins
phenothiazines
phenytoin
sulfonamides

**Leukocytoclastic vasculitis:**
allopurinol
benzothiazides
food additives
naproxen
penicillin
phenytoin
propylthiouracil
sulfonamides

**Linear IgA bullous dermatosis:**
captopril
diclofenace
lithium
vancomycin

**Pemphigus foliaceous:**
captopril
nifedipine

penicillamine
rifampine

**Pemphigus vulgaris:**
captopril
cephalexin
enalapril
penicillamine
penicillin
rifampin

**Pseudoporphyria:**
furosemide
nalidixic acid
naproxen
piroxicam
tetracycline

**Toxic epidermal necrolysis:**
allopurinol
aminopenicillins
phenobarbital
phenylbutazone
phenytoin
sulfonamides

*Bullous pemphigoid*
amoxil
fluorouracil (topical)
furosemide
penicillin
PUVA
sulfasalazine
*Candidiasis*
tetracyclines
*Dermatomyositis*
acetylsalicylic acid
*Dry lip*
accutane
etretinate

**Drug Hypersensitivity Syndrome:**
Usually occurs on primary exposure 1–8 weeks
     after initial ingestion. Fever is initial
     sypmtom, followed by rash, and internal
     organ involvement (most commonly liver,
     kidney, & bone marrow)

abacavir
azathioprine
carbamazepine

lamotrigine
minocycline
phenobarbital
phenytoin
sulfamethoxazole
timethoprim

**Eczematous eruptions**
aminophylline
antibiotics (neomycin, penicllin, streptomycin, sulfonamides)
arsenicals
disulfiram
diuretics
hypoglycemic agents
meprobamate
mercurials
phenothiazines
quinacrine
resorcin

**Elastosis perforans serpiginosa**
penicillamine (for Wilson's disease)

**Erythema annulare centrifugum**
cimetidine
chloroquine
estrogens
penicillin
plaquinel
progesterones
salicylates

**Erythema multiforme-like**
barbiturates*
hydantoins*
minoxidil
non-steroidal anti-inflammatory drugs
penicillin
phenolphthalein
phenothiazines
rifampin
sulfonamides*
sulfonylureas*

**Erythema nodosum**
accutane
halogens
oral contraceptive pills*
penicillin
phenacetin
sulfonamides*
sulfones
sulfonyreas
tetracycline
thiazide derivatives

**Exfoliative dermatitis**
allopurinol

arsenicals
barbiturates
captopril
chloroquine
cimetidine
gold salts
griseofulvin
hydantoins
isoniazid
lithium
mercurials
penicillin
phenothiazine
phenylbutazone
phenytoin
pyrazolon derivatives
quinacrine
septra
sulfonamides

**Fixed Drug Eruption**
acetylsalicylic acid
aspirin
barbiturates
gold
minocin
non-steroidal anti-inflammatory drugs
oral contraceptive pills
phenacetin
phenolphthaline
phenylbutazone
quinidine
salicylates
tetracycline*
trimethoprim–sulfamethaxazole*

**Folliculitis**
Tar

**Grover's disease**
Interleukin-4
Pyrimethamine (fansidar)
sulfadoxine

**Hirsutism**
ACTH
astezolamide
corticosteroids
cyclosporine
diaxoxide
dilantin
hexachlorobenzene
minoxidil
penicillamine
steroid drugs containing androgens

tamoxifen
**Keloid**
insulin
**Keratoderma**
gold salts
**Lichenoid**
antimalarials
arsenicals
β-blockers
captopril
chloroquine
dapsone
demeclocycline
color film processors*
furosemide
gold salts*
isoniazid
levamisole
methyldopa
penicillamine
phenothiazines
phenytoin
pyrithamine
quinidine
streptomycin
sulfonylurea
thiazides
**Linear IgA bullous dermatosis**
amipcillin
Captopril
cefamandole
diclophenac
interferon gamma
interlukin-2
iodine
lithium
penicillin
phenytoin
PUVA
somatostatin
vancomycin
**Lipoatrophy**
insulin
**Livedo reticularis**
amantadine quinidine
**Longitudinal melanonychia**
AZT
bleomycin
cyclophosphamide
ketoconazole
minocin
psoralen
**Loss of hair pigmentation**

chloroquine
quinacrine
**Maculopapular (exanthematous)**
allopurinol
ampicillin
barbiturates
chloroquine
dilantin
dolobid
gentamicin
gold salts
isoniazid
meclomen
penicillin (especially if involves palms and soles
   as well)
phenothiazines
phenylbutazones
piroxicam
quinidine
septra
streptomycin
sulfonamides
thiazides
thiouracil
**Melasma**
oral contraceptive pills
**Morbilliform**
acetylsalicylic acid
ampicillin*
barbiturates
benzodiazepines
chlorpromazine
erythromycin
gentamicin
griseofulvin
gold salts
isoniazid
phenothiazines
thiazides
**Morphea**
penicillamine
**Ochronosis**
antimalarials
phenol
resorcin
**Onycholysis**
doxycycline
minocin
tetracycline
thiazides
**Paraneoplastic pemphigus**
Interferon alfa
**Pellagra-like eruption**

anticonvulsant drugs
antidepressants
5-fluorouracil
isoniazid
6-mercaptopurine
sulfonamides

### Pemphigoid (ocular)
demecarium bromide
epinephrine
idoxuridine
pilocarpine
timolol

### Pemphigus (foliaceus*)
aspirin with penicillin/rifampin/ampicillin/indocin
captopril
penicillamine

### Pemphigus vulgaris
penicillin
penicillamine

### Photoallergic drug eruption
griseofulvin
musk ambrette, 6-methylcoumarin
PABA esters
phenothiazines
sulfonamides
sulfonyreas
thiazides

## PIGMENTARY CHANGE SECONDARY TO DRUGS

BLUE-GRAY: gold (chrysoderma)
BROWN: ACTH, Bleomycin, oral contraceptives, zidovudine
RED: Clofazamine
SLATE-BLUE: Amiodarone
SLATE-GRAY: chloroquine, hydroxychloroquine, Minocycline, phenothiazines
YELLOW: Beta-carotene, Quinacrine

### Phototoxic drug eruption
All drugs are capable of causing photoallergic reaction, when a high enough concentration of the drug is given

amiodrone
anthracene
chloroquine
doxycycline
fluorouracil
methotrexate
nalidixic acid
naproxen

para-aminobenzoic acid
piroxicam
psoralens
quinidine
sulfonamides
sulfonyreas
tetracyclines
thiazides
vinblastine

### Pigmentation
ACTH: brown
amiodrane: slate blue
antimalarials: blue–gray or yellow
argyria: slate blue
arsenic: brown, diffuse macular eruption
bismuth: blue–black pigmentation on gingival margin
bleomycin: flagellate pigmentation
chloroquine: blue-gray discoloration over shins
chlorpromazine: slate gray
chrysiasis: slate blue
clofazamine: red to purple–black
diltiazem: reticulated slate-gray hyperpigmentation on sun-exposed areas.
mercury: slate gray
methysergide: red
minocycline: blue–black (in acne scar), blue–gray, muddy brown
quinacrine: yellow
plaquenil (hydroxychloroquine): blue–black
rifampin: red man syndrome (with very high dose)
tetracycline: blue cutaneous osteomas

### Pityriasis rosea-like
Herald's patch absent, and distribution of the eruption may not be classic

arsenicals
barbiturates
β-blockers
bismuth
captopril
clonidine
gold salts
griseofulvin
isotretinoin
ketotifen
methoxypromazine
metronidazole
penicillin
pyribenzamine
tripelennamine

### Porphyria cutanea tarda

chloroquine
dapsone
estrogens
ethyl alcohol
furosemide
hexachlorobenzene
nalidixic acid
naproxen
pyridoxine
tetracycline
2, 4, 5-trichlorophenol
**Pseudolymphoma**
dilantin
**Pseudoporphyria**
Amiodarone
Bumetanide
Carisoprodol/aspirin
chlorthalide
chronic renal failure\dialysis
coca-cola
cyclosporine
dapsone
diflunisal
etretinate
excessive sun exposure
5-fluorosemide
flutamide
furosemide
hydrochlorothiazide/triamterene
isotretinoin
ketoprofen
lasix
mefenamic acid
nabumetone
nalidixic acid
naproxen
NSAIDs
oxaprozine
PUVA
pyridoxine
retinoids
tetracycline
UVA tanning beds
lasix
**purpura pigmentosa chronica**
sedatives
**Purpuric eruption**
barbiturates
carbamides
chlorothiazide
chlorpromazine
gold
griseofulvin

iodides
phenylbutazones
quinidine
sulfonamides
**Pustular eruption**
bromoderma
iododerma
**Rosacea**
aminophylline
amyl nitrite
cyclosporine
diazoxide
ethyl alcohol
glutamate
hydralazine
iodides
isoprel
isordil
nicotinic acid
nitrate
papaverine
persantin
reserpine
theophyline
vasodilators
**Scleroderma-like eruption**
Vitamin k1 (phytonadione)
**Seborrheic dermatitis**
gold
**Serum sickness vasculitis**
cephalosporins
penicillin*
sulfa
thiazides
**Subacute cutaneous lupus**
alpha-methyldopa
chlorpromazine
cotrimoxazole
diphenylhydantoin
ethosuximide
gold salts
griseofulvin
hydantoins
hydralazine
hydrochlorothiazide
isoniazid
lithium
mephenytoin
methyldopa
methylthiouracil
minocin
oral contraceptive pills
para-aminosalicylic acid

penicillin
d-penicillamine
phenothiazines
phenylbutazone
phenylethylacetylurea
practolol
procainamide
propylthiouracil
quinidine
reserpine
streptomycin
sulfasalazine
sulfonamides
tetracycline
trimethadione

**Sweet's syndrome**
bactirum
BCG
Furosemide
Granulocyte colony stimulating factor
Hydralazine
Minocycline
Oral contraceptive
Pneumococcal vaccine

*Systemic lupus erythematosus*
anticonvulsants (dilantin*)
cimetidine
hormonal contraceptives
hydralazine*
methyldopa
penicillins
procainamide* (pleuropericarditis most
    common manifestation)
sulfonamides
tetracycline
thiouracil
trimethadione

*Thrombocytopenic purpura*
non-steroidal anti-inflammatory drugs
phenothiazines
quindines
thiazides

*Toxic epidermal necrolysis*

allopurinol
anticonvulsants (phenytoin)
barbiturates
hypoglycemic agents
non-steroidal anti-inflammatory drugs
penicillins
sulfonamides

*Vasculitis*
ampicillin*
chlorothiazide*
phenylbutazone*
phenytoin
sulfonamides*
thiazides
thiouracil

*Vesiculobulous eruption*
arsenic
bromides
captopril
iodides
mercury
penicillamine
phenolphthalein
phenytoin
salicylates

**Vitiligo**
Chloroquine
clofazimine

*Urticarial*
ACTH
barbiturates
chloramphenicol
griseofulvin
indomethacin
insulin
opiates
penicillin
phenolphthalein
phenothiazines
salicylates
streptomycin
sulfonamides
tetracycline

# Dermatosis exacerbated by medications

*Dermatitis herpetiforms*
potassium iodide
*Lupus erythematosus*
alpha-methyldopa
diphenylhydantoin
griseofulvin
hydralazine
isoniazid
mephenytoin
methylthiouracil
minocin
oral contraceptive pills
*para*-aminosalicylic acid
penicillin
phenylbutazone
procainamide
propylthiouracil
reserpine
streptomycin
sulfonamides
tetracycline
trimethadione
*Mastocytosis*
alcohol
amphotericin B
aspirin
codeine
decamethonium
dextran
estrogens
gallamine
iodine-containing contrast media
morphine (and other narcotics, but not
    meperidine)
non-steroidal anti-inflammatory drugs

polymyxin B
quinine
scopolamine
succinylcholine
tubocurarine
vancomycin
vitamin B (thiamine)
*Porphyria (cutaneous)*
alcohol
androgens
barbiturates
chloroquine
estrogens
griseofulvin (can also precipitate acute
    intermittent porphyria)
oral contraceptive pills
sulfonamides
sulfonylureas
*Porphyria cutanea tarda*
chlorinated hydrocarbons
estrogens
ethyl alcohol
iron
*Psoriasis*
antimalarials
beta-adrenergic blockers
cimetidine
clonidine
gold salts
ibuprofen
indomethacin
iodide (flares pustular psoriasis)
lithium
*Pyoderma grangrenosum*
iodides

# SECTION FIVE

## General dermatological and dermatopathological pearls

# General dermatological pearls

*Actinic keratosis*
UVB/UVA
*Actinic reticuloid*
UVA/UVB, visible light
*Argon laser = 488–514 nm*
hemoglobin
*Argon pumped tunable dye*
488–630 nm
*Berloque dermatitis*
UVA
*Carbon dioxide laser = 10600 nm*
water
*Fine wrinkling of face*
UVA/UVB
*Hydroa vacciniforme*
UVA
*Immediate tanning*
UVA
*Lupus erythematosus photosensitivity*
UVB, rarely UVA
*ND : YAG laser*
1064 nm
*Persistent light reaction*
UVB
*Photoallergic drug reaction*
UVA
*Photocontact dermatomyositis*
UVB
*Phytophotodermatitis*
UVA
*Polymorphous light eruption (action spectrum)*
UVA (primarily, but also UVB, UVC, and visible
    light)
*Porphyrins*
400–410 nm (Soret band)
*Ruby laser*
694 nm
Solar urticaria
UVA/B, visible (light)
*Sunburn*
UVB

*Tunable dye*
variable

UV RADIATION:

UVA1 (340–400nm)
UVA2 (320–340nm)
UVB (290–320nm)
NARROW BAND UVB 311nm
UVC (200–290nm)
VISIBLE LIGHT (400–760nm)

Acneiform eruptions:
acne keloidalis nuchae
gram-negative folliculitis
Rosacea
Steroid acne

Childhood acne:
Infantile ace
Neonatal acne

Extrinsic acne:
acne aestivalis
acne cosmetica
acne excori'ee des jeunes filles
acne mechanica
acne tropicalis
chloracne
drug induced acne
Favre-Racouchot syndrome
Occupational acne
Pomade acne

Intrinsic acne:
Acne conglobata
Acne fulminans
Acne vulgaris

hidradenitis suppurativa
perioral dermatitis
pyoderma faciale

## ANHIDROSIS OR HYPOHIDROSIS

### Infectious
leprosy

### Traumatic
central nervous system lesions (or tumors)
heat stroke
miliaria
poral occlusion

### Medicinal
acetylcholine inhibitors (e.g. atropine)
other drugs

### Metabolic
alcoholism
dehydration
diabetes mellitus
hypothyroidism
neuropathy
systemic disease
toxic reaction

### Idiopathic
atrophic skin disorders
autonomic insufficiency syndrome
Bazex syndrome
Guillain–Barré syndrome
ichthyosis and inflammatory or hyperkeratotic
   skin disorders
idiopathic
morphea
psoriasis
scars
Sjögren's syndrome
Sweat gland dysfunction or atrophy
Systemic sclerosis
Tropical anhidrotic asthenia
ulcers
xerosis

### Neoplastic
tumors

### Congenital
anhidrotic ectodermal dysplasia
autonomic insufficiency syndrome
central nervous system lesions
congenital absence of or dysfunction ofsweat
   glands
Fabry's disease (XR)
Naegeli's syndrome (AD)
Riley–Day syndrome (AR)
Ross syndrome

## ANGIOID STREAKS

Cowden's disease (AD)
Ehler's–Danlos syndrome
hyperphosphotemia
intracranial disorders
lead poisoning
Paget's disease
pituitary disorders
pseudoxanthoma elasticum
sickle cell anemia
trauma

## ANTIPHOSPHOLIPID ANTIBODY MANIFESTATIONS

acrocyanosis
blue toe
capillaritis
digital ischemia/gangrene
hemorrhage
livedo reticularis
necrosis
nodules
porcelain-white scars/atrophie blanche
Raynaud's phenomenon
splinter hemorrhages
thrombophlebitis
ulceration

## APPLE-JELLY COLOR (yellow–brown color of lesion on diascopy)

leishmaniasis
lupus miliaris disseminatus faciei
lupus vulgaris (cutaneous tuberculosis)
sarcoidosis

## AXILLARY FRECKLING

Moynahan's syndrome
progeria
Von Recklinghausen's syndrome (considered a *pathognomonic* finding)

## BLUEBERRY MUFFIN LESIONS (A Reflection of Dermal Erythropoiesis)

AIDS
congenital rubella
congenital toxoplasmosis
congenital varicella
cytomegalic virus inclusion disease

## BORRELIA MANIFESTATIONS

acrodermatitis chronica atrophicans
eosinophilic fasciitis
erythema chronica migrans
Jessner's lymphocytic infiltrate
lichen sclerosis et atrophicus
Lyme disease
lymphadenosis benigna cutis (Spiegler–Fendt sarcoid)
morphea (some types)
progressive facial hemiatrophy (Perry–Romberg syndrome)

## BURNING SENSATION (or strange sensation) IN SUN-EXPOSED AREAS

delusional parasitosis
diabetes mellitus

erythropoietic protoporphyria
flushing syndrome
herpes simplex (prodrome)
herpes zoster (prodrome)
neurologic disease
pruritus

## CAFE-AU-LAIT SPOTS

Albright's syndrome
ataxia telangiectasia
Bloom's syndrome
dyskeratosis congenita
epidermal nevus syndrome
Fanconi's syndrome
Niemann-Pick disease
normal (10% of people have 1–3)
nevus spilus
silver-Russel syndrome
tuberous sclerosis
Von Recklinghausen's syndrome
Watson's syndrome
Westerhof's syndrome

## CALCIFICATION IN THE BRAIN

basal cell nevus syndrome (AD)
Cockayne syndrome
Papillon–Lefèvre syndrome
rubella
Sturge–Weber syndrome
toxoplasmosis
tuberous sclerosis

## CALCINOSIS CUTIS

**Dystrophic Calcinosis Cutis**
Deposit of calcium in previously-damaged skin (normal serum calcium and phosphorous)

*Calcinosis universalis*
Dermatomyositis (subcutaneous and periarticular calcification, particularly common in children)
Systemic scleroderma (occasionally)

*Calcinosis circumscripta*
CREST syndrome

folliculitis
lupus erythematosus
mixed connective tissue disease
morphea (widespread)
neurologic diseases (head injury, hemiplegia,
    paraplegia)
parasitic infections
pseudoxanthoma elasticum
rheumatoid arthritis
skin trauma (injection site, physical, thermal)
skin tumors (basal cell carcinoma, callus,
    chondroid syringoma, chondroma,
    epidermal cyst, hemangioma,
    neurilemmoma, nevi, pilomatrichoma,
    sclerosing hemmangioma, senile keratosis,
    trichoepithelioma)
subcutaneous fat necrosis of the newborn
subcutaneous nodules in Ehlers–Danlos
    syndrome
systemic scleroderma
venous stasis

**Idiopathic Calcinosis Cutis**
No underlying disease

*Idiopathic calcinosis of scrotum*

*Tumoral calcinosis*
usually familial and associated with
    hyperphosphotemia

**Metastatic Calcinosis Cutis**
Results from hypercalcemia and
    hyperphosphotemia

excessive milk and alkali intake
extensive bone destruction secondary to
    osteomyelitis or metastasis of cancer
hyperparathyroidism
hypervitaminosis D
hypoparathyroidism
pseudo-hypoparathyroidism
pseudo-pseudo-hypoparathyroidism
renal failure
sarcoidosis

**Subepidermal Calcified Nodule
(Cutaneous Calculous)**
Most common in children and on the face

## CANDIDA INFECTIONS

erosio interdigitalis blastomycetica
intertrigo
paronychia
perleche
thrush

## COLD EXACERBATED CONDITIONS

Cold panniculitis
Cutis marmorata
{erythromelalgia improves with cold}
Frost bites
Glomus tumor
Leiomyomas (may also contract when irritated)
Livedo reticularis
Perniosis
Raynaud's phenomenon

## CERVICAL ADENOPATHY/ADENITIS

**Vascular**
hemangioma
lymphangioma

*Infectious*
*Bacterial*
    brucellosis
    streptococcal pharyngitis
*Parasitic*
    toxoplasmosis
*Viral*
    adenovirus
    coxsackievirus (herpangina)
    cytomegalovirus
    herpes simplex
    Epstein–Barr virus (mononucleosis)
    rubella

**Metabolic**
Grave's disease
Hashimoto's thyroiditis
thyroid goiter

**Neoplastic**
Benign
    branchial cleft cyst
    dermoid cyst
    esophageal diverticulum
    laryngocele
    teratoma
    thyroglossal duct cyst
Malignant
    Hodgkin's disease
    leukemia
    non-Hodgkin's disease
    rhabdomyosarcoma
    thyroid carcinoma

## COLLAGEN TYPES AND LOCATIONS

I: bone, skin, tendon
II: cartilage, vitreous
III: blood vessels, gastrointestinal tract, skin
    (wound healing)
IV: basement membrane, lamina densa, (for
    lamina lucida, laminin)
V: ubiquitous, minor component of skin
VI: cartilaginous and non-cartilaginous
VII: anchoring fibrils of basement membrane
VIII: endothelial cells
IX. X: cartilage
XI, XII: hyaline cartilage

## CUTANEOUS ERYTHROPOIESIS

anemia secondary to twin–twin transfusion
congenital leukemia
intrauterine anemia due to spherocytosis
rubella

## CYSTS ASSOCIATED WITH DISEASES

*Epidermal cyst*
Gardner's syndrome
pachyonychia congenita
*Fibrocystic disease of the breast*
Cowden's disease
*Odontogenic cyst*

basal cell nevus syndrome
*Syringocystadenoma papilliferum*
nevus sebaceus

## DARIER'S SIGN

congenital smooth muscle hamartoma
    (pseudo-Darier's sign)
infantile leukemia cutis
mastocytosis
papular urticaria (insect bite)

## DERMATOSIS GENERALLY SPARING THE FACE

dermatitis herpetiformis
lichen planus
parapsoriasis
pityriasis rosea
psoriasis
scabies
tinea versicolor

## DERMATOSIS WITH SCALES AS A PROMINENT FEATURE

atopic dermatitis
exfoliative dermatitis (adherent; small and thin
    or large sheets)
eczematous dermatitis
ichthyosis (fish-like scales)
keratosis pilaris
lichen planus (scanty, adherent scales)
parapsoriasis (brownish or yellowish scaling)
pellagra
pityriasis alba (fine, adherent scales)
pityriasis rosea (collarette scales)
pityriasis ruba pilaris (yellowish pink scaling)
psoriasis (grayish white or silvery white,
    imbricated and lamellar scales)
seborrheic dermatitis (scanty, loose, dry, moist,
    or greasy scales)
secondary syphilis
superficial dermatophytosis

## DERMOGRAPHISM

acute urticaria
mastocytosis (one third to one half of patients)
normal population (5%)

## DESQUMATION

Kawasaki syndrome
Scarlet fever (post strep)
Staphyococcal scalded skin syndrome
Toxic shock syndrome

## DOWN'S SYNDROME

acute myelogenous leukemia
alopecia areata
deep folliculitis of the posterior neck
ears low-set and small
elastosis perforans serpiginosa
furunculosis
keratosis pilaris
macroglossia
micropenis
scalp hair fine and sparse
scrotal tongue
single horizontal palmar crease
syringoma (seen in 18% of adult patients)
tinea palmaris, pedis and ungium
vitiligo

## DRUG ABUSE, CUTANEOUS SIGNS

abscesses with ulcerations
camptodactylia
fixed drug eruption
hyperpigmentation
keloids, and cutaneous fibrosis
soot tattoos
thrombosis
urticaria

## ELEPHANTIASIS NOSTRANS VERRUCOSA

congenital disruption of lymphatic system

Infections
Localized infections:
　Lymphangitis
　staphylococcal cellulites
　streptococcal
　Parasitic:
　filariasis
　malaria
　schistosomiasis
morphea
radiation dermatitis
scleredema
surgical disruption of lymphatic channels
traumatic disruption of lymphatic channels
venous stasis

## ECZEMA HERPETICUM

(Coxsackie A16, herpes simplex virus-1*,
　herpes simplex virus-2, vaccina virus)

atopic dermatitis
congenital ichthyosiform erythroderma
Darier's disease (AD)
ichthyosis vulgaris (AD)
mycosis fungoides
pemphigus foliaceus
seborrheic dermatitis
second-degree burn
Wiskott–Aldrich syndrome

## ENZYME DEFICIENCIES

*Alkapotonuria (Ochronosis)*
homogentisic acid oxidase

*Chronic Granulomatous Disease*
glutathione peroxidase

*Ehlers–Danlos syndrome*
Type V: lysyl oxidase
Type VI: lysyl hydroxylase
Type VII: procollagen aminoprotease
Type IV (X-linked cutis laxa): lysyl oxidase

*Farber's disease (Lipogranulomatosis)*
ceramidase

**Febry's disease**
α-galactosidase A

**Fucosidosis (AR)**
α-L-fucosidase

**Gaucher's disease (AR)**
glucocerebrosidase

**Hartnup disease**
neutral amino acid (tryptophan) transport
    defect

**Hereditary Angioedema**
C1 esterase inhibitor (decreased level or
    nonfunctional)

**Homocystinuria**
Beta-cystathionine synthetase

**Huler's syndrome (Mucopolysaccharidosis II, XR)**
iduronate sulfatase

**Hunter's syndrome (Mucopolysaccharidosis I, AR)**
α-L-iduronidase

**Ichthyosis**
lamellar ichthyosis: transglutaminase I
Refsum's disease: α-phyanic acid α-hydroxylase
X-linked ichthyosis: (arylsulfatase C) steroid
    sulfatase

**Lipodystrophy**
C3 deficiency

**Lipogranulomatosis (Farber's disease)**
ceramidase

**Niemann-Pick disease (AR)**
shingomyelinase deficiency

**Oculocutaneous Albinism**
tyrosinase

**Phenylketonuria**
phenylalanine hydroxylase

**Porphyrias**
Acute intermittent porphyria
uroporphyrinogen I synthetase
*Congenital erythropoietic porphyria (Günther's
    disease)*
uroporphyrinogen III cosynthetase
*Erythropoietic protoporphyria*
ferrochelatase (heme synthetase)
*Hepatoerythrocytic porphyria*
uroporphyrinogen decarboxylase
*Hereditary coproporphyria*
coproporphyrinogen oxidase
*Porphyria cutanea tarda*
uroporphyringoen decarboxylase
*Variegate porphyria*
protoporphyrinogen oxidase

**Severe Combined Immunodeficiency**
adenosine deaminase

**Sjögren's–Larsson Syndrome**
fatty alcohol
$NAD^+$ oxidoreductase deficiency

**Tyrosinemia II (AR, Richner–Hanhart Syndrome)**
(hepatic) tyrosine aminotransferase

**Xeroderma Pigmentosum**
DNA endonuclease
DNA ligase
DNA polymerase

## ERYTHEMA NODOSUM

**Infectious**

*Fungal*
blastomycosis
coccidioidomycosis
histoplasmosis
*Trichophyton* fungal infection

*Bacterial*
*Campylobacter jejuni*
cat-scratch disease
leptospirosis
lymphogranuloma venereum
*Streptococcus** (erysipelas, rheumatic fever,
scarlet fever, streptococcal pharyngitis
and tonsilitis

*Yersinia*

*Parasitic*
American leishmaniasis

**Medicinal**
bromides
iodides
sulfonamides*
oral contraceptive pills*

**Idiopathic**
Behçet's disease
inflammatory bowel disease
sarcoidosis*

**Hematologic**
leukemias

## FEVER WITH AN ERUPTION

***Fever With An Erythematous Eruption***
**Infectious**

*Bacterial*
brucellosisdisseminated gonococcal
infection, ecthyma gangrenosum, rheumatic
fever, Rocky mountain spotted fever
scarlet fever , staphylococus endocarditis
toxic shock syndrome

*Spirochetal*
Lyme disease

secondary syphilis

*Viral*
enteroviruses

Atypical measles
erythema infectiosum

dengue

hand foot & mouth disease
hepatitis B

herpes simplex
infectious mononucleosis
measles
roseola infantum
rubella

varicella-zoster

**Medicinal**
drug eruption

**Idiopathic**
erythema marginatum
erythema multiforme
erythema nodosum
juvenile rheumatoid arthritis
Kawasaki's disease
systemic lupus erythematosus

***Fever With Arthritis or Arthralgia***
acute meningococemia infection
allergic purpura
disseminated gonococcal infection
erythema marginatum(acute rheumatic fever)
erythema infectiosum (parvovirus B19)
hepatitis B virus (prodromal phase)
lyme disease
Reiter's syndrome
Rocky Mountain spotted fever
roseola(especially in adults)
rubella
serum sickness
Still's disease
Systematic lupus erythematosus

***Fever With Desqumation***
corynebacterium haemolyticum infection
drug hypersensitivity
graft-versus-host-reaction
kawaski syndrome
measles

Rocky Mountain spotted fever
scarlet fevers
staphylococcal scalded skin syndrome
Stevens-Johnson syndrome
toxic epidermal necrolysis
toxic shock syndrome
von Zumbusch pustular psoriasis

### Fever With Lymphadenopathy
Cervical adenopathy
    Kawasaki syndrome
    rubella
    scarlet fever
Generalized adenopathy
    infectious mononucleosis
    sarcoidosis
    secondary syphilis
    serum sickness
    systematic lupus erythamatosus
    toxoplasmosis
Hilar adenopathy
    atypical measles
    sarcoidosis
Local adenopathy
    cat-scratch disease
    tularemia

### Fever with meningitis
acute meningococcemia
cryptococcosis
enterivirus(coxsackieviruses,echoviruses)
leptospirosis
lyme disease
Rocky Mountain spotted fever
Secondary syphilis

### Fever With A Purpuric Eruption
**Infectious**
*Bacterial*
    epidemic typhus
    gonococcemia
    meningococcemia
    *Pseudomonas*/staphylococcal sepsis
    Rocky Mountain spotted fever
    subacute bacterial endocarditis
*Viral*
    atypical measles
    echovirus
    TORCHS viral infections

### Medicinal
drug eruption

### Idiopathic
Henoch–Shönlein purpura

### Fever With A Vesiculopustular Eruption
**Infectious**
*Bacterial*
    rickettsialpox
    staphylococcal scalded skin syndrome
*Spirochetal*
    congenital syphilis
*Viral*
    enterovirus
    hand–foot–mouth disease
    herpes simplex virus
    herpes zoster
    varicella

### Medicinal
drug eruption

## FLAP types

Advancement flap: O to T, V to T, U flap, O to U, double advancement flap

Rotation flap: glabellar flap, O to Z

Transposition flap: Bilobed flap, Labial-ala flap, Limberg or rhomboid flap, nasolabial flap, Z-plasty

Pedicle flap: Island pedicle flap, paramendian forehead flap

## FLUSHING

### Allergic
seborrheic dermatitis

### Medicinal
aminophylline
amyl nitrate

cyclosporine
diazoxide
ethyl alcohol
glutamate
hydralazine
isoprel
isordil
nicotinic acid
nitrate
papaverine
persantin
reserpine
theophylline

**Metabolic**
carcinoid syndrome
emotional
hormonal (menopausal, menstrual)
Zollinger–Ellison's syndrome

**Idiopathic**
rosacea
systemic lupus erythematosus
systemic mastocytosis

**Neoplastic**
pheochromocytoma

**Hematologic**
polycythemia vera

## FOOD ALLERGIES

Majority of food-allergic reactions are due to:
In adults/older children: fish, peanut, shellfish,
    tree nuts (cashew, walnut, etc.)
In children: cow's milk, eggs, fish,
    peanut,shellfish, soy, tree nuts, wheat
In infants: cow's milk, eggs, peanut, soy

## GENE MUTATION

epidermolysis bullosa dominant dystrophic: type
    VII collagen

epidermolysis bullosa junctional: laminin 5
epidermolysis bullosa recessive dystrophic: type
    VII collagen
Epidermolysis bullosa simplex: keratin 1 or 5
Epidermolytic hyperkeratosis: keratin 1 or 10
Epidermolytic palmoplantar keratoderma
    (localized palmoplantar epidermolytic
    hyperkeratosis): keratin 9
Piebaldesim: mutation in c-kit protooncogene

## HELIOTROPE RASH

aldosterone-producing tumors
dermatomyositis
toxoplasmosis
trichinosis

## HEPATITIS B MANIFESTATIONS

erythema multiforme
essential mixed cryoglobulinemia
jaundice
palpable purpura
papular acrodermatitis
polyarteritis nodosa
urticaria

## HYPERESTHESIA

erythema nodosum
erythromelalgia
herpes zoster
Melkersson–Rosenthal syndrome
paroxysmal finger hematoma
Raynaud's phenomenon
temporal arteritis
thrombophlebitis (acute)

## HYPERHIDROSIS

***Generalized***
**Vascular**
heart failure
shock
syncopal states

**Infectious**
any infectious disease
brucellosis
tuberculosis

**Traumatic**
cold exposure
peripheral neuropathy
post-sympathectomy
post-traumatic hypertension
post-traumatic syringoma
spinal cord injury
trauma to hypothalamus

**Medicinal**
alcohol intoxication (or alcohol withdrawal)
antipyretic agents
cholinergic agents
emetic agents
insulin overdose

**Metabolic**
anxiety
carcinoid syndrome
diabetes mellitus
dumping syndrome
emotional stress
febrile illness
gout
heat
hyperpituitarism
hyperthyroidism (thyrotoxicosis)
hypoglycemia
intense pain
menopause
obesity
poisoning with insecticides or mercury
porphyria
pregnancy
rickets
scurvy (in infants)
systemic illness

**Idiopathic**
carcinoid syndrome
compensatory
hypothermia
idiopathic

intrathoracic processes
olfactory hyperhidrosis
Parkinson's disease
paroxysmal unilateral hyperhidrosis

**Neoplastic**
brain lesions
lymphoma
pheochromocytoma

**Congenital**
Chediak–Higashi syndrome
Congenital autonomic dysfunction with
    universal pain loss
phenylketonuria (AR)
Riley–Day syndrome (familial autonomic
    dysfunction, AR)

*Localized*
**Vascular**
arteriovenous malformation
blue rubber bleb
erythrocyanosis
Klippel–Trenauney–Weber syndrome
Maffucci's syndrome

**Infectious**
encephalitis
herpes zoster
parotid abscess
parotitis
pitted keratolysis
tabes dorsalis

**Traumatic**
chilblains
frostbite
local heat or pressure
syringomyelia
thoracic sympathectomy
trauma to central nervous system

**Metabolic**
anxiety
diabetic neuropathy
fear

pain
pretibial myxedema

### Idiopathic
burning feet syndrome
causalgia
epidermolysis bullosa (localized epidermolysis
    bullosa simplex [Weber–Cockayne)
granulosis rubra nasi
Horner's syndrome
idiopathic
keratolysis exfoliativa (lamellar dyshidrosis)
pachydermoperiostosis
POEMS syndrome
rheumatoid arthritis
symmetrical lividities of palms and soles

### Neoplastic
blue rubber bleb nevus
eccrine nevus
glomus tumor

### Congenital
auriculotemporal or Frey's syndrome
epidermolysis bullosa (localized epidermolysis
    bullosa simplex [Weber–Cockayne
    syndrome])
Gopalan's syndrome (burning feet syndrome)
hereditary palmoplantar keratoderma
    (Unna–Thost)
Jadssohn–Lewandowsky syndrome

## HYPESTHESIA/ ANESTHESIA

congenital sensory neuropathia
congenital total analgesia
familial acroosteolysis
leprosy
peripheral neuropathies (infectious or toxic)
schizophrenia
syringomyelia
tabes dorsalis

## HYPOPIGMENTATION

actinic reticuloid

addison's disease
Albinism OCA type I,II,III
Alopecia areata
Alpert's syndrome
Ataxia telangiectasia
Burns
canities
chloroqiun
Chromosomal 5p defect
Chronic protein loss
Halo nevus
Hypopituitarism
hypothyroidism
Horner's syndrome
Idiopathic guttate hypomelanosis
kwashirkor
Leprosy
Leukoderma acuisitum centrifugum
Malabsorbsorbtion
Medication:
    Chloroquin
    Glucocorticoids
    Hydroquinone
    Hydroxchloroquin
    mercaptoethylamines
    Monobezylether of hydroquinone
    Para-substituted phenols
    Retinoids
    Sulfhydryls
melanoma
Mycosis fungoides
Nevus anemicus
Nephrosis
Onchocerciasis
Osteopathic striase
piebaldism
Pinta
Pityriasis alba
Pityriasis lichenoides chronicus
Post dermabrasion
Post-Kal-azar
Post-laser
Postinflammatory
Prolidase deficiency
Sarcoidosis
sceloderma
Syphilis
Tinea versicolor
trauma
Ulcerative colitis
Vagabond's leukoderma
Vit. B12 deficiency
Vitiligo

Waardenburg's syndrome
Woolf's syndrome
Wornoff's ring
Xeroderma pigmentosa
Yaws
Zipokowski-Margolis syndrome

## IMPAIRED OLFACTION & SKIN DISEASES

atopy
Cushing's syndrome
Diabetes mellitus
Hypothyroidism
Kallmmann's syndrome
leprosy
pseudohypoparathyroidism
Sjorgren's syndrome
Turner's syndrome
Wegener's granulomatosis

## INTRACRANIAL CALCIFICATIONS

basal cell nevus syndrome
lipoid proteinosis ('bean-shaped' calcification in
    the hippocampus)
Papillon-Lefevre syndrome
Sturge–Weber syndrome ('railroad track'
    calcification in the outer layers of the
    cerebral cortex, and in the area of
    meningeal angiomatosis)
toxoplasmosis
tuberous sclerosis (calcification within tubers in
    the basal ganglia)

## KELOID FORMATION

acne conglobata/vulgaris
dissecting cellulitis of scalp
hidradenitis suppurativa
localized infection with herpes, smallpox,
    vaccina
pilonidal cyst
trauma

## KOEBNER PHENOMENON

autosensitization dermatitis ('-id reaction')
contact dermatitis
Darier's disease
dermographism
eruptive xanthoma
erythema multiforme
Henoch–Schönlein purpura
Kyrle's disease
lichen nitidus*
lichen planus*
lichen sclerosis et atrophicus
molluscum contagiosum
pellagra
perforating disorder of renal disease
pityriasis rubra pilaris
porokeratosis
psoriasis*
reactive perforating collagenosis
Rhus (poison ivy) dermatitis (pseudo-Koebner
    phenomenon)
verruca
vitiligo

## KOPLIK SPOTS

coxsackievirus A16
echovirus 9
measles*

## LACRIMAL & SALIVARY GLANDS SYMMETRICAL ENLARGEMENT

cancers
Infectious:
Encephalitis
Hepatitis C
Mumps

gout
Grave's disease
leukemia
Lupus erythematosus
Lymphoprolifative disease:
Hodgkin's disease
Leukemia
Lymphoid hyperplasia

Lymphosarcoma
Non-Hodgkin's disease

Poisoning (iodine, lead)
Saroid
Sickle cell anemia
Sjogren's syndrome
syphilis
tuberculosis
uveoparothid fever (Heerford''s syndrome)

## LEONINE FACIES

actinic reticuloid
amyloidosis
follicular mucinosis (alopecia mucinosa)
leprosy
leukemic infiltrate
multicentric reticulohistiocytosis
mycosis fungoides
pachydermoperiostosis
scleromyxedema (a variant of lichen
    myxedematosus, also known as papular
    mucinosis)

## LESIONS CLEARING FROM THE CENTER

dermatophytosis
erythema annulare centrifigum
erythema chronicum migrans
erythema marginatum
granuloma annulare
impetigo
psoriasis
urticaria

## LESIONS OCCURRING IN SCAR

amyloidosis
basal cell carcinoma
Crohn's disease
cutaneous endometriosis
lichen planus
lichen sclerosis et atrophicus
milia
pityriasis rubra pilaris
psoriasis

sarcoidosis
squamous cell carcinoma
verruca
xanthoma

## LESIONS PREDOMINANTLY OCCURRING IN WOMEN

acne excoriee dés jeunes filles
acrogeria (transparent, thin, atrophic
    skin of dorsum of hands and feet of
    young female)
acrokeratoelastoidosis of Costa
adiposis dolorosa
atrophoderma of Pasini and Pierini
autoerythrocyte sensitization (painful
    bruising/Gardner–Diamond syndrome)
cutaneous endometriosis
dermatosis of pregnancy
desmoid tumor
Fox–Fordyce disease
generalized essential telangiectasia
hidradenoma papilliferum
keratoderma climacterium
lichen sclerosis et atrophicus (greatest
    frequency in menopausal women)
lupus erythematosus profundus (LE panniculitis)
melasma
multiple miliary osteoma of the face
nevus of Ota (80% in women)
Paget's disease
pigmented preribuccal erythema of Brocq
    (erythrose peribuccale Brocq)
progesterone dermatosis
proliferating trichilemmal cyst (80%)
pyoderma faciale (postadolescent female)
subacute nodular migratory panniculitis
    (Vilanova's disease)
syringoma

## LESIONS THAT MAY FOLLOW LINES OF BLASCHKO

Becker's melanosis
CHILD syndrome
chondrodysplasia punctata(Conradi disease)
focal dermal hypoplasia

hypohidrotic ectodermal dysplasia
incontinentia pigmenti
incontinentia pigmenti achromians
    (hypomelanosis of Ito, AD)
lichen striatus
linear epidermal nevus
linear lichen planus
linear nevus sebaceus
linear porokeratosis
linear psoriasis
linear scleroderma
nevoid telangiectasia
nevus angiolipomatosis
nevus comedonicus
proteus syndrome

## LESIONS THAT MAY HAVE HALOS

basal cell carcinoma
blue nevus
congenital and acquired nevus
histiocytoma
involuting flat wart
malignant melanoma (primary of metastatic)
neurofibroma
neuroma
seborrheic keratosis

## LESIONS THAT MAY LEAD TO SQUAMOUS CELL CARCINOMA

actinic keratosis (20% chance)
Bowen's disease (squamous cell carcinoma
    in situ)
chronic sinus tract
cutaneous horn
leukoplakia
lichen sclerosis et atrophicus
osteomyelitis
radiation dermatitis
thermal burn scars

## LESIONS THAT MAY PRODUCE SCAR

acne and other follicular occlusion disorders

any deep infection
cicatricial pemphigoid
epidermolysis bullosa
keratoacanthoma
leishmaniasis
lichen sclerosis et atrophicus
mixed connective tissue disease
nevus comedonicus
porphyria
sarcoid
syphilis
systemic lupus erythematosus
trauma
ulerythema ophryogenes

## LEUKOCYTOCLASTIC VASCULITIS

drug eruptions
erythema elevatum diutinum
hypergammaglobulinemic purpura of
    Waldenstrom
Sjögren's syndrome
systemic rheumatoid vasculitis
systemic lupus erythematosus
urticarial vasculitis

## LUPUS ANTICOAGULANT (Antiphospholipid Antibody)

acute rheumatic fever
Addison's disease
autoimmune hemolytic anemia
Behçet's syndrome
chronic active hepatitis
Hashimoto's thyroiditis
HIV infection
idiopathic thrombocytopenic purpura
lymphoreticular malignancies
medication: hydralazine, quinidine,
    phenothiazines, procainamide
rheumatoid arthritis
Sneddon's syndrome
systemic lupus erythematosus*
Takayasu's syndrome
ulcerative colitis

## LYMPHEDEMA

### Vascular
arteriovenous fistula
lymphangioma
post-thrombophlebitis

### Infectious
*Bacterial*
   chronic recurrent erysipelas
   pyogenic infections
   tuberculosis
*Parasitic*
   filariasis
*Spirochetal*
   syphilis
*Viral*
   cat-scratch fever

### Traumatic
lymph-node excision
post-paralytic
post-trauma
surgical scar
X-ray overexposure

### Allergic
immune response to bacteria or fungi

### Medicinal
methysergide (causes retroperitoneal fibrosis)

### Idiopathic
idiopathic
idiopathic retroperitoneal fibrosis
localized myxedema
panniculitis
stasis
yellow-nail syndrome

### Neoplastic
lymphangiosarcoma
   malignant infiltration of lung, ovary, prostate, uterus

### Congenital
Milroy's disease
neurofibromatosis (AD)
Turner's syndrome

## MASQUERADERS (IMITATORS)

### General Imitators
AIDS
drug eruption
Hansen's disease
sarcoidosis
syphilis

### Specific Imitators
*Atopic Dermatitis-like eruptions*
acrodermatitis enteropathica
agammaglobulinemia (Swiss type)
ataxia telangiectasia
chronic granulomatous disease
contact dermatitis
Darier's disease
dermatitis herpetiformis
histiocytosis X (Letterer–Siwe disease, Hand–Schüller–Christian disease)
hyperimmunoglobulin E syndrome
nummular eczema
phenylketonuria
psoriasis
scabies
seborrheic dermatitis
selective IgA deficiency
Wiskott–Aldrich syndrome

Child abuse-like conditions
accidental bruising(also haematological disease)
dermatitis artefacta
Ehlers-danlos syndrome
epidermolysis bullosa
growth ('whiplash') stirae
hypersensitivity to aluminun(causes nodules at vaccination sites on upper arm or buttock)
lichen sclerosus et atrophicus of vulva
linear epidermal nevus affecting enital region
localized vulval pemphigoid
molluscum contagiosum in genital area(a common site normally)
Mongolian spot
Napkin rashes of various causes

Plant contact dermatitis or phytophotocontact
 reaction

Pityriasis lichenoids acuta
Psoriasis (of genital area)

*Condyloma acuminatum-like lesions*
angiokeratoma
granuloma inguinale
lichen nitidus
lichen planus
nevi
pearly penile papules
sarcoidosis
seborrheic keratosis

**Cutaneous T-cell lymphoma-like eruptions**
actinic reticuloid
eczema
Norwegian scabies
Parapsoriasis

Dermatofibroma-like lesions:
histoid type of leprosy

*Hemorrhagic pyogenic granuloma-like lesions*
Oroya fever (Barton's bacillus)

*Ichthyosis-like Eruptions*

**Infectious**
AIDS
leprosy

**Medicinal**
butyrophenones
nicotinic acid
triparanol

**Metabolic**
hypothyroidism
hypo/hyper-vitaminosis A
other nutritional deficiencies

**Idiopathic**
dermatomyositis
lupus erythematosus
sarcoidosis

**Neoplastic**
*Malignant*
 carcinomas
Hodgkin's and non-Hodgkin's lymphoma
multiple myeloma
mycosis fungoides

*Keloid-like lesions*
lobomycosis
sarcoidosis

LEISHMANIA-LIKE LESIONS
paracoccidiosis

## LUPUS-LIKE ERUPTIONS OF THE FACE

**Vascular**
telangiectasia macularis eruptiva perstans

**Allergic**
contact dermatitis
erythrosis pigmentata faciei (erythrose
 peribuccale pigmentaire of Brocq)
perioral dermatitis
phototoxicity
polymorphous light eruption
seborrheic dermatitis

**Medicinal**
fixed drug eruption
poststeroid atrophy

**Idiopathic**
dermatomyositis
discoid lupus erythematosus
granuloma faciale
Jessner's lymphocytic infiltrate
pemphigus erythematosus
rosacea
scleroderma
systemic lupus erythematosus

**Congenital**
Bloom's syndrome (AR)
Cockayne's syndrome (AR)
Rothmund–Thomson syndrome (AR)

*Malignancy-like lesions (pseudomalignancies)*
*Pseudocarcinomas*
Bowenoid papulosis
condyloma acuminatum recently treated with
    podophyllin
inflamed seborrheic keratosis
keratoacanthoma
proliferating trichilemmal cyst

## MALIGNANT MELANOMA-LIKE LESIONS

Angiokeratoma (thrombosed)
Appendegeal tumors
Atypical fibroxanthoma
Blue nevus (especially cellular type)
Calcaneal petechiae
Congenital nevus (with change)
Dermatofibroma
Dysplastic nevus
Hemangioma pseudomelanoticum
Large cell acanthoma
Pigmented actinic keratosis
Pigmented basal cell carcinoma (nodular type)
Pigmented spindle cell tumor of Reed
Pyogenic granuloma
Recurrent nevus
Seborrheic keratosis
Solar lentigo
Spitz's nevus
Tinea nigra palmaris

## METASTATIC TUMORS MASQUERADING AS SKIN DISEASES

Breast- alopecia areata, erysipelas
    (inflammatory type, keratoacanthoma,
    lymphangiomas, morphea

Congenital leukemia- "blueberry muffin baby"
Lymphoma- chancre, gumma
Nasopharyngeal transitional cell-chancre
Neuroblastoma- "blueberry muffin baby"
Prostate-multiple cylindromas, pilar or
    sebaceous cyst
Rectal adenocarcinoma- hidradenitis
    suppurativa
Renal cell- kaposi sarcoma, pyogenic granuloma
Salivary gland adenocarcinoma- kerion

## MOLLUSCUM-LIKE LESIONS
cryptococcosis
Penicillum marneffeii

## Mycosis fungoides-like lesion
lithium

## ONYCHOMYCOSIS-LIKE LESIONS
aging
alopecia areata
chronic onycholysis
chronic paronychia
hemorrhage/trauma
lichen planus
median canalicular dystrophy
onychogryposis
pincer nail
psoriasis
subungual malignant melanoma
subungual squamous cell cacinoma
yellow nail syndrome

## Perlèche-like lesions
avitaminosis
glucagonoma syndrome
iron deficiency states
secondary syphilis

Pseudo-Hutchinson's sign

AIDS patients
Bowen's disease of nail
Congenital nevus
Ethnic pigmentation
Laugier-Hunziker syndrome
Malnutrition
Minocycline
Peutz-Jegher syndrome
Pigment recurrence post biopsy
Radiation therapy
Regressin nevoid melanosis in children
Subungal hematoma post trauma

*Pseudolymphomas*
actinic reticuloid
antioimmunoblastic lymphadenectomy
arthropod bites and stings
borrelial lymphocytoma

Jessner's lymphocytic infiltrate
lymphomatoid papulosis
persistent nodules of scabies
penytoin-induced drug eruption

*Pseudo-ochronosis*
*Antimalarials (chloroquine)*

*Pseudosarcomas*
angiolymphoid hyperplasia with eosinophilia
atypical fibroxanthoma
fibromatoses
intravascular papillary endothelial hyperplasia
nodular fasciitis

Sarcoid-like skin changes
*Local sarcoidal reactions*
mercury
quartz
silica
talc
zirconium

*Systemic sarcoidal reactions*
beryllium
bruncellosis
giant cell arteritis
leprosy
syphilis

*Scleroderma-like skin changes*
acromegaly
ataxia telangiectasia (AR)
augmentation mammoplasty (silicon)
carcinoid syndrome
chemicals: bleomycin, chlorethylene, epoxy
    resins, paraffin injection, pentazocine,
    pesticides, vinyl chloride
chronic graft versus host disease
congenital poikiloderma
dermatomyositis
eosinophilic fasciitis
erythropoietic protoporphyria
Hurler's syndrome (AR)
Hunter's syndrome (XR)
leprosy
lipoid proteinosis (AR)
morphea
myxedema
phenylketonuria (AR)
POEMS syndrome
porphyria cutanea tarda (late manifestation)
primary systemic amyloidosis

progeria (AR)
scleromyxedema
Sezary's syndrome
Sjögren's syndrome
systemic lupus erythematosus
vitamin K injections (Texier's syndrome)
Werner's syndrome

*Seborrheic dermatitis-like eruptions*
ataxia telangiectasia
biotin deficiency
chronic granulomatous disease
deficiency of vitamin $B_2$ (ribogflavin), $B_6$
    (pyrixodine), E
diabetes mellitus (especially in obese patients)
drug eruption secondary to arsenic and gold
histiocytosis X (Letterer–Siwe*)
keratosis lichenoides chronica (Nekam's
    disease)
Leiner's disease
malabsorption disorders
psoriasis
seizure disorder
severe combined immunodeficiency syndrome
sprue

*Thrombophlebitis-like eruptions*
cutaneous polyarteritis nodosa
dermatophyte cellulitis in saphenous
    phlebotomy site
hyperalgesic pseudotheombophlebitis
    associated with Kaposi's sarcoma in
    HIV-positive patients
sarcoidal granuloma

Urticaria-like eruptions
bullous pemphigoid
dermatitis herpetiforms
erythema multiforme
herpes simplex/zoster
PUPPP(pruritic urticarial papules and plaques of
    pregnancy
Schnitzler's syndrome

## MEASUREMENTS

Skin is 16% of total body weight.
Adult body fat is 15–20% of total body weight.
Surface are = weight × height × 71.84

## Epidermal turnover time:

From basal layer to stratum cornium- 14 days

Through stratum cornium & desqumation- 14 days

Total epidermal turnover time 70 days

## Percutaneous absorption from least to greatest:

1–Dorsal feet & hands
2–Lower arms & legs
3–Upper arms & legs
4–Back & chest
5–Face
6–Eyelids
7–Scrotum
8–Mucous membranes

## Dermal thickness in mm

| | |
|---|---|
| abdomen | 2.2 |
| back | 4.0 |
| eyelid | <.1 |
| forehead | 1.7 |
| palm & soles | 1.5 |
| scalp | 1.3 |
| thigh | 2.3 |
| wrist | 1.7 |

## SKIN AVERAGE THICKNESS

| Region | % body surface area | Thickness in mm |
|---|---|---|
| anterior trunk | 18 | 2.2 |
| arms | 18 | 1.5 |
| head | 9 | 1.5 |
| lower legs | 18 | 1.5 |
| posterior trunk | 18 | 4.0 |
| thighs | 18 | 2.3 |

## HAIR MEASUREMENTS:

In general: anagen length 2–5 years
Catagen length 35 days
Telogen length 100–150 days

Total number of scalp hair follicules= 100,000
(blonds average 120,000; brunettes about 100,000; redheads about 80,000)
50–150 hairs fall from scalp on daily basis

| Body region | % anogen | Anogen duration | % Telogen | Telogen duration | Daily growth |
|---|---|---|---|---|---|
| arms | 20 | 13 wks | 80 | 18 wks | 0.3mm |
| axillae | 30 | 4 mths | 70 | 3 mths | 0.3mm |
| breasts | 30 | | 70 | 0 | 35mm |
| cheeks | 50–70 | | 30–50 | | 0.35mm |
| chin | 70 | 1 yr | 30 | 10 wks | 0.35mm |
| ear | 15 | 4–8 wks | 85 | 3 mths | |
| eyebrows | 10 | 4–8 wks | 90 | 3 mths | 0.16mm |
| legs/thigh | 20 | 16 wks | 80 | 24 wks | 0.21mm |
| pubic | | 30mths | 70 | 12 wks | |
| scalp | 85 | 2–6 yrs | 13 | 3–4 mths | 35mm |
| trunk | | | | | 0.3mm |
| upper lip | 65 | 16 wks | 35 | 6 wks | |

## NAIL MEASUREMENTS:

Nail growth .5–1.2 mm per week
Fingernail growth from matrix to free edge of nail about 5.5 months.

Nail growth in general:

| FASTER | SLOWER |
|---|---|
| Day | night |
| Fingers | toes |
| Men | women |
| Middle (index,ring) | thumb, little |
| Minor trauma (nail biting) | |
| Pregnancy | first day of life |
| Right hand | left hand |
| Young age | old age |

Nail growth in diseases, or use of medication:

| FASTER | SLOWER |
|---|---|
|  | Azathioprine |
| A-V shunts | Beau's lines |
| bullous ichthyosiform erythroderma | denervation etretinate |
| etritanate-rarely | fever |
| hyperthyroidism | finger immobilization |
| idiopathic onycholysis of women | hypothyroidism |
| L-dopa | kwashiorkor disease |
|  | Methotrexate |
| pytriasis rubra pilaris | poor nutrition |
| psoriasis | relapsing polychondritis |
|  | yellow nail syndrome |

## MELASMA

cosmetics
genetic and racial predisposition
hepatic disease
nutrition
oral contraceptive pills
parasitosis
pregnancy

## MIGRATORY ERUPTIONS

bronchial carcinoma
celiac disease
cirrhosis
erythema annulare centrifigum
Erythema marginatum
Glucagonoma
Gluten sensitive enteropathy
hepatitis
Hepatocellular carcinoma
Inflammatory bowel disease
Juvenile rheumatoid arthritis
Necrolytic migratory erythema
pancreatitis

## MILIA FORMATION

acne
bullous lichen planus
burn (second degree)
congenital
dermabrasion
epidermolysis bullosa

herpes zoster
porphyria cutanea tarda
post radiation therapy
post treatment with flouorouracil
scar
steroid (topical)

## MITE INFESTATIONS IN HUMANS

Canine scabies- dogs
Cheyletiella- cats, dogs, rabbits
Dermanyssus gallinae- chickens
Feline scabies- cats
Ornithonyssus bacoti- rats
Ornithonyssus bursa- sparrows
Ornithonyssus sylviarum- chickens

## MITTEN DEFORMITY OF HANDS AND FEET

characteristic of recessive dystrophic
    epidermolysis bullosa

## MONGOLIAN SPOTS (CONGENITAL DERMAL MELANOCYTOSIS)

seen in:
96% of blacks
45% of hispanics
10% of whites

## MNEMONICS

CREST SYNDROME
C–Calcinosis cutis
R–Raynaud's phenomenon
E–Esophageal dysfunction
S–Sclerodactyly
T–Telangiectasia

FUNGI RESPONSIBLE FOR FLUORESCENT
    TINEA CAPITIS
See Cats And Dogs Fight
See– T.Schoenleinii
Cats–M.Canis

And–M.Audouinii
Dogs–M.Distortum
Fight–T.Ferrugineum

## LEOPARD SYNDROME
L–Lentigines
E–Electrocardiographic conduction
   abnormalities
O–Ocular hypertelorism
P–Pulmonic stenosis
A–Abnormal genitalia
R–Growth Retardation
D–Deafness

## LICHEN PLANUS PRIMARY LESIONS
"P"s Papular, planar, plentiful, polished,
   polygonal, Pruritic, Purple

## PAINFUL NODULE
(Mnemonic = C/O BENGAL)
Cutaneous endometriosis
Osteoma cutis
Blue rubber bleb nevus
Eccrine spiradenoma
Neurilemmoma, Neuroma
Glomus tumor
Angiolipoma
Leiomyoma

## PELLAGRA
4 "D'S" Diarrhea, Dementia, Dermatitis, Death

## NERVE INVOLVEMENT

enlarged, hard, and tender nerves of limbs with
   signs of peripheral neuropathy

chronic diffuse amyloidosis
hereditary familial hypertrophic neuropathy
leprosy

## NIKOLSKY'S SIGN

bullous impetigo
bullous pemphigoid (may or may not be
   present)
epidermolysis bullosa (dystrophic and junctional
   types only)
graft versus host disease (acute)
intracutaneous bulla formation
pemphigus erythematosus

pemphigus foliaceus
pemphigus vulgaris
staphylococcal scalded skin syndrome
Stevens–Johnson disease
toxic epidermal necrolysis

## NODULAR B CELL LYMPHOID HYPERPLASIA

acupuncture
antigen injection
Borrelia infection
Drug reaction
Herpes zoster scars
Persistent insect bite reactions
tattoos

## OSTEOMA CUTIS

Primary osteoma cutis:
Albright's hereditary osteodystrophy
fibrodysplasia ossificans progressiva
military osteoma in women
platelike osteoma cutis
progressive osseous heteroplasia

Secondary osteoma cutis:
acne vulgaries
actinic keratosis
appendageal and fibrous proliferations
atypical fibroxanthoma
basal cell carcinoma
bronchogenic carcinoma,metastatic
calcification
chondroid syringoma
chondroma
chronic venous insufficiency
dermatofibroma
dermatomyositis
desmoid tumor
desmoplastic melanoma
epidermal nevus
folliculitis
Gardner's syndrome
Hemangioma
inflammation
infundibular cyst
lipoma
lupos erythematosus
morphea

myositis ossificans
neurilemmoma
nevi
pilar cyst
pilomatricoma
pyogenic granuloma
scars
scleroderma
syphilis
trauma
trichoepithelioma

**Fetid odor seen in:**
bromhidrosis
cutis vertis gyrata
Darier's disease
epidermoid cyst
epidermolytic hyperkeratosis
mal de meleda
pitted keratolysis
Vincent's infection (fusospirochetal gingivitis)

**Others:**
diphtheria-sweet
favus-"Mousy"
isovaleric academia-sweaty feet;cheesy
maple syrup urine disease-maple syrup
pellagra-sour or musty bread
pemphigus-foul;unpleasant
phenylketonuria-sweaty locker room towel
pseudomonas-musty
rubella-freshly plucked feathers
scrofula-stale beer
scurvy-putrid
subpreputial discharge- gardnerella vaginitis
    infection (fishy odor)
trimethylaminuria-fishy

lichen planus–pemphigoides
lupus erythematosus–lichen planus overlap
    syndrome
mixed connective tissue disease (cutaneous
    lupus erythematosus and scleroderma
    features)
systemic lupus erythematosus and
    dermatomyositis
systemic lupus erythematosus and systemic
    scleroderma

Kawasaki's disease
scarlet fever

Behçet's syndrome
bowel bypass syndrome (bowel-associated
    dermatitis–arthritis syndrome)
pyoderma gangrenosum
Wegener's granulomatosis

**Darier's disease:** "sandwich of red & white
    lines with a peripheral notch or split"
**dermatitis herpetiformis:** IgA in granular
    pattern in the dermal papillae of the normal
    skin
**dermatomyositis:** Gottron's papules,
    Gottron's sign
**Fabry's disease:** subcapsular cataracts
**Gardner's syndrome:** congenital
    hypertrophy of retinal pigment epithelium
**Goltz syndrome** (NEVOID BASAL CELL
    CA): PALMOPLANTAR PITS
**HIV infection:** proximal subungal
    onychomycosis
**lipoid proteinosis:** intracranial calcifications
    (bilateral "bean-shaped" calcifications of
    hippocampus
**lymphogranuloma venereum:** Groove's
    sign
**mastocytosis:** Darier's sign
**measles:** Koplik''s spots
**nail–patella syndrome:** bilaterally
    symmetrical osseous horns that arise from
    posterior aspect of iliac wings
**multicentric reticulohistiocytosis:**
    periungal papules
**neurofibromatosis:** axillary freckeling
    (Crowe's sign)
**pityriasis rubra pilaris:** follicular papules on
    dorsal aspect of fingers
**porphyria cutanea tarda** or **pseudo
    porphyria:** caterpillar bodies
**Sturge-Weber syndrome:** opaque
    double-contoured ("railroad track")
    sinusodal lines that follow convolutions of

the brain, which represent calcium deposits on X-ray

**Sulzberger-Garbe syndrome:** penile & scrotal lesions

**Syphilis, late congenital:** Hutchinson's triad

**tuberus sclerosis:** Hypopigmented macules; periungal (Koenen's tumors) subungal & gingival fibromas; shagreen's patches; tooth pits

**Wegenr's granulomatosis:** Strawberry gingivitis

## PERFORATED NASAL SEPTUM

leishmaniasis
leprosy
sniffing cocaine
syphilis

## PERIAURICULAR SKIN TAGS

Cri-du-chat syndrome

## PERIODONTITIS

Ehlers–Danlos syndrome (type VIII)
Papillon–LeFevre syndrome

## PERIORBITAL EDEMA

contact dermatitis
dermatomyositis
Epstein–Barr virus infection
Fabry's disease
trichinosis

## PERIOROFACIAL DERMATITIS

acrodermatitis entropathica
chronic granulomatous disease
cystic fibrosis
eosinophilic granuloma
glucoganoma syndrome
seborrheic dermatitis

## PETECHIAE AND FEVER

acute bacteremia and endocarditis
acute hypersensitivity vasculitis
enteroviral infections (coxsackie, echo 9 viruses)
meningococcal infection
Rocky Mountain spotted fever
toxic shock syndrome

## PHAKOMATOSES

ataxia telangiectasia (AR)
basal cell nevus syndrome (AD)
neurofibromatosis (AD)
nevus sebaceus
Sturge–Weber syndrome
tuberous sclerosis
Von Hippel–Lindau's syndrome (angiomatosis retinae)

## PHYTOPHOTO-DERMATITIS ASSOCIATED PLANTS

bergomot
buttercup
celery
dill
fennel
fig
garden carrot
lemon
lime
mustard
parsley
parsnip
Persian lime
Wild carrot

## POIKILODERMA VASCULARE ATROPHICANS

achrodermatitis chronica atrophicans
amyloidosis cutis (macular amyloidosis)
ataxia telangectasia

Bloom's syndrome
dermatomyositis
dyskeratosis congenita
Fanconi's syndrome
hereditary sclerosing poikiloderma
Hodgkin's disease
Kindler's syndrome (combination of
    poikiloderma congenitale and epidermolysis
    bullosa)
large-plaque parapsoriasis
lichen planus erythematosus
lymphoma
mycosis fungoides
pityriasis lichenoides et varioliformis acuta
pityriasis lichenoides chronica
poikiloderma congenitale (Rothmund–Thomson
    syndrome)
post-inflammatory
reticuloses
rosacea
scleroderma
systemic lupus erythematosus
thermal radiation
Werner's syndrome
xeroderma pigmentosum
X-irradiation

## PRURITUS

### Anal Pruritus
adenomas
anal fissure
cancer
contact dermatitis (allergic/irritant)
dermatophytosis
diabetes mellitus (rare)
drug eruption
dyspeptic stool
folliculitis
hemorrhoids
leukemia (rare)
pinworm (and other parasites)
psoriasis
psychogenic (depression, phobia)
systemic disease

### Generalized Pruritus
### Vascular
mastocytosis
urticaria

### Infectious
brain abscess
echinococcosis
folliculitis
herpes zoster
hookworm
onchocerciasis
pediculosis
scabies (usually with excoriations)
tabes dorsalis
trichinosis

### Traumatic
caffeine ingestion
insect bites
miliaria
sunburn

### Allergic
atopic diathesis
contact dermatitis
fiberglass dermatitis
lichen simplex chronicus

### Medicinal
drug eruption

### Metabolic
anhidrosis (secondary to central nervous
    system disease, endocrine disease, metal
    poisoning)
carcinoid syndrome
cholestatic liver disease
chronic renal failure
diabetes insipidus
diabetes mellitus
gout
hyperthyroidism
hypo- or hyperparathyroidism
hypothyroidism
iron deficiency anemia
obstructive biliary disease
pregnancy
thyrotoxicosis
uremia

## Idiopathic
bullous pemphigoid
dermatitis herpetiformis (usually with
    excoriations)
juvenile rheumatoid arthritis
lichen planus
multiple sclerosis
pruritic papules and plaques of pregnancy
psoriasis
psychogenic
senile pruritus
Sjögren's syndrome
systemic lupus erythematosus
xerosis

## Neoplastic
carcinoma of breast/lung
Hodgkin's disease
intra-abdominal malignancies
leukemia
lymphoma
multiple myeloma
mycosis fungoides
Waldenstrom's macroglobulinemia

## Hematologic
polycythemia vera

### Localized Pruritus

*Eyes and nose*
contact allergens
hay fever

*Other localized pruritus*
contact dermatitis
eczematous dermatitis
infestations
lichen simplex chronicus
psoriasis
seborrheic dermatitis
stasis dermatitis
xerosis

*Vagina/vulva*
see Genital

*Without an eruption*
atopic dermatitis

cholestatic liver disease
chronic renal failure
debilitated skin
elderly skin
fiberglass
lymphomas
polycythemia vera
systemic pruritogens
thyroid disorders

### Intensely Pruritic Eruptions
confluent and reticulated papillomatosis
dermatitis herpetiformis (papulovesicular)
eosinophilic folliculitis of scalp
Fox–Fordyce (bilateral axillae)
herpes gestationis
impetigo (pustular)
insect bites
lichen amyloidosis
lichen planus
lichen sclerosis et atrophicus
mastocytosis
prurigo nodularis
ragweed dermatitis
scabies
Sezary syndrome
urticaria

## PSEUDOMONAS INFECTION

cellulitis
ecthyma gangrenosum
external otitis (swimmer's ear"); malignant
    external otitis (seen in elderly diabetic
    patients)
folliculitis (hot-tub dermatitis)
gram negative toe-web infection
green-nail syndrome (onycolysis)
necrotizing fasciitis
paronychia
wound infection(especially in burns)

## PSYCHOCUTANEOUS DERMATOSIS

### Artefactial Dermatitis
*With conscious purpose*
automutilation
dermatitis artefacta

*Without conscious purpose*
dermatothlasia (uncontrollable desire to rub or pinch oneself to form bruised areas)
lichen simplex chronicus
neurotic excoriations
prurigo nodularis

### Delusional States
acarophobia
bromidrosiphobia
delusional parasitosis
dysmonophobic states
syphilophobias

### Diseases Influenced by Psychic State
acne vulgaris
alopecia areata
anogenital pruritus
atopic dermatitis
autoerythrocyte sensitization (painful bruising/Gardner–Diamond syndrome)
chronic urticaria
dyshidrotic eczema
generalized pruritus
hyperhidrosis
lichen planus
psoriasis
psychogenic purpura syndrome
recurrent herpes simplex
seborrheic dermatitis

### Tics
compulsive behaviors such as hand washing
lip licking
onychodystrophy mediana canaliformis (onychotillomania)
onychotillomania
trichotillomania

## RAPIDLY EVOLVING (growing) LESIONS

atypical fibroxanthoma
chondrodermatitis helicis (arises in 2–8weeks & is painful)
keratoacanthoma
malignant granular cell tumor
merkel cell carcinoma

metastasis (in order of incidence: breast, gastrointestinal tract, lung, kidney)
nodular malignant melanoma
nodular pseudocarcinomatous fasciitis
pilomatricoma (as a result of hematoma formation)

## RAYNAUD'S PHENOMENON

### Vascular
arterial embolism
arteriosclerosis obliterans
arteriovenous fistula
Burger's disease
coronary artery disease
panarteritis nodosa
Wegener's granulomatosis

### Infectious
kala azar
malaria
subacute bacterial endocarditis
viral

### Traumatic
intraarterial injections
occupational ([vibratory tools], jackhammering, meat cutting piano playing, typewriting)
post-injury
with Sudeck's atrophy (post-trauma osteoporosis)
without Sudeck's atrophy (as acute attack)
post-surgery

### Medicinal
amphetamine
β-adrenergic blockers
bleomycin
bromcriptine
clonidine
cyclosporine
methysergide
poisoning (alcohol, arsenic, cyanamide, ergotamine, heavy metals, vinyl chloride)
oral contraceptive pills
tobacco
vinblastine

**Metabolic**
cirrhosis
hypothyroidism

**Idiopathic**
*Collagen vascular diseases*
dermatomyositis (30%)
mixed connective tissue disease (85%)
rheumatoid arthritis
scleroderma (80–90%)
Sjögren's syndrome
systemic lupus erythematosus (10–35%)
hepatitis B antigenemia
*Neurologic*
carpal tunnel syndrome
cervical rib syndrome
hemiplegia
multiple sclerosis
poliomyelitis
syringomyelia
vasculitis

**Neoplastic**
lymphocytic leukemia
lymphosarcoma
multiple myeloma

**Hematologic**
cold agglutinins
cryofibrinogenemia
cryoglobulinemia
paroxysmal hemoglobinuria
polycythemia vera

## RED COLOR, SHADES OF

Brown Red:
granuloma
Bright Hot Red:
Active congestion
boil
emotional flush
inflammatory
vascular
Carmine Red:
discoid lupus erythematosus
Cooked Ham:
secondary syphilis on palms and soles

Deep Red:
end stage of inflammatory red
passive congestion
Flat Purple Red:
dermatomyositis
systematic lupus erythematosus
Papular Purple Red:
Lymphocytic accumulations

## RED TRANSIENT ERUPTIONS (disappear within 24 h)

carcinoid syndrome
cholinergic urticaria
erythromelalgia
juvenile rheumatoid arthritis
pheochromocytoma
Raynaud's phenomenon
rheumatic fever
transient erythema in the newborn
urticaria
urticaria pigmentosa

## RHEUMATOID NODULES

Jaccoud's arthritis (a non-erosive arthritis
following repeated bouts of rheumatic fever
or systemic lupus erythematosus)
rheumatoid arthritis* (20–30% of adult patient)
scleroderma
seronegative ankylosing spondylitis
systemic lupus erythematosus (5–7% of
patients)

## SADDLE-NOSE DERFORMITY

anhidrotic ectodermal dysplasia
congenital syphilis
Hurler's syndrome (AR)
lepromatous leprosy
relapsing polychondritis

## SCALING PATTERN

CONGENITAL ICHTHYOSIFORM
    ERYTHRODERMA: FINE WHITE SCALE
Epidermolytic hyperkeratosis: thick scales,
    corrugated pattern
Erythema annulare centrifugum: trailing scale at
    the inner border of the annular erythema
Erythema craquele: dense scale
Ichtyosis linearis circumflexa: double edged
    scale
Ichtyosis vulgaris: fish-like, scales attached to
    the center, translucent adherent ("pasted
    on") scales
Lamellar ichtyosis: large plate-like scales
Lichen planus: scanty adherent scales
Lupus erythematosus: carpet tack, adhrent
    thick scales
Parasporiasis: brownish-yellow scale
Pityriasis alba: fine adherent scale
Pityriasis rosea: collarette; peripherally attached
    thin, cigarette-paper-like
Pityriasis rubra pilaris: yellowish pink scales
Psoriasis: silvery-white scales, imbricated &
    lamellar, micacious
Seborrheic dermatiotis; yellowish brown-red
    greasy scales
Tinea versicolor: fine scaling
X-linked ichtyosis: adherent, "dirty" brown
    scale

## SKIN PHOTOTYPES

I    Always burns, never tans White color skin
II   Always burns,minimal tan White color skin
III  Minimal burn, tans gradually
                             White color skin
IV   Minimal burn, always tan Light brown skin
V    Rarely burns, tans darkly Brown color skin
VI   never burns, tans darkly Dark brown skin

## SPIDER NEVUS

alcoholism
chronic liver disease
estrogen treatment
oral contraceptive pills
pregnancy
rheumatoid arthritis
thyrotoxicosis

## STAPHYLOCOCCAL MANIFESTATIONS

botryomycosis
bullous impetigo
carbunculosis
cellulitis
furunculosis
pyogenic paronychia (acute paronychia)
pyomyositis
scarlet fever
septicemia
staphylococcal scalded skin syndrome
superficial pustular folliculitis (impetigo of
    Bockhart)
sycosis barbae
toxic shock syndrome
wound infection

## STREPTOCOCCAL MANIFESTATIONS

### Diseases Associated
erythema elevatum diutinum
erythema multiforme
erythema nodosum*
guttae psoriasis
leukocytoclastic vasculitis
pustulosis acuta generalisata
scarlet fever
sclerederma

### Infections Associated
blistering distal dactylitis
cellulitis
ecthyma
erysipelas
impetigo contagiosum
meningitis
necrotizing fasciitis
sepsis (purpura fulminans)

## STRIAE

adolescence
Cushing's disease
Marfan's syndrome
obesity

pregnancy
steroids (oral/topical)

## SUNLIGHT EVOKED OR AGGRAVATED DERMATOSIS (light sensitivity)

### Vascular
purpura solaris
solar urticaria

### Infectious
herpes simplex
lymphogranuloma venereum

### Allergic
atopic dermatitis
persistent light reaction
polymorphous light eruption

### Medicinal
chlorpromazine
coal tar derivatives
demeclocycline
doxycycline
5-fluorouracil
furocumarines
griseofulvin
musk ambrette
phenothiazines
psoralen
sulfanilamide
thiazides

### Metabolic
carcinoid syndrome
pellagra (nicotinic acid deficiency)
panhypopituitarism
porphyrias (porphyria cutanea tarda, congenital
  erythropoietic porphyria, erythropoietic
  protoporphyria, variegate porphyria)
pyridoxine (vitamin B6) defciency

### Idiopathic
*Collagen vascular diseases*
  dermatomyositis
  systemic lupus erythematosus
*Other diseases*
  acne aestivalis
  actinic comedonal plaque
  actinic granuloma
  actinic reticuloid
  bullous pemphigoid
  citrine skin of Milian
  colloid degeneration (colloid milium)
  cutis rhomboidalis nuchae
  Darier's disease
  diffuse elastoma of Dubreuih
  disseminated actinic porokeratosis
  elastotic nodules of the ear
  erythema multiforme
  Favre–Racouchot syndrome (nodular
    elastolysis)
  Grover's disease
  Hailey-Hailey disease
  hydroa vacciniforme
  Jessner's lymphocytic infiltrate
  lichen planus tropicus (actinicus or actinic
    lichen planus)
  melasma
  pemphigus erythematosus, foliaceous,
    vulgaris
  pityriasis rubra pilaris
  reticular erythematous mucinosis
  vitiligo

### Neoplastic
*Benign*
  ephelis
  nevus
*Pre-malignant*
  actinic cheilitis
  actinic keratosis
  Bowen's disease
  disseminated superficial actinic
    porokeratosis
  keratoacanthoma
*Malignant*
  basal cell carcinoma
  squamous cell carcinoma
  malignant melanoma

**Congenital**
acrokeratoelastoidoses marginalis
albinism (AD, AR)
Bloom's syndrome (AR)
Cockayne's syndrome (AR)
Darier's disease (AD)
Hailey–Hailey disease (AD)
Hartnup disease
hydroxykynureninuria
piebaldism (AD)
phenylketonuria (AR)
Rothmund–Thompson syndrome (poikiloderma congenitale, AR)
trichothiodystrophy
xeroderma pigmentosum (AR)

## SWEAT RETENTION

dyshidrotic eczema (pompholyx)
Grover's disease (transient acantholytic dermatosis)
miliaria crystallina
miliaria rubra
miliaria pustulosa
tropical anhidrotic asthenia

## UNUSUALLY FRAGILE SKIN

congenital ichthyosis
corticosteroid use (oral or topical)
Ehlers–Danlos syndrome
epidermolysis bullosa
porphyria cutanea tarda
senile skin

## TATTOO ASSOCIATED PROBLEMS

allergic reaction
folliculitis
hepatitis C
keloid formation
loss of pigmentation
sarcoidal reaction

## TEETH FINDINGS

anhidrotic ectodermal dysplasia: hypo-anodontia, peg-shaped/ conical
Cockayne syndrome: caries
Congenital Syphilis: Hutchinson teeth
Down syndrome: dental abnormalities, periodontal disease
Dystrophic epidermolysis bullosa: caries, dysplastic
Erythropoietic porphyria (Gunther's disease): Erythrodontia
Gardner syndrome: odontomas, supernumerary teeth
Hidrotic ectodermal dysplasia: Tiger teeth
Hypomelanosis of ito: anodontia, dental dysplasia
Incontinentia pigmenti: anodontia, peg/conical teeth
Minocin, tetracycline: pigmentation
Osteogenesis Imperfecta: dentinogenesis imperfecta
Rothmund-Thomson syndrome: dysplasia
Sjogren-Larsson Syndrome: dental dysplasia with enamel defects
Tuberus sclerosis: Tooth pits
Waardenburg syndrome: caries

## XEROSIS (DRY SKIN)

atopic dermatitis
carcinoma(breast, cervix, lung, Kaposi sarcoma, leiomyosarcoma)
connective tissue diseases(especially SLE)
Drug-induced:
    clofazamine
    cimetidine
    diazocholesterol
    flutamide
    kava ingestion
    nicotinic acid
    retinoids
    triparanol
essential fatty acid deficiency
hepatic dysfunction
human immunodeficiency
human T-cell lymphotropic virus type II
hypervitaminosis A
hypoparathyroidism
hypothyroidism

Ichthyosis syndromes:
    epidermolytic hyperkeratosis(bullous
    congenital ichthyosiform erythroderma)
    ichthyosis vulgaris
    lamellar ichthyosis
    nonbullous congenital ichtyosiform
    Refsum's,KID syndromec
kwashiorkor
leprosy
lympoma(Hodgkin's and CTCL)
malabsorption syndromes
radiotherapy
renal failure
sarcoidosis
Sjorgen's syndrome
stasis dermatitis (venous or arterial
    insufficiency)
zinc deficiency(including acrodermatitis
    enteropathica and cystic fibrosis)

## ZINC LEVELS DECREASED

acrodermatitis entropathica
glucagonoma syndrome

## ZOSTERIFORM SKIN METASTASIS

Angiosarcoma
Basal cell carcinoma
Bladder carcinoma
Breast cancer
Bronchogenic adenocarcinoma
Cutaneous adnexal neoplasm
Cutaneous plasmacytoma
Eccrine porocarcinoma
Kaposi's sarcoma
Leukemia cutis
Lymphoplasmocytoid lymphoma
Melanoma
Mycosis fungoides
Ovarian cancer
Prostate carcinoma
Squamous cell carcinoma
Tonsil carcinoma

# General dermatopathological pearls

## ACANTHOLYSIS

The loss of coherence between epidermal or
    epithelial cells

### Primary Acantholysis
Occurs among undamaged cells as a result of
    dissolution of the intercellular cement

Darier's disease
Grover's disease (transient acantholytic
    dermatosis)
Hailey–Hailey disease
herpesvirus infections
pemphigus foliaceus and vulgaris
staphylococcal scalded skin syndrome
warty dyskeratoma

### Secondary Acantholysis
Occurs among damaged cells

actinic keratosis
adenoid dyskeratotic squamous cell carcinoma
impetigo
subcorneal pustular dermatosis
viral vesicles

## ACANTHOLYTIC INVASIVE DERMAL LESION

acantholytic squamous cell carcinoma
warty dyskeratoma

## ATROPHY OF EPIDERMIS

acrodermatitis chronica atrophicans
actinic keratosis (atrophic type)
atrophoderma
dermatomyositis
graft versus host disease (chronic type)
lentigo maligna
lichen planus (atrophic type)
lichen sclerosis et atrophicus
lupus erythematosus
necrobiosis lipoidica diabeticorum
poikilodermas
radiodermatitis
scleroderma
steroid atrophy

## BALLOONING DEGENERATION OF EPIDERMIS

Degeneration of epidermal cells resulting in their marked swelling and loss of intercellular bridges. Subsequently, acantholysis and bullae formation occurs. It is a diagnostic feature of viral infections.

epidermolytic hyperkeratosis
herpesvirus infections (simplex, varicella–zoster)
smallpox
verruca

## BIREFRINGENCE

amyloidosis
gout

## CATERPILLAR BODIES

elongated & sometimes segmented eosinophilic bodies seen in epidermis forming roof of the blister in porphyrias

## CARTWHEEL (Storiform) PATTERN

Elongated cells radiate from a central hub of fibrous tissue in a whorl-like pattern.

Dermatofibrosarcoma protuberans
Elongated cells radiate from a central hub of fibrous tissue in a whorl-like pattern.

dermatofibrosarcoma protuberans

## CLEAVAGE (Separation) LEVEL

### Intra-epidermal
eczematous dermatitis
epidermolysis bullosa simplex
    generalized (Köbner)
    herpetiformis (Dowling–Meara)
    localized (Weber–Cockayne)
epidermolytic hyperkeratosis
erythema multiforme (epidermal type)
friction blister
herpes simplex/zoster
incontinentia pigmenti
miliaria rubra
variola

### Intra-Lamina Lucida
bullous pemphigoid
cicatricial pemphigoid
heat (mild)
herpes gestationis
junctional epidermolysis bullosa
    generalized, gravis (Herlitz variant)
    generalized, mitis (non-Herlitz variants)
liquid nitrogen
porphyria cutanea tarda
pseudoporphyria
suction blister

### Subcorneal
bullous diabeticorum
bullous impetigo
epidermolysis bullosa simplex (superficialis)
erythema toxicum neonatorum
friction blister
miliaria crystallina

pemphigus foliaceus and pemphigus
   erythematosus
staphylococcal scalded skin syndrome
subcorneal pustular dermatosis

### Subepidermal
bullous pemphigoid
cicatricial pemphigoid
dermatitis herpetiformis
erythema multiforme (dermal type)
herpes gestationis
lichen planus
lichen sclerosis et atrophicus
linear IgA dermatosis
lupus erythematosus
porphyria cutanea tarda
urticaria pigmentosa

### Sub-Lamina Densa
dermatitis herpetiformis
dystrophic erpidermolysis bullosa (all types)
erythema multiforme (dermal type)
lichen sclerosis
porphyria cutanea tarda

### Suprabasal
Darier's disease
Hailey–Hailey (familial benign pemphigus)
pemphigus vulgaris and pemphigus vegetans
transient acantholytic dermatosis (Grover's
   disease)

## CORNOID LAMELLA

A parakeratotic column seen in the center of a
   keratin-filled invagination. It is a
   characteristic feature of porokeratosis of
   Mibelli. Also seen in:

disseminated superficial actinic porokeratosis
pachyonychia congenita
punctate keratoderma

## CORPS RONDS

An individual keratinocyte which is prematurely
   keratinized or has faulty keratinization
   (dyskeratosis)

### Acantholytic Dyskeratosis
Darier's disease
focal acantholytic dyskeratoma
Grover's disease (transient acantholytic
   dermatosis, rare)
lichen striatus
warty dyskeratoma

### Neoplastic Dyskeratosis
actinic keratosis
Bowen's disease
keratoacanthoma
proliferating trichilemmal cyst
squamous cell carcinoma

## DILAPIDATED-BRICK-WALL APPEARANCE

Hailey–Hailey disease

## ELASTIC FIBER ABNORMALITIES

actinic elastosis
anetoderma
Buschke–Ollendorff syndrome
cutis laxa
DeBarsay syndrome
elastoderma
Elastofibroma dorsi
Elastomas (isolated)
Elastosis perforans serpiginosa
Marfan's syndrome
mid dermal elastolysis
pseudoxanthoma elasticum
The wrinkly-skin syndrome

## ELASTIN ACCUMULATION

Buschke–Ollendorff syndrome
elastoderma
elastofibroma
pseudoxanthoma elasticum
solar elastosis

## EOSINOPHILS IN INFILTRATE (in significant numbers)

angioedema
autoimmune progesterone dermatitis
eosinophilic spongiosis
herpes gestationis
hypereosinophilic syndrome
infestations
insect bite
papular dermatitis of pregnancy
pruritic urticarial papules and plaques of
    pregnancy

## EOSINOPHILS IN TISSUE

angiolymphoid hyperplasia with eosinophilia
    (Kimura's disease)
eosinophilic cellulitis (Well's syndrome)
eosinophilic ulcer of the tongue
erythema toxicum neonatorum
granuloma faciale
Ofuji's disease

## EOSINOPHILIC SPONGIOSIS

allergic contact dermatitis
bullous dermatosis
bullous pemphigoid
cicatricial pemphigoid
dermatitis herpetiformis
eosinophylic cellulitis (Well's Syndrome)
epidermolysis bullosa (epidermolytic)
erythema toxicum neonatorum
erythromelanoderma
fixed drug eruption
herpes gestationis
hypereosinophilic syndrome
incontinentia pigmenti
insect bite
Milker's nodule
pemphigus foliaceus
pemphigus vegetans
pemphigus vulgaris
polycythema rubra vera
porokeratosis of Mibelli

pustular folliculitis (Ofuji's syndrome)
scabies
subcorneal pustular dermatosis

## EPIDERMAL NECROSIS

erythema multiforme
glucagonoma syndrome
graft versus host disease
hydroa vacciniforme
ischemia (vascular occlusion)
toxic epidermal necrolysis

## EPIDERMOTROPISM

Mononuclear cells in epidermis without or with
    little spongiosis, seen in mycosis fungoides

## EPITHELIAL MEMBRANE ANTIGEN

SEBACEOUS CARCINOMA
SEBACEOUS EPITHELIUM

## ERYTHROPHAGOCYTOSIS

cytophagic histiocytic panniculitis
malignant histiocytosis

## EXOCYTOSIS

Mononuclear cells in epidermis with spongiosis
    and micro-vesiculation

eczema
mycosis fungoides
parapsoriasis en plaque
pityriasis lichenoides et varioliformis acuta
pityriasis rosea

## EXTRACELLULAR CHOLESTEROLOSIS

erythema elevatum diutinum
North American blastomycosis

## EXTRAVASATION OF RED BLOOD CELLS IN EPIDERMIS

allergic contact dermatitis
drug eruptions
eczematous dermatitis
graft rejection
insect bite
leukocytoclastic vasculitis
lymphamatoid papulosis
pityriasis lichenoides et varioliformis acuta
pityriasis rosea
polymorphous light eruption

## FIBRINOID DEPOSITS

dermatomyositis
leukocytoclastic vasculitis
rheumatoid nodules
subcutaneous granuloma annulare
systemic lupus erythematosus

## FLAME FIGURES

Aggregation of degranulated eosinophil granules on collagen fibers

arthopad bite
bullous pemphigoid
dermatophytosis
drug eruption
eczematous dermatitis
eosinophilic cellulitis (Well's syndrome)
hypereosinophilic syndrome
prurigo nodularis

## FLORET TYPE GIANT CELLS

pleomorphic lipoma

## FOAM CELLS

Histiocytes that have absorbed lipid and have a bubbly appearance

juvenile xanthogranuloma

leishmaniasis (acute cutaneous)
lepromatous leprosy
reticulohistiocytic granuloma
Weber–Christian disease
xanthoma

## GIANT MELANIN GRANULES

cafe-au-lait spots
eruptive nevi
generalized lentigenies
melanoderma of metastatic malignant melanoma
xeroderma pigmentosum

## GHOST (shadow) CELLS

fat necrosis
pilomatricoma

## GRANULOMA

### Foreign Body Granuloma
calcium
mineral oil
ruptured follicular cyst
silica
splinter
suture
tattoo

### Necrotizing Granuloma
allergic granulomatosis
Wegener's granulomatosis

### Palisading Granuloma
gout
granuloma annulare
necrobiosis lipoidica diabeticorum
necrobiotic xanthogranuloma
pseudorheumatoid nodule
rheumatic fever nodule
rheumatoid nodule

### Sarcoidal Granuloma
sarcoidosis
silica
zirconium

### Tuberculous or Tuberculoid (Infiltrate) Granuloma
deep fungal infections (some)
foreign-body reactions not associated with hypersensitivity (e.g. cactus spine, silk, or nylon sutures, starch, talc)
hypersensitivity to foreign substances (e.g. beryllium, zirconium, and certain dyes in tattoos)
leishmaniasis (chronic cutaneous)
leprosy
lupus miliaris disseminatous faciei
rosacea (papular type)
syphilis
tuberculoid leprosy
tuberculosis and atypical tuberculosis

## GRENZ ZONE
achrodermatitis chronica atrophicans
granuloma faciale*
leukemia cutis
lepromatous leprosy*
lymphoma cutis
parapsoriasis en plaque
sarcoidosis

## GROUND-GLASS APPEARANCE
multicentric reticulohistiocytosis

## HORN CYST
seborrheic keratosis
squamous cell carcinoma
trichoepithelioma

## HYDROPIC (liquefaction, vacuolar) DEGENERATION
A degenerative process in which vacuolization of the basal cells occurs

dermatomyositis
discoid lupus erythematosus
erythema dyschromicum perstans
erythema multiforme
fixed drug eruption
lichen planus (early lesions)
lichen sclerosis et atrophicus
poikiloderma atrophicans vasculare
poikiloderma congenitale
subacute cutaneous lupus erythematosus
systemic lupus erythematosus

## HYPERGRANULOSIS
epidermal nevus
epidermolytic hyperkeratosis
ichthyosis (X-linked)
lichen planus
lichen simplex chronicus
verruca vulgaris

## HYPOGRANULOSIS
ichthyosis vulgaris (AD)
mucous membrane (normal)
psoriasis

## IMMUNE DEPOSITS
Location and type of immune deposits

**Behçet's syndrome** – IgA and complement component deposits within and around blood vessel walls or in the subepidermal zone

***bullous lupus erythematosus*** – granular IgG and IgM at dermal–epidermal junction, sublamina densa. Autoantibodies to type VII collagen within anchoring fibrils

**bullous pemphigoid** – C3 and IgG and other immunoglobulins in linear pattern in basement membrane zone, lamina lucida. Auto antibodies to bullous pemphigoid antigen I

### chronic bullous dermatosis of childhood

(linear IgA bullous dermatosis) – linear IgA in basement membrane zone, sublamina densa, or lamina lucida

### cicatricial pemphigoid – linear

immunoglobulins and complement components in basement membrane zone, lamina lucida. Autoantibodies to Laminin 5

dermatitis herpetiformis – IgA in a stippled or granular pattern in the tips of dermal papillae, within lamina lucida, sublamina densa

erythema multiforme – IgM and C3 in walls of superficial dermal vessels – epidermolysis bullosa acquisita – linear IgG and C3 in basement membrane zone, sub-lamina densa, auto-antibodies to anchoring fibrils (type VII collagen)

Henoch–Schönlein purpura – IgA in blood vessel walls

herpes gestationis – C3 and occasionally IgG in linear pattern in basement membrane zone, lamina lucida. Autoantibodies to bullous pemphigoid antigen2 or collagen type XVII

leukocytoclastic vasculitis – granular IgM and C3 in vessels

linear IgA dermatosis – linear IgA in dermal–epidermal junction, lamina lucida, or sub-lamina densa

### paraneoplastic pemphius: autoantibodies to Desmoplakin II & periplakin

### pemphigus erythematosus –

immunoglobulins and complement components at dermal–epidermal junction, intercellular IgG and C3

pemphigus foliaceus – like pemphigus vulgaris, but immune deposits are more superficial, IgG on the surface of keratinocytes

pemphigus vegetans – IgG and C3 at intercellular spaces of epidermis

### pemphigus vulgaris – IgG and C3 at

intercellular spaces of epidermis. Autoantibodies to plakoglobin & Desmoglein I

porphyria cutanea tarda – IgG and occasionally complement components in the walls of blood vessels at dermal–epidermal junction of light-exposed skin

rheumatoid arthritis – IgM and C3 in vesel walls

subcorneal pustular dermatosis (Sneddon–Wilkinson disease) – intraepidermal deposits of IgA

toxic epidermal necrolysis – intercellular deposits of IgG, IgM, IgA and C3 around epidermal basal cells

## IMMUNOPEROXIDASE STAIN

cytotoxic T-cell: CD8
dermatofibrosarcoma protuberans: CD34 & antifactor XIIIa
desmoplastic malignant melanoma: S-100
granular cell tumor: S-100
Hodgkin's cells: CD-15
lymphomatoid papulosis: CD-30
macrophages: CD-68
Merkel cell ca: cytokeratin

## INCLUSION BODIES

### Asteroid and Schaumann Bodies

asteroid bodies consist of collagen. Schaumann bodies are round or oval, laminated, calcified cells, probably resulting from laminated residual bodies of lysosomes

berylliosis
foreign body granuloma
leprosy
sarcoidosis*
sporotrichosis
tuberculosis

### Banana-shaped Bodies

Seen within the Schwann cells in Farber's disease (lipogranulomatosis)

### Cigar-shaped Bodies

sporotrichosis

### Civatte (Colloid or Cytoid of Hyaline) Bodies

Round or ovoid with a homogeneous eosinophilic appearance. Present in the lower epidermis or in the papillary dermis, they are the result of dyskeratosis of individual epidermal cells (necrotic keratinocytes)

benign lichenoid keratosis
discoid lupus erythematosus
fixed drug eruption
graft versus host disease
lichenoid keratosis
lichen nitidus
lichen planus*
lupus erythematosus
poikiloderma

### Councilman Bodies
Cytoplasmic inclusions containing cellular
remnants seen in basal cell carcinoma

### Cowdry Type A Bodies
herpes simplex virus

### 'Crystal Ghosts'
Needle-shaped tyrosine crystals seen in
Richner–Hanhart syndrome

### Curvilinear (Farber) Bodies
Found within the cytoplasm or phagosomes of
fibroblasts, histiocytes, or endothelial cells in
Farber's disease (lipogranulomatosis)

### Donovan Bodies
Diagnostic of granuloma inguinale,
intracytoplasmic inclusion bodies within
histiocytes (macrophages) which stain with
Wright or Giemsa stain

### Guarneri Bodies (Paschen Bodies)
Diagnostic eosinophilic, intracytoplasmic
inclusion body seen in smallpox

### Henderson–Patterson Bodies
molluscum contagiosum

### Intracellular Inclusion Bodies, Parasitized Macrophages
granuloma inguinale
histoplasmosis
leishmaniasis

nocardiosis
rhinoscleroma

### Kamino Bodies
Red globules resembling colloid bodies seen in
epidermis of 60–80% if patients with Spitz
nevus*, but occasionally seen in other
patients with melanocytic lesions

### Lamella Bodies
Fabry's disease (lipid deposits, seen on electron
microscopy)

### Medlar Bodies (sclerotic bodies)
An intermediate between yeast and hyphae

chromoblastomycosis

### Metchnikoff Bodies
tuberculosis

### Michaelis–Gutmann Bodies (intracellular calcified lamellated bodies)
malakoplakia

### MULBERY CELLS
Multivacuolated cells containing lipid droplets,
seen in brown fat (embryonic fat) & in
hibernoma.

### Papillary Mesenchymal Bodies
trichoepithelioma

### Psammoma Bodies
Concentrically laminated, hyaline bodies with
varying degrees of calcification, seen in
cutaneous meningioma

### Russel Bodies, Mikulicz Cells
Russel bodies, round to ovoid in shape and
twice the size of normal plasma cells, arise
within plasma cells as a result of excess
synthesis of immunoglobulins. Mikulicz cells
are large histiocytes with pale vacuolated

cytoplasm, within which are found many
*Klebsiella rhinoscleromatis* or Frisch bacilli.

Granuloma inguinale
Multiple myeloma
Rhinoscleroma*
syphilis, early

### Verocay Bodies
A highly characteristic feature of
neurilemmoma, where nuclei are arranged
in two parallel rows and enclose
homogenous anucleate material

### Virchow (Lepra) Cells
Macrophages with abundant foamy or
vacuolated cytoplasm, seen in lepromatous
leprosy

### Weibel–Palade Bodies
Vascular endothelial cells

### Zebra Bodies
Seen within endothelial cells and neurons in
Farber's disease (lipogranulomatosis)

## INDIAN FILING

Single rows of cells extending between and
around collagen fibers

cutaneous metastasis from breast carcinoma
granuloma annulare (occasionally)
lymphocytic lymphoma (non-Hodgkin's
lymphoma)
lymphocytoma cutis

## INTRAEPIDERMAL NEUTROPHILIC MICRO-ABSCESSES

candidiasis
deep fungal infection
granuloma inguinale
halogenoderma
impetigo

psoriasis
tuberculosis verrucosa cutis

## INTRAEPIDERMAL BLISTER

### Acantholytic
Darier's disease
familial benign pemphigus
pemphigus foliaceus
pemphigus vulgaris
transient acantholytic dermatosis

### Spongiotic
eczema
incontinentia pigmenti
miliaria rubra

### Viral
herpes simplex
herpes zoster
variola

## JIGSAW-PUZZLE APPEARANCE

cylindroma

## LICHENOID INFILTRATE

graft versus host disease
lichenoid drug eruption
lichenoid keratosis
lichen planopilaris
lichen planus
lupus erythematosus
poikiloderma vasculare atrophicans

## MAST CELLS INCREASED

atopic dermatitis
lichen planus
lichen simplex chronicus
mastocytoma
neurofibroma
spindle cell lipoma

## MAX–JOSEPH'S SPACES

Small areas of separation between epidermis and dermis in lichen planus

## MIESCHER'S MICROGRANULOMA

A collection of histiocytes within the septa of subcutaneous tissue, possibly pathogonmonic of erythema nodosum. Also seen in Sweet's syndrome and other panniculitides

## MULBERRY CELLS

Multi-vacuolated cells seen in hibernoma

## MUNRO MICRO-ABSCESSES

Neutrophils located within parakeratotic areas of horny layer

psoriasis*
seborrheic dermatitis

## NECROBIOSIS, PALISADING GRANULOMA

acne rosacea
actinic granuloma
AIDS
Allergic granulomatitis
Cat-scratch disease
Collagen implant-induced granuloma
Connective tissue disease
Epitheloid cell carcinoma
Foreign body granulomas
granuloma annulare
necrobiosis lipoidica diabeticorum
necrobiotic xanthogranuloma
Rheumatoid nodule
Syphilis
Wells' syndrome

## NEUTROPHILIC DERMATOSIS

### Dermal Infiltrate
Behçet's syndrome
cellulitis with abscess
familial Mediterranean fever
intestinal bypass syndrome
neutrophilic eccrine hidradenitis
pyoderma gangrenosum
rheumatoid nodule
Sweet's syndrome

### Epidermal Infiltrate
infantile acropustulosis
impetigo herpetiformis
neutrophilic spongiosis
pustular psoriasis
Reiter's syndrome
subcorneal pustular dermatosis

## NON-SPECIFIC CHRONIC DERMATITIS

lichen planus
mycosis fungoides (early)
parapsoriasis en plaque
pellagra
pityriasis rosea
pityriasis rubra pilaris
psoriasis

## NUCLEAR DUST

Scattered nuclear fragments which result from disintegration of neutrophils

acute febrile neutrophilic dermatosis (Sweet's syndrome)
leukocytoclastic vasculitis

## PAGETOID SPREADING

Bowen's disease
colonal seborrheic keratosis
malignant eccrine poroma
Paget's disease (mammary or extra-mammary)*

sebaceous carcinoma
superficial spreading malignant melanoma*

## PANNICULITIS

The predominant site of the inflammatory
infiltrate is denoted by (L) = lobular or
(S) = septal

### In Association with Another Disease
cutaneous periarteritis nodosa
sarcoidosis (subcutaneous)
scleroderma
superficial thrombophlebitis

### Non-Specific (Indefinite) Panniculitis
Rothmann–Makai
Weber–Christian (L)

### Primary Panniculitis
cytophagic histiocytic panniculitis
erythema induratum (nodular vasculitis) (L)
erythema nodosum (S)
fasciitis with eosinophilia (S)
lipodystrophy (L)
necrobiosis lipoidica diabeticorum (S)
sclerema neonatorum (L)
subcutaneous fat necrosis of the newborn (L)

### Secondary Panniculitis
*Secondary to disease process*
$\alpha_1$-antitrypsin deficiency (L)
connective tissue panniculitis (L)
infection (L)
leukemia (L)
lupus panniculitis (lupus profundus) (L)
lymphoma (L)
pancreatic disease (L)

*Secondary to physical agent*
blunt trauma (L)
cold (L)
factitial
post-steroidal (L)
sclerosing lipogranuloma

## PAPILLARY MICRO-ABSCESSES

bullous lupus erythematosus
dermatitis herpetiformis

## PAUTRIER MICROABSCESSES

Intraepidermal mononuclear cells located
within a vacuole

contact dermatitis (dermal type)
drug eruptions
leukemia cutis
mycosis fungoides*
pityriasis lichenoides et varioliformis acuta
pityriasis rosea
poikiloderma vasculare atrophicans

## PIGMENTARY INCONTINENCE

Melanin lost from basal cells accumulates in the
upper dermis within melanophages

fixed drug eruption
erythema dyschromicum perstans
erythema multiforme
incontinentia pigmenti
lentigo
lichen planus
lichenoid reactions
lupus erythematosus
poikiloderma
post-inflammatory hyperpigmentation

## PLASMA CELLS

actinic keratosis
basal cell carcinoma
folliculitis (chronic)
foreign body granuloma
granuloma inguinale
mycosis fungoides
necrobiosis lipoidica diabeticorum
periorificial inflammatory infiltrates
plasmacytoma*

rhinoscleroma
secondary syphilis*
syringocystadenoma papilliferum*
Zoon's balanitis*

## POLYMORPHONUCLEAR CELLS AROUND VESSELS

cellulitis
eriseplas
neutrophilic urticaria
Still's disease
Sweet's syndrome

## PSEUDOCARCINOMATOUS (Pseudoepitheliomatous) HYPERPLASIA

blastomycosis
blastomycosis-like pyoderma (pyoderma
  vegetans)
bromoderma
chronic ulcers
  basal cell carcinoma
  burns
  granuloma inguinale
  gumma
  lupus vulgaris
  osteomyelitis
  pyoderma gangrenosum
  scrofuloderma
granular cell tumor
hidradenitis suppurativa
iododerma
mycobacterial infections
pemphigus vegetans

## PSORIASIFORM DERMATITIS

contact dermatitis
dermatophytosis
epidermal nevus
geographic tongue
incontinentia pigmenti (verrucous stage)
lamellar ichthyosis
lichen simplex chronicus
mycosis fungoides

necrolytic migratory erythema
nummular dermatitis (chronic)
pellagra
pityriasis rosea (Herald's patch)
pityriasis rubra pilaris
prurigo nodularis
psoriasis
Reiter's syndrome
scabies (Norwegian)
seborrheic dermatitis (chronic)
syphilis (secondary)

## PURPURA, NON-INFLAMMATORY

**With Vascular Occlusion**
coumarin or heparin necrosis
monoclonal cryoglobulinemia
purpura fulminans
thrombotic thrombocytopenic purpura

**Without Vascular Occlusion**
autoerythrocyte sensitization syndrome
lupus anticoagulant
scurvy
senile purpura
thrombocytopenia
trauma-induced

## SATELLITE CELL NECROSIS

Mononuclear inflammatory cells seen in
  association with individually necrotic
  keratinocytes

erythema multiforme
graft versus host disease
toxic epidermal necrolysis

## SEZARY CELLS

actinic reticuloid
atopic dermatitis
B-cell lymphoma
basal cell carcinoma
chronic dermatoses
discoid lupus erythematosus

lichen planus
lymphomatoid papulosis
mycosis fungoides
normal individuals
parapsoriasis en plaques
pityriasis lichenoides et varioliformis acuta
solar keratosis
psoriasis

## SPONGIFORM PUSTULES

Intercellular aggregation of neutrophils within a sponge-like network composed of flat, degenerated keratinocytes

candidiasis
geographic tongue (superficial migratory glossitis)
halogenodermas
impetigo
psoriasis (including pustular type)
Reiter's disease
subcorneal pustular dermatosis

## SPONGIOSIS

Allergic contact dermatitis (acute, subacute and chronic)
Atopic dermatitis
Bullous pemphigoid
Dyshidrotic dermatitis
Evolving erythema multiforme
Id reaction
Irritant dermatitis
Lichen striatus
Mycosis fungoids, patch and plaque stages
Nummular dermatitis
Photoallergic contact dermatitis
Pityriasis rosea
Psoriasis
Seborrheic dermatitis
Spongiotic drug eruptions

## SQUAMOUS EDDIES

Eosinophilic, flattened squamous cells

actinic keratosis
irritated seborrheic keratosis
keratoacanthoma

squamous cell carcinoma
warty dyskeratoma

## STELLATE ABSCESSES

cat-scratch disease
lymphogranuloma venereum
melioidosis
sporotrichosis

## SUBCORNEAL PUSTULES

candidiasis
dermatophytosis
impetigo
miliaria crystallina
pemphigus erythematosus
pemphigus foliaceus
psoriasis (guttate, pustular)
pyoderma gangrenosum
staphylococcal scalded skin syndrome
subcorneal pustular dermatosis (Sneddon–Wilkinson disease)
toxic erythema of the newborn

## SUBEPIDERMAL BULLOUS DISEASE

### With Dyskeratosis or Necrosis
burn (chemical or thermal)
coma blister
erythema multiforme
fixed drug eruption
graft versus host disease (acute)
insect bite
leukocytoclastic vasculitis
radiodermatitis (acute)
septic emboli
toxic epidermal necrolysis

### With Eosinophil Predominance
chronic bullous dermatosis of childhood
drug eruption
herpes gestationis
insect bite
pemphigoid

**With Lymphocyte Predominance**
erythema multiforme
fixed drug eruption
graft versus host disease (acute)
lichen planus
lichen sclerosis et atrophicus
lupus erythematosus
polymorphous light eruption
toxic epidermal necrolysis

**With Mast-Cell Predominance**
bullous mastocytosis

**With Neutrophil Predominance**
chronic bullous dermatosis of childhood
dermatitis herpetiformis
leukocytoclastic vasculitis
linear IgA dermatosis
lupus erythematosus
septic emboli

## SULFUR GRANULES

actinomycosis
botryomycosis
mycetoma

## T HELPER LYMPHOCYTES INCREASED

alopecia areata
atopic dermatitis
erythema multiforme (in the dermis)
granuloma annulare
Kawasaki disease
leprosy (tuberculoid)
lichen planus (early)
lymphomatoid granulomatosis
lymphomatoid papulosis
sarcoidosis
scleroderma
Sézary syndrome
Sjögren's syndrome
urticarial vasculitis

## T SUPPRESSOR LYMPHOCYTES INCREASED

actinic reticuloid
erythema multiforme (in the epidermis)
filariasis
fungal infections
graft versus host disease
leprosy (lepromatous)
lichen planus (late)
pityriasis lichenoides et varioliformis acuta
viral disease (e.g. cytomegalovirus, Epstein–Barr virus, measles, varicella)

## VASCULITIS

**Histiocytic (Granulomatous) Vasculitis**
allergic granulomatosis
giant-cell arteritis
lethal midline granuloma
necrobiosis lipoidica diabeticorum
Wegener's granulomatosis

**Lymphocytic Vasculitis**
*With Epidermal Changes*
atypical pityriasis rosea
collagen vascular disease (lupus erythematosus)
lymphomatoid papulosis
pityriasis lichenoides et varioliformis acuta
pityriasis lichenoides chronica

*Without Epidermal Changes*
drug eruption
Lyme disease
purpura pigmentosa chronica
viral infections

**Neutrophilic Vasculitis**
*Leukocytoclastic Vasculitis*
allergic granulomatosis (Churg–Strauss disease)
cryoglobulinemia
drug eruption
erythema elevatum diutinum
granuloma annulare
granuloma faciale
Henoch–Schönlein purpura

infections (herpes)
leprosy (erythema nodosum leprosum, Lucio's
   phenomenon)
necrobiosis lipoidica diabeticorum
polyarteritis nodosa
rheumatoid arthritis
systemic lupus erythematosus
Waldenstrom's macroglobulinemia
Wegener's granulomatosis

*Non-Leukocytoclastic Vasculitis*
erythema induratum (nodular vasculitis)

infections (gonococcus, meningococcus,
   *Pseudomonas*, staphylococcus, *Treponema*)
migratory thrombophlebitis
Mondor's disease
scleroderma

**Other Vasculitis**
Degos' disease (malignant atrophic papulosis)
hyperparathyroidism
livedo vasculitis and atrophie blanche
lymphomatoid granulomatosis

# SECTION SIX

## Malignancies associated with skin disorders

In this section, different dermatological diseases are listed according to their classifications. Malignant diseases seen associated with these dermatologic diseases are then cited. The symbols below are used to 'quantify' these associations:

\* Most common
+ High incidence
++ Very high incidence, almost certain

# Bullous diseases

Dermatitis herpetiformis
intestinal lymphoma
Epidermolysis bullosa acquisita
carcinoma of bronchus
multiple myeloma
Erythema multiforme
acute leukemia
Herpes gestationis
hydatiform mole (can evolve into
    choriocarcinoma)
Paraneoplastic pemphigus
most commonly tumors of
    lymphoreticular origin
bronchogenic squamous cell ca
Castleman's tumor

Colon ca
Sarcoma
Thymoma
Waldenstrom's macroglobulinemia

Pemphigus erythematosus
bronchial carcinoma
malignant thymoma

Pemphigus vulgaris
colon* carcinoma
Hodgkin's disease
Kaposi's sarcoma
thymoma

# Collagen vascular diseases

Dermatomyositis
*bronchogenic carcinoma
carcinoma of breast, ovary, cervix,
    gastrointestinal tract

Progressive systemic sclerosis
*carcinoma of lung
Systemic lupus erythematosus
lymphoma

# Congenital disorders

Ataxia telangiectasia
biliary, gastric, ovarian carcinoma
lymphoreticular malignancies*
Bloom's syndrome
adenocarcinoma of sigmoid colon
leukemia
lymphosarcoma

Sigmoid's adenoma
squamous cell carcinoma
Chediak–Higashi syndrome
lymphoma+
Cowden's disease
carcinoma of breast*+ (30%) or thyroid
    (7%)

*Dyskeratosis congenita*
leukemia
rectal adenocarcinoma
squamous cell carcinoma (skin and
    systemic)
*Fanconi's syndrome*
leukemia
squamous cell carcinoma of
    mucocutaneous junction
*Gardner's syndrome*
carcinoma of colon *++
other gastrointestinal carcinomas
*Hyperkeratosis (palmar)*
1 – Diffuse (keratoderma, tylosis)
    eosphageal carcinoma++
2 – Punctate
carcinoma of
    bladder/breast/colon*/lung/uterus
*Maffucci's syndrome*
carcinoma of pancreas
sarcomas (chondrosarcomas*)
*Muir–Torre syndrome*
carcinoma of
    colon*+/endometrium/larynx/other
    gastrointestinal carcinomas
*Multiple mucosal neuroma syndrome
    (multiple endocrine neoplasia type 2b,
    Sipple's syndrome)*
medullary carcinoma of the thyroid++
pheochromocytoma
*Nevoid basal cell syndrome*
astrocytoma
crainophrangioma
fibrosarcoma
medulloblastoma*

meningioma
*Peutz–Jeghers syndrome*
carcinoma of duodenum*/other
    gastrointestinal carcinomas
*Porokeratosis of Mibelli*
Bowen's disease
basal cell carcinoma
squamous cell carcinoma
*Tuberous sclerosis*
sarcomas
*Von Hippel–Lindau disease*
hypernephroma
pheochromocytoma
*Von Recklinghausen's syndrome*
acute and chronic myelogenous leukemia
fibrosarcoma
malignant schwannoma
nephroblastoma (Wilm's tumor)
rhabdomyosarcoma
(increased incidence of ocular melanoma)
*Werner's syndrome*
fibrosarcoma
leiomyosarcoma
meningioma
*Wiskott–Aldrich syndrome*
astrocytoma
leiomyosarcoma
leukemia
lymphosarcoma
reticulum cell sarcoma
*Xeroderma pigmentosum*
basal cell carcinoma
malignant melanoma
squamous cell carcinoma

# Endocrine disorders

*Acne*
adrenal tumor
carcinoma of breast (severe acne and in
    females)
*Cushing's syndrome*

carcinoma of lungs*/pancreas
*Gynecomastia* (in males)
carcinoma of the lung/testicle
*Hirsutism*
carcinoma of the ovary/testicle

# Infections and infestations

*Herpes simplex (generalized)*
leukemia
lymphoma
mycosis fungoides
*Herpes zoster (disseminated)*
leukemia
lymphoma

*Lupus vulgaris*
squamous cell carcinoma > > basal cell
  carcinoma
*Norwegian scabies*
leukemia
lymphoma

# Vascular disorders

*Chilblains*
chronic myelomonocytic leukemia
*Erythema (palmar)*
primary/metastatic liver carcinoma
*Flushing*
carcinoid tumors
*Polyarteritis nodosa*
acute lymphocytic leukemia
hairy-cell leukemia
multiple myeloma
*Purpura*
leukemia
lymphoma
multiple myeloma
*Raynaud's phenomenon (or frank gangrene)*
carcinoma of kidney/ovary/pancreas/small
  intestine/stomach
*Telangiectasia*
adenoma of hepatic bile duct
carcinoma of the breast (local or
  metastatic)

carcinoid tumors
malignant angioendotheliomatosis
*Thrombophlebitis (superficial migratory;*
  *Trousseau syndrome)*
carcinoma of breast/colon/gallbladder/
  liver/lung/ovary/pancreas*/prostate/
  stomach/leukemia/lymphoma
Mondor's disease (thrombophlebitis of
  anterior chest wall = carcinoma of the
  breast
*Urticaria (chronic)*
cancer
leukemia
lymphoma
*Vasculitis*
hairy-cell leukemia
leukemia
lymphoma
paraproteinemia
squamous cell carcinoma of the
  bronchus*

# Miscellaneous

Acanthosis nigricans
intra-abdominal adenocarcinomas
tumors of APUDoma group
ACQUIRED HYPERTRICHOSIS
  LANUGIONOSA
Carcinoma of bladder, breast*, bronchus,
  colon, gallbladder, ovary, pancreas,
  rectum, uterus
Hypertrophic osteoarthropathy
Alopecia neoplastica
metastatic breast carcinoma in the
  female; metastatic lung or kidney
  carcinoma in the male
Amyloidosis (systemic)
multiple myeloma*+
Arsenical keratosis
Bowen's disease (within ten years)
hepatic angiosarcoma
invasive squamous cell carcinoma (after
  20 years)
leukemia
pulmonary malignancy (after 30 years)
Balanitis xerotica obliterans
penile carcinoma
Clubbing
bronchogenic carcinoma*
Hodgkin's disease
intestinal lymphoma
mesothelioma
Eczema craquele (generalized)
adenocarcinoma of the stomach
angioimmunoblastic lymphadenopathy
Hodgkin's disease
Eosinophilic fasciitis
cutaneous T-cell lymphoma
Hodgkin's lymphoma
leukemia
Epidermodysplasia verruciformis
Bowen's disease
squamous cell carcinoma
Erythema gyratum repens++
carcinoma of the bladder/breast/cervix/
  esophagus/lung/prostate/stomach
  multiple myeloma

Erythroderma
carcinoma of the
  colon/liver/lung/pancreas/
  prostate/stomach/thyroid
leukemia
lymphoma
mycosis fungoides
Sézary syndrome
Florid cutaneous papillomatosis
internal malignancy (gastrointestinal,
  ovarian, etc.)
Follicular mucinosa (alopecia mucinosa)
lymphoma or mycosis fungoides (40%)
Hemochromatosis
hepatocellular carcinoma
Horney spicules
multiple myeloma
Hypereosinophilic syndrome
eosinophilic leukemia
Hypertrichosis lanuginosa acquisita
carcinoma of the bladder/breast/colon/
  gallbladder/lung/uterus
lymphoma
Ichthyosis (acquired)
carcinoma of the breast/cervix/lung

Kaposi's sarcoma
Angiofollicular lymphoid hyperplasia
Angioimmunoblastic lymphadenopathy
Hairy cell leukemia
Hodgkin's disease
Leiomyosarcoma
leukemia
lymphoma
multiple myeloma
mycosis fungoides
Non-Hodgkin's lymphoma
Sezary syndrome
Waldenstorm's macroglobulinemia

Icterus
carcinoma of the gallbladder/bile
  duct/pancreas/adjacent bowel
Leukoderma

carcinoma of the thyroid
malignant melanoma
*Lichen planus (ulcerative and in foot)*
carcinoma+
*Lichen planus pemphigoides*
craniopharyngioma
lymphosarcoma
neuroblastoma
stomach carcinoma
*Lichen sclerosis et atrophicus*
genital carcinoma
*Lymphomatoid papulosis*
lymphoma (10–20% of patients)
*Melanosis*
adrenal insufficiency secondary to tumor
malignant melanoma
*Multicentric reticulohistiocytosis*
adenocarcinoma of axilla/rectum
carcinoma of the
    breast/cervix/colon/lung/
    ovary/stomach
lymphoma
sarcoma
*Necrolytic migratory erythema
    (GLUCAGONOMA SYNDROME)*
α-2-glucagon-producing islet cell tumor
    of the pancreas
*Neutrophilic eccrine hidradenitis*
acute myelogenous leukemia*
Cytarabine associated chemotherapy
<u>Hodgkin's and non-Hodgkin's lymphoma</u>
osteogenic sarcoma
testicular carcinoma
*Pachydermoperiostosis (acquired)*
carcinoma of lung
*Paget's disease*
1 – Extra-mammary
carcinoma of the gastrointestinal
    tract/genitourinary tract
    (25–50%)/sweat gland
2 – Mammary
carcinoma of the breast++
*Paraneoplastic acrokeratosis of Bazex++*
carcinoma of the
    esophagus/lung/tongue/upper
    respiratory tract++

metastatic cancer of the lymph node
*Pityriasis rotunda*
cancer
leukemia
myeloma
*Porphyria cutanea tarda*
carcinoma of the liver
*Pruritus*
carcinoma of the central nervous
    system/pancreas/stomach
leukemia
lymphoma
polycythemia vera
*Pyoderma gangrenosum (atypical)*
acute myelogenous leukemia
*Seborrheic keratosis (multiple eruptive;
    Leser–Trelat's sign)(67% abdominal
    adenocarcinoma)*
carcinoma of the breast/colon/lung/
    prostate/stomach
lymphoma
*Sister Mary Joseph's nodule*
intra-abdominal adenocarcinoma
*Sjögren's syndrome*
lymphoreticular malignancies (e.g.
    non-Hodgkin's lymphoma)
*Subcutaneous fat necrosis*
acinar cell carcinoma of the pancreas
*Sweet's syndrome*
adenocarcinoma and embryonal
    carcinoma of the testes
acute myelogenous leukemia*
*Systemic mastocytosis*
leukemia
*Triple palm*
Thickened, moss-like or velvety textured
    exaggeration of the normal
    dermatoglyphics, with prominent
    ridges and furrows and/or cobbled or
    honeycomb configuration. In 94% of
    cases, associated with cancer, most
    commonly, gastric carcinoma (27%)
    and pulmonary carcinomas (22%)
*Xanthomas*
multiple myeloma
myelocytic leukemia

# SECTION SEVEN

## Special states and skin

# Black skin

DERMATOSIS MORE
COMMON IN BLACK SKIN

acne cosmetica
acne keloidalis
acral lentiginous melanoma
acropustulosis of infancy
African histoplasmosis
ainhum
blue nevus
bullous lupus erythematosus
Buruli ulcer
Chancroid
Dermatitis cruris pustulosa et
  atrophicans
dermatosis papulosa nigra (seen in 35% of
  Blacks)
dissecting cellulitis of scalp
disseminate infundibulofolliculitis (almost
  exclusively in Blacks)
drancunculiasis (guinea worm)
filariasis
follicular pustular syphilis (unique to
  Blacks)
granuloma inguinale
granuloma multiforme
hamartoma moniliformis
hyper/hypopigmentation
hypertensive ulcer
idiopathic guttate hypomelanosis
impetigo
infundibulofolliculitis
keloid
Kaposi's sarcoma
keratosis punctata
kwashiorkor
leishmaniasis
leprosy
lichen nitidus
lichen simplex chronicus
loiasis

longitudinal melanonychia (melanonychia
  striate)
madura foot
mongolian spot
nevus of Ito/Oto
onchocerciasis
papular pityriasis rosea (Black children in
  particular)
periumbilical perforating
  pseudoxanthoma elasticum
  (perforating calcific elastosis) (in
  multiparous Black women)
pityriasis alba
pityriasis rotunda
pomade acne
porphyria cutanea tarda
post-inflammatory
  hyper/hypo-pigmentation
pseudofolliculitis barbae
pseudomonas toe web infection
reticulated papillomatosis of Gougerot
  and Carteaud
sarcoidosis (more in females)
segmental folliculitis
sickle cell ulceration
sycosis barbae
tinea capitis (tinea tonsurans*)
traction alopecia
transient neonatal pustular melanosis
  (unique to Blacks)
tropical ulcer
trypanosomiasis

NON-PATHOLOGIC
CHANGES

Futcher's lines (abrupt linear color
  dermarcation)
hair lines in infants
hyperpigmentation of palms and soles
  and perifollicular hyperpigmentation

293

linea alba
linea nigra
localized hyperpigmentation in infants
luxtaclavicular beaded lines

mucous membrane hyperpigmentation
(lips and others)
nailfold hyperpigmentation

# Nutritional disorders

## DEFICIENCIES

*Biotin*
alopecia
blepharitis
depigmentation of the hair and skin
geographic tongue
scaly eczematous eruption
seborrheic dermatitis

*Copper*
Menkes' kinky-hair syndrome
in infants, defective pigmentation of hair
and skin

*Essential Fatty Acids (Linoleic Acid)*
Eruption similar to acrodermatitis
enteropathica. Dry scaly skin, diffuse
alopecia of scalp and eyebrows, and
lightening of the remaining hair.
Thrombocytopenia, poor wound
healing

*Folic Acid*
anemia
cheilitis
glossitis
peripheral neuropathies
recurrent aphthous ulcers and
glossodynia
sialorrhea
stomatitis

*Iron*
angular stomatitis and glossodynia

glossitis
koilonychia
Plummer–Vinson syndrome
recurrent folliculitis

*Pantothenic Acid*
'burning feet' syndrome
cheilosis and glossitis

*Protein–Energy (Malnutrition)*
anorexia nervosa
(Russel's sign – thickened scar on knuckle
pads)
chronic renal failure
fad diets
kwashiorkor
low protein diet, and high calories from
sugar or starch; associated dermatosis
(referred to as 'enamel paint spots') –
hyper- and hypopigmentation, scaling
of skin, skin ulcers, hyperkeratosis, and
petechial hemorrhage;
depigmentation of hair; flag sign
(alternating bands of dark and pale
hair)
Marasmus
deficiency of protein and caloric intake;
dry, thin, wrinkling and inelastic skin
metastatic cancer
protein-losing enteropathies
short bowel syndrome

*Selenium*
Loss of pigmentation of hair and skin;
thinning of hair
Terry's nail

*Vitamins*
**Vitamin A**
Bitot's spots (discrete plaques of keratinizing epithelium on the conjunctival surface); extreme xerosis*; keratomalacia; phrynoderma (follicular keratosis, pigmented keratotic papules); xerosis of conjunctiva and cornea; leading cause of blindness in Third World countries; night blindness
*Vitamin B1 (thiamine)*
Beriberi; skin edema, and a burning red tongue; burning soles; vesicles on buccal mucosa, palate or tongue; Wernicke's encephalopathy and Korsakoff's syndrome
*Vitamin B2 (riboflavin)*
cheilitis, glossitis, oral mucosal pain, paraesthesia, and burning sensation; oro–oculo–genital syndrome (corneal vascularization, flattened lingual papillae, inflammation of lips, interstitial keratitis, seborrheic dermatitis-like eruption, scrotal dermatitis)
*Vitamin B3 (niacin)*
Casal's necklace (symmetric hyperpigmented plaques in sun-exposed areas); glossitis and glossodynia; pellagra ('3 D's': dementia, dermatitis, diarrhea); stomatitis (atrophic, red, and ulcerated mucosa)
*Vitamin B6 (pyridoxine)*
angular cheilosis; glossitis; seborrheic dermatitis-like eruption; also, combined features of pellagra and fatty acid deficiency
*Vitamin B12 (cobalamin)*
severe atrophic glossitis; severe stomatitis with recurrent ulcers; symmetrical hyperpigmentation (because of tyrosinase increase) of extremities (especially over joints of hands and feet)
*Vitamin C (ascorbic acid)*
follicular hyperkeratosis with 'corkscrew hair'; gingivitis; peripheral edema; petechiae and later purpura; poor wound-healing; scurvy
*Vitamin D*
alopecia; rickets
*Vitamin E (tocopherol)*
seborrheic dermatitis-like eruption
*Vitamin K*
ecchymosis

*Zinc*
acrodermatitis enteropathica (AR, circumorificial and acral dermatitis (a range of dry, scaly, eczematous plaques to pustular, vesiculobulous, and erosive lesions), alopecia, and diarrhea); epithelial thickening of oral mucosa; Beau's lines frequently found

## EXCESSES

*Iron*
hemochromatosis; hyperpigmentation

*Selenium*
alopecia; exfoliative dermatitis

*Vitamin A*
acute toxicity: cutaneous exfoliation
chronic toxicity: alopecia; bleeding of marginal gingiva; generalized scaling; sore tongue and mouth; fissuring of lips

*Vitamine B3 (Niacin)*
flushing

*Vitamin D*
metastatic calcification

# Old age and skin

## DECLINED FUNCTIONS

cell replacement and tissue repair
  (wound healing)
immunological response
sebum production
sensory perception
temperature regulation
vitamin D production
sweat production

## NEOPLASTIC CHANGES

acrochordons
actinic cheilitis
actinic keratosis
basal cell carcinoma
cherry angiomas
Fordyce's condition
keratoacanthoma
pleomorphic lipoma (predominantly in
  males)
sebaceous hyperplasia
seborrheic keratosis
squamous cell carcinoma
spindle cell lipoma (predominantly in
  males)

## PREMATURE AGING
## (Skin and Hair)

acrogeria
ataxia telangiectasia
Cockayne syndrome
Down's syndrome
Klinefelter's syndrome
metageria
myotonia congenita
progeria
Rothmund–Thompson syndrome
  (poikiloderma congenitale)
Werner's syndrome
xerodermic idiocy

## PREMATURE CANITIES

dystrophia myotonia
pernicious anemia
progeria

## SKIN CHANGES

actinic granuloma (Miescher's
  granuloma)
alopecia
atrophy
bulla formation
cadidiasis
cellulitis
colloid milium (special form of senile
  elastosis)
cutis rhomboidalis nuchae
delusions of parasitosis
diffuse and focal solar elastosis
dyspigmentation
easy bruisability
elastotic nodule of the ear
Favre–Racouchot syndrome
folliculitis
idiopathic pruritus
increased susceptibility to injuries
increased susceptibility to superficial
  dermatophytosis and herpes zoster
increased terminal hair
keratoelastoidosis marginalis
miliaria
nail: decreased linear growth; fragile;
  increased nailplate thickness;
  longitudinal striations*; soft
neurotic excoriation
poikiloderma of Civatte
prurigo nodularis
solar elastotic bands of the forearm
wrinkling
xerosis

296

# Pregnancy and skin

*Poorly Defined Dermatosis of Pregnancy*
linear IgM dermatosis
papular dermatosis of pregnancy
prurigo gestationis of Besnier
pruritic folliculitis of pregnancy

*Well-Defined Dermatosis of Pregnancy*
autoimmune progesterone dermatitis of
   pregnancy
herpes gestationis (pemphigoid
   gestationis, 1/3000–5000)
impetigo herpetiformis (pustular
   psoriasis of pregnancy)
pruritus gravidarum (recurrent
   cholestasis of pregnancy, 0.02–2.5%)
pruritic urticarial papules and plaques of
   pregnancy (1/200–1/300)

*Connective Tissue*
striae distensae

*Glandular Tissue*
decreased apocrine gland action
   (improvement of Fox–Fordyce disease,
   and hidradenitis suppurativa)
increased eccrine gland activity (except
   in palms) near end of pregnancy
   (increased dyshidrotic eczema,
   hyperhydrosis and miliaria)
sebaceous gland: variable, decreased or
   increased

*Hair*
hirsutism

increased anagen hair follicles in scalp
   during pregnancy
male pattern baldness and hypotrichosis
   (postpartum)
telogen effluvium after delivery

*Mucous Membrane*
pregnancy gingivitis (marginal gingivitis,
   80%)

*Nail*
brittleness
distal onycholysis
subungal hyperkeratosis
transverse grooving

*Other*
dermatographism
Goodell's sign
Jacquemier-Chadwick sign
localized or generalized pruritus (20%)
non-pitting edema of ankles, eyelids
   (50%), face, feet, hands
urticaria (last half of pregnancy)

*Pigmentation*
hyperpigmentation (90%) (areolae,
   external genitalia, inner thighs, linea
   alba, nipples)
jaundice
melasma (chloasma, 50–75%), (face)

*Tumors*
dermatofibromas, desmoid tumors
   (occur following pregnancy),
   leiomyomas
molluscum fibrosum gravidarum
   (resembles skin tags clinically and
   histologically)

pyogenic granuloma of pregnancy
    (granuloma gravidarum, gingivitis,
    gravidarum, 2%)

*Vascular Changes*
cutis marmorata (of legs)
glomangiomas
hemangiomas (5%)
hemorrhoids
palmar erythema (one third of Black
    females, two thirds of White females)
purpura (of legs)
varicosities (> 40%)
vascular spiders (67% of White females)
vasomotor instability

## MEDICATIONS SAFE IN PREGNANCY

*Antibiotics*
ampicillin
cephalosporins
clindamycin
dapsone (may be used for maintenance
    treatment of dermatitis
    herpetiformis)
erythromycin
penicillin

*Antihistamines*
cimetidine (found to cause
    hypoandrogenization in adult life of
    fetal rats)
cyproheptadine (no problems in animals;
    human study not done)
diphenhydramine (Benadryl⁻)
hydroxyzine (Atarax⁻) (no reported
    problems in humans)

*Analgesics*
acetaminophen (Tylenol⁻)

*Other*
chlorhexidine maleate
chlorpheneramine
lidocaine
methylprednisolone
prednisone
providine–iodine (short term, healthy
    skin)

## PREGNANCY RISK CATEGORY

CATEGORY A: Studies did not show a
    risk to the fetus in the first trimester
    of pregnancy, and there is no risk in
    later trimesters.
CATEGORY B: No adverse effect on
    fetus noted in animal studies in the
    first trimester of pregnancy. No
    adequate clinical trials in pregnant
    women.
CATEGORY C: Adverse effect on fetus
    seen in animal studies. No adequate
    studies in human.
CATEGORY D: There is risk to human
    fetus (potential benefits inpregnant
    women may be acceptable despite
    potential risks.)
CATEGORY X: Animal & human studies
    show fetal abnormalities, or other
    risks. (The risks outweigh potential
    benefits).

## VIRUSES CROSSING THE PLACENTA

herpes simplex
measles (rubeola)
rubella
vaccinia
variola
varicella

# Smoking & Skin

acute necrotizing ulcerative gingivitis
("Trench mouth", Vincent's disease)
Burger's disease(thromboangitis
obliterans)
Crohn's disease
Decreased flap & graft survival
Decreased incidents of aphtus ulcers
Harlequin nail (quitter's nail)
keratoacanthoma
Leukokeratoris nicotima gloni
Leukokeratoris nicotima palati

Lip cancer
Leukoplakia
Nicotine sign (yellow–brown
discoloration of fingernails)
Oral cancer
Palmoplantar pustulosis
Premature aging and wrinkling
Psoriasis flare
Squamous cell ca
vasoconstriction

# Sport-related dermatosis

## ENVIRONMENTAL RELATED ERUPTIONS:
actinic damage
    acute: painful sunburn
acitinic keratosis
allergic contact dermatitis
basal cell carcinoma
frostbite
frostnip
insect bites
malignant melanoma
photoaging
phototoxcity
squamous cell carcinoma
xerosis

## EXACERBATED SKIN ERUPTIONS:
acne mechanica
cholinergic urticaria
essential cold urticaria
exercise-induced urticaria / anaphylaxis
solar urticaria

## INFECTIOUS RELATED ERUPTIONS:
Herpes gladiatorum
Impetigo
Pitted keratolysis
Seabather's eruption
Swimmer's ear
Swimmer's itch
Tinea corporis & pedis

## SWIMMING RELATED ERUPTIONS:
Aquagenic acne
Bikini bottom(deep bacterial folliculitis of
    the inferior buttocks)
Catfish stings
Cercarial dermatitis(swimmer's itch)
Coral and sea anemone injury
Cutaneous larva migrans
Goggles dermatitis
Green hair (in hair of blond-,gray-or
    white haired swimmers)

Increase melanoma risk
Jellyfish stings
Seabather's eruptions
Swimmer's ear (external otitis)
Swimmer's shoulder (mechanical irritant dermatitis)
Swimmer's xerosis

## TRAUMA RELATED ERUPTIONS:

Athlete's nodules
Atrophic striae (secondary to anabolic steroids)
Black palm (tache noir)
calcaneal petechiae (black heel)
callus formation
chilblains
corn
follicular keloidalis
friction blister
golfer's nails (splinter hemorrhages or linear dark streaks of fingernails)
hooking thumb (abrasions, hematomas, bullae,calluses, denudation, subungal hematoma on distal 3$^{rd}$ of thumb in weight lifters)
inrown toenail
jazz ballet bottom (natal cleft abscess in the absence of a pilonidal cyst in in a young female ballerina)

jogger's nipples (painful, fissured, eroded nipples)
linear keloid (secondary to anabolic steroids)
Mogul
skier' palm (hypothenar ecchymosis)
piezogenic papules
ping pong patches ( erythematous macules 2–3cm in diameter on forearms & dorsal hands from high velocity impact of the ball)
pulling boat hands
punctate hyperkeratosis
rower's rump (a frictional form of lichen simplex chronicus from rowing while sitting on an unpadded seat for prolonged periods)
runner's rump (small ecchymosis on the superior area of gluteal cleft in long distance runners)
striae distenase
surfer's ear (exostoses in the external auditory canal)
surfer's nodule (over the tibial prominence)
tennis toe (subungual hemorrhages of the first& 2ed toes)
turf toe acute tendonitis of the flexor & extensor tendons)

# SECTION EIGHT

## Dermatological Trivial Pursuit

Dermatological diagnosis is often based on *simple observation*; thus, this 'trivial pursuit' is of the utmost importance to the clinician in order to arrive at a diagnosis. This section is divided into two subsections: Eruptions Qualified, and Eruptions Trivialized

# Eruptions qualified

**Morphologic and/or other features highly characteristic and/or diagnostic of different eruptions are alphabetically presented. The most crucial diagnostic features are printed in bold type**

## ACANTHOSIS NIGRICANS

**Velvety**, light brown to black verrucous or papillomatous hypertrophic plaques, most commonly seen in axillae, neck and groin

## ACROKERATOSIS PARANEOPLASTICA (BAZEX SYNDROME)

Progressive psoriasiform symmetrical eruption with a bluish hue involving hands, feet, ears and nose

## ACNE

Comedones, papules, pustules, cysts, nodules, and scar

### Clinical Variants
*Acne astivalis*
Small, hard, red papules (absent or sparse comedones and pustules), almost exclusively in women of 25–40 years of age; starts in the spring, progresses in the summer, and resolves in the fall

*Acne conglobata*
Characterized by many comedones, large abscesses with interconnecting sinuses, and grouped inflammatory nodules.
**Suppuration** is a characteristic finding

*Acne cosmetica*
Papulopustules, and comedones on the chin and the cheeks of women

*Acne detergicans*
Closed comedones occur as a result of overwash with soaps

*Acne éxcoriée des jeunes filles*
Common in girls who have a compulsive neurotic habit of picking the face and squeezing the tiny comedones, thus producing secondary lesions

*Acne fulminans*
Very inflammatory nodules and plaques which quickly suppurate and leave ragged ulcerations. Fever and leukocytosis commonly occur

*Acne keloidalis nuchae*
Commonly seen in Black and Oriental men; secondary pyogenic infection in and around pilosebaceous structures leads to keloidal scarring in the back of the neck

*Acne mechanica*
Due to mechanical forces (friction, pressure, tension, etc.); an **unusual distribution pattern** is characteristic

*Acne miliaris necrotica (acne varioliformis)*
**Pruritic follicular** vesicopustules on the **scalp** or adjacent areas. Lesions rupture and dry up after a few days

*Acne neonatorum*
Transient facial papules and pustules which
clear spontaneously

*Acne tropicalis*
Occurs in the hot and humid seasons in the
tropics, in **older** patients. Pustules, cysts,
and nodules occur on the back, buttocks,
and thighs, but characteristically, the **face is
spared**

*Acne venenata*
Comedones produced as a result of contact
with acnegenic chemicals (toiletries,
cosmetics, chlorinated hydrocarbons, cutting
oils, petroleum oil, and coal tar)

*Dissecting cellulitis of the scalp (perifolliculitis capitis
abscendens et suffodiens)*
A suppurative disease of the scalp with
numerous follicular and perifollicular
nodules which interconnect after
suppuration, and form sinuses. Alopecia and
scarring, and an indefinite seropurulent
drainage occur

*Gram-negative folliculitis*
Follicular pustules or cystic nodules that appear
suddenly as a complication of long-term
treatment of acne; may appear as
**worsening of acne which was under
control**

*Pomade acne*
Almost exclusively in Blacks; due to use of
various oils and greases on the scalp and
face; mostly comedones

*Pyoderma faciale*
Mild acne suddenly erupts, producing purulent
nodulocystic lesions with superficial and
deep abscesses. Most commonly affects the
**face**, and in **post-adolescent women
(20–40 years old)**

*Solar (Senile) comedones*
Seen in periorbital areas of older paeople who
have had high exposure to ultraviolet light

*Steroid acne*
Monomorphous papules and pustules;
comedones are absent or rare

## ACNE ROSACEA

Papules, pustules, erythematosus patch, flushing
and telangiectasia; but **very rarely
comedones**. Rhinophyma (hypertrophic,
hyperemic, large nodular masses around the
distal half of the nose, which is almost
exclusively seen in men; also see Rosacea)

## ACRODERMATITIS CHRONICA ATROPHICANS

Initially red and slightly edematous plaques.
Later the plaques become atrophic, blue,
red or brown with a wrinkled appearance,
with visible subcutaneous veins. Almost
always occur on the extremities and often
on the extensor aspects

## ACRODERMATITIS ENTEROPATHICA

Acral and periorificial vesiculobullous, pustular,
and eczematoid eruptions; associated with
serum zinc deficiency

## ACROKERASTOE-LASTOIDOSIS OF COSTA (AD)

Small, round, firm, shiny papules which occur
on the dorsum of the hands, knuckles, and
lateral aspect of the palms and soles

## ACROPUSTULOSIS OF INFANCY

Noted predominantly over the **distal
extremities**, are recurrent (every few
weeks) very pruritic pustules or
vesiculopustules (1–3 mm). Begin at birth or
during the first year of life and
spontaneously clear by age 3

## ACTINIC CHEILITIS

Lips (especially lower lip) scaly, fissured, and swollen. Painful erosions may be present (cf. cheilitis grandularis)

## ACTINIC (Solar) KERATOSIS

Poorly circumscribed, discrete, flat or elevated; verrucous or keratotic; pink to red; pigmented or skin-colored, usually < 1 cm in diameter eruption which on palpation is rough-surfaced with adherent scales

## ACTINOMYCOSIS

Draining sinus with yellow **sulfur granules** in the pus. Also, there is a characteristic **purple–red** color of the skin, and a 'wooden' hardness
Three forms:
  abdominal
  cervicofacial
  thoracic

## ACTINIC PRURIGO

Common among American Indians. Onset is before puberty and involves both **covered and exposed** areas of skin. Lesions are primarily **prurigo-like** papules; eczematous patches are also noted

## ACTINIC RETICULOID

Most commonly seen in elderly men. At first, lesions are **severely pruritic**, infiltrated, lichenified papules and plaques on the sun-exposed areas of the skin, but lesions gradually spread to cover most of the skin. Skin may thicken and result in deep furrows. Episodes of erythroderma and lymphadenopathy may occur

## ALBINISM

Generalized congenital depigmentation, and light blue iris which transilluminates (cf. piebaldism, vitiligo)

## ALBRIGHT'S SYNDROME

**Albright dimpling sign**: Because of absence of several knuckles in patients with Albright's syndrome, when fist is clenched, a depression or dimple is apparent.
'Coast of Maine': Serrated or irregular jagged margins of macules in Albright's syndrome (cf. neurofinromatosis)
The cafe-au-lait spots are usually unilateral and stop abruptly at the midline

## ALLERGIC GRANULOMATOSIS (Churg–Strauus syndrome, necrotizing angiitis with granulomata)

Petechiae to ecchymotic plaques, sometimes accompanied by necrotic ulcers. Subcutaneous, usually tender, nodules. Skin lesions are present in two thirds of the patients, and most commonly on the extremities; usually preceded by asthma of many years' duration, and marked eosinophilia, and pulmonary infiltrates

## ALOPECIA AREATA

Sudden onset of oval or round sharply defined patch(es) of complete hair loss, most commonly affecting the scalp. Affected area may be peach- or ivory-colored. Sharply defined, focal areas of hair loss; **exclamation mark** hairs found within or at the margins of alopecia areata (a sign of active disease)

### Clinical Variants
alopecia totalis
alopecia universalis

## AMYLOIDOSIS

### Cutaneous Amyloidosis
*Primary cutaneous amyloidosis*
Common Types:
Lichenoid or papular amyloidosis:
Closely set, discrete, firm, hyperkeratotis, scaly papules, which are **very pruritic**. Most commonly on the shins and the extensor surface of the forearms. Lichenified or verrucous plaques may form, resembling lichen simplex chronicus or hypertrophic lichen planus
macular amyloidosis:
Dark brown macules with a reticulated or rippled or occasionally spotty follicular pattern, located in the upper back, characteristically in the **interscapular** area. Moderately pruritic
Biphasic amyloidosis:
Papules and macules are associated
Rare types:
Nodular (tumefactive) amyloidosis:
One to several 1–3 cm nodules on the legs and face. The center of the nodule may be atrophic because of amyloid involution. About 50% of cases represent the initial stage of systemic amyloidosis
anosacral amyloidosis
bullous amyloidosis
poikiloderma-like cutaneous amyloidosis
vitiliginous amyloidosis

*Secondary localized cutaneous amyloidosis*
In epithelial tumors (actinic keratosis, basal cell carcinoma, Bowen's disease, pilomatricoma, porokeratosis, seborrheic keratosis)
solar elastosis
post PUVA therapy

### Systemic Amyloidosis

*Primary systemic amyloidosis*
Translucent, shiny, smooth, firm, flat-topped or spherical, waxy papules, commonly located on the face
familial
idiopathic
multiple myeloma-associated

*Secondary systemic amyloidosis*
No cutaneous manifestations. Most commonly secondary to osteomyelitis and rheumatoid arthritis

## ANETODERMA (Macular Atrophy)

Thin, blue–white atrophic patches which on palpation may feel like a herniation. The upper trunk is mainly involved

## ANGIOFIBROMAS (Adenoma Sebaceum)

Many red, smooth, small papules, symmetrically located on the nasolabial folds, on the cheeks, and on the chin; associated with tuberous sclerosis

## ANGIOKERATOMA CIRCUMSCRIPTUM

Unilateral discrete papules and cystic nodules that may become verrucous and coalesce into plaques (resemble lymphangioma)

## ANGIOKERATOMA CORPORIS DIFFUSUM (Fabry's Disease, Generalized Systemic Angiokeratoma) (XR)

Numerous widespread telangiectatic papules, some with hyperkeratosis. Most commonly seen on lower extremities, the scrotum and penis, the lower trunk, the axillae, and the hips

## ANGIOKERATOMA OF FORDYCE

Multiple 2–4 mm vascular papules on the scrotum and sometimes the vulva of the middle-aged and the elderly

## ANGIOKERATOMA OF MIBELLI (Telangiectatic warts; AD)

Several dark red, 1–5 mm papules which with time become dull red or purplish black and verrucous. Usually occur on the dorsum of the fingers and toes, the elbows and knees, in childhood or adolescence

## ANGIOKERATOMA, SOLITARY PAPULAR

One or occasionally several 2–10 mm bright red, soft papules which later become blue–black, firm and hyperkeratotic, and most commonly occur on the lower extremities

## ANGIONEUROTIC EDEMA

*Evanescent* swelling without evidence of infection

## ANTHRAX

**Malignant pustule**, (gangrenous pustule) a dark eschar surrounded by vesicles and pustules situated upon a red, hot, swollen, non-tender, and indurated area of the skin. A characteristic **brawny gelatinous non-pitting edema** surrounds the lesion

## APHTHOSIS (Recurrent Aphthous Stomatitis)

Often start with prodromal symptoms of pain, burning, and tingling followed by maculopapular erythematous lesions which within hours develop into typical shallow, erosive ulceration with a yellow–gray membrane, a **regular** border, and a surrounding ring of hyperemia. Most commonly buccal and labial mucosa are affected. Recurrence is a frequent feature

### Clinical Variants
Aphthosis in association with Behçet's syndrome – 16% of aphthosis; features similar to those of minor aphthae
Herpetiform aphthae – 9% of aphthosis; 1–2 mm in size; 10–100 shallow, grouped ulcers which are **very painful**
Major aphthae – 12% of aphthosis; > 10 mm in size; 1–10 deep **crateriform ulcers**
Minor aphthae – 63% of aphthosis; < 10 mm in size; 1–5 shallow ulcers with an erythematous halo

## ASCHER'S SYNDROME

An inherited condition, where **swelling** of the **lips** and **edema** of the **eyelids** occur (cf. Melkersson–Rosenthal syndrome)

## ATROPHODERMA OF PASINI AND PIERINI

Irregularly demarcated 1–10 cm brownish, oval, round, atrophic patches with a '**cliff-drop**' border. Most commonly seen in young females and on the trunk

## BACILLARY ANGIOMATOSIS

Firm, non-tender, non-blanching, 2–3 mm red, violaceous or skin-colored papules or nodules which may be solitary to > 100 and rarely > 1000. Lesions spare palms and soles and the oral cavity. Almost exclusively seen in HIV+ patients

## BALANITIS CIRCUMSCRIPTA PLASMACELLULARIS (Zoon's Balanitis)

Seen on the inner surface of prepuce and the glans penis of uncircumcized male. Clinical appearance is the same as Bowen's disease of the penis, but erosions with a tendency to bleed may be present as well

## BASAL CELL CARCINOMA

### Clinical Variants
Fibroepithelioma of Pinkus
One or several raised, moderately firm, skin-colored or slightly red, sessile or slightly pedunculated nodules, most commonly located on the trunk, groin or thigh, and often resembling fibroma or papilloma
Morphea-like (fibrosing)
Solitary, flat or slightly depressed, waxy, white or yellowish sclerotic plaque with prominent telangiectasia. It generally lacks a rolled border, ulceration or crusting. Most commonly seen on the head and neck regions
Nodulo-ulcerative
Most common type. Small, waxy, semi-translucent nodule which is formed around a central depression with a **pearly, rolled border** and surface telangiectasias. As the lesion grows in size, ulceration and crusting occur
Pigmented
Like nodulo-ulcerative, but in addition, brown or black pigmentation is present
Superficial
Predominantly on the trunk. Psoriasiform, scaly, slightly infiltrated plaques with telangiectasia and a thread-like, pearly border. Smooth, atrophic scarring may be present in the center of the lesion; small areas of

superficial ulcerations and crusts may be seen as well
Other Clinical Variants
Bazex syndrome
AD, multiple small basal cell carcinomas, follicular atrophoderma, localized anhidrosis or generalized hypohidrosis and congenital hypotrichosis of the scalp
Linear unilateral basal cell nevus
Basal cell carcinomas are present since birth in a linear or zosteriform pattern
Nevoid basal cell epithelioma syndrome
AD, hundreds to thousands of small nodules, epidermal cysts, and palmar pits

## BECKER'S MELANOSIS (Nevus)

Unilateral, few to many centimeters, uniformly fair to dark brown patch, at times slightly elevated with a verrucous surface with a **sharp**, but **irregular** border. Hyperkeratosis is often present and always follows the onset of pigmentation. More commonly seen in males (M : F 5 : 1) and appears in the **second** or **third decade** of life, on the shoulder or the chest

## BENIGN LICHENOID KERATOSIS

Solitary papule or slightly indurated plaque (5–20 mm) with smooth or slightly verrucous surface. Bright red to violaceous to brown color. Lesions are not pruritic, and involute spontaneously

## BERLOCQUE DERMATITIS

**Drop-like, pendant-like, geometric configuration**; streaky, brown macule/patch

## BLASTOMYCOSIS

### Verrucous Lesions
An erythematous plaque which is boggy and indurated and studded with pustules on its

advancing verrucous border. Central healing and scarring occurs

### Ulcerative Lesions
Start as pustules and rapidly develop into ulcers

## BLUE RUBBER-BLEB NEVUS SYNDROME

Solitary or many blue–purple, soft, rubbery, painful and tender nodules of 1–5 cm with a wrinkled surface. A diagnostic sign is that blood can be expressed with pressure on the lesion, leaving an empty wrinkled sac

## BOWENOID PAPULOSIS

Multiple small (2–10 mm) **red–brown**, dome-shaped verrucous papules; seen in men on the glans and shaft of the penis, and in women in the perianal and vulvar regions. Clinical appearance is similar to genital warts, and spontaneous resolution is common

## BOWEN'S DISEASE

**Sharply defined**, slowly enlarging, erythematous patch/plaque, slightly scaly and crusted with slight or no infiltration, and **irregular outline** (cf. basal cell carcinoma, no pearly border, and does not heal with central atrophy)

## BREAST CARCINOMA METASTATIC TO THE SKIN

### Clinical Variants
Cancer erythema nodosum crurasse
Diffuse induration of the skin of the diseased breast and its surrounding area
Hematogenous spread
Commonly involves the scalp, initially resemble patches of alopecia areata, thus referred to as alopecia neoplastica; later cutaneous nodules are formed

Inflammatory carcinoma
Well demarcated, slightly indurated, warm, red plaque, mimicking **erysipelas**
Nodular carcinoma
Firm asymptomatic nodules. Most common form of metastasis via lymphatic route
Telangiectatic carcinoma
Purpuric papules or plaques with occasional pseudovesicles

## BULLOUS PEMPHIGOID

Tense bullae on an erythematous base, but if seen on **normal skin**, are highly diagnostic

## CALLUSES

Localized, yellowish **thickened**, (more diffusely than in corn) skin in area of repeated trauma or pressure; especially **over the bony prominences** of the joints

## CANDIDIASIS OF MUCOCUTANEOUS AREAS

**Loosley adherent**, white, crud-like patchy mucous membrane, which, after removal, characteristically reveals a raw surface with pinpoint bleeding

## CANDIDIASIS OF SKIN

Erythematous, scaly patch or plaque with **satellite pustules or papules**
In infants three variants are noted:
1. Patches or plaques with beet red color and with satellite pustules
2. Erythematous patches with peripheral scale
3. Small, discrete papules with superimposed scales

## CARBUNCLE

Two or three confluent furuncles

## CELLULITIS

**Erythematous** eruption with a non-elevated, **not well-demarcated border** (cf. erysipelas which has a well-demarcated border), with **swelling and tenderness**

## CHANCROID (Soft Chancre)

Initially starts with a macule or papule which becomes a vesiculopapule. Single or multiple round or oval ulcers with a sharply circumscribed 'punched out' appearance or **undermined and irregular and ragged** edges, and surrounded by an erythematous halo. The base of the ulcer is covered with a purulent, yellowish exudate. Characteristically, the incubation period is very short (**12 hours to 3 days**) and the ulcer is very **tender** and bleeds easily. Lymphadenopathy is usually **unilateral**. Multiple lesions are usually present and extend into each other

*Clinical Variants*
autoinoculation chancroid
follicular chancroid
giant chancroid
papular chancroid
phagedenic chancroid
transient chancroid

## CHEILITIS GLANDULARIS

Enlargement of lips, swelling and eversion of the lower lips and enlarged mucous glands which feel like pebbles when palpated (cf. actinic cheilitis)

## CHONDRODERMATITIS NODULARIS CHRONICA HELICIS

Slightly reddish, small (2–4 mm) **tender** nodule (on the outer helix of ear). Most common in men

## CHONDROMYCOSIS

Verrucous nodules or plaques, most commonly on the lower extremities

## CHRONIC BULLOUS DISEASE OF CHILDHOOD (Linear IgA Bullous Dermatosis)

Annular and serpiginous patches with bullae arranged at their periphery like a '**string of pearls**', or '**cluster of jewels**'; often severe pruritus is present and usually it is a self-limited disorder

## CLEAR-CELL ACANTHOMA

Well-demarcated reddish, **moist** nodular plaque of 1–2 cm with some crusting and peripheral scales. It has a 'stuck on' appearance similar to seborrheic keratosis and a vascular appearance similar to pyogenic granuloma. Most commonly seen after age 40 and on the legs

## CLEAR-CELL HIDRADENOMA

Solitary, solid or cystic, 0.5–3 cm flesh-colored or reddish nodule which may be lobulated. Superficial ulceration and a discharge of serous material may be present. Most commonly occurs on the head, but may be found anywhere on the body. Most commonly occurs in ages 20–50, and is twice as common in women than in men

## COMEDONE

If this is nicked, a cheesy material is released (cf. sebaceous cyst)

## CONDYLOMA ACUMINATUM

Gray, pale yellow or pinkish, small, pointed, verrucous papules that occasionally coalesce into cauliflower-like masses or may multiply to form large vegetating clusters

## CORN

Circumscribed, conical thickening of the skin with a **horny core** which arises at the sites of friction or pressure (cf. callus)

*Clinical Variants*
Hard corn
Occurs on dorsa of the toes, or on the soles
Soft corn
Occurs between the toes (softened by the macerating action of sweat), usually in the fourth web-space of the foot

## CUTANEOUS LARVA MIGRANS

Erythematous, serpiginous papular or vesicular linear lesions, 2–3 mm wide, most commonly on the feet and the buttocks

## CUTIS LAXA (Elastolysis)

Loose, redundant skin, hanging in folds; usually the entire skin is involved. Skin **slowly** returns to normal position after stretching

## CUTIS RHOMBOIDALIS NUCHAE

Thickened and furrowed skin of the neck region secondary to years of sun exposure

## DARIER'S DISEASE (Keratosis Follicularis)

Symmetrical, dirty, warty, red–brown, scaly, waxy papules **around hair follicles** in a seborrheic distribution. Papules become covered with a greasy, gray, brown or black crust. Oral papules with cobblestone appearance

*Clinical variants*
hypertrophic
linear or zosteriform
vesiculobullous

## DEGOS' DISEASE (Malignant Atrophic Papulosis)

Eruption is composed of pale rose or yellowish red, rounded, edematous papules occurring mostly in the **trunk and the proximal extremities**. Later, the lesions become umbilicated, with a central depression. The center becomes distinctively **atrophic porcelain-white**; however, the periphery becomes livid red and telangiectatic

## DERMATITIS HERPETIFORMIS

Grouped, tense, vesicles/bullae on an erythematous base with frequent excoriations and crusts. The eruption is characteristically polymorphous, thus papules, papulovesicles, vesiculobullae or urticarias may be present. Also, the eruption is characteristically symmetrically distributed and is seen in the scalp, scapulae, sacrum, buttocks, posterior axillary folds, elbows and knees. **Extreme pruritis** is almost always present. Presence of IgA in a granular pattern in the dermal papillae of the normal skin is a **pathognomonic** finding

## DERMATOFIBROMA

Flesh-colored, red, red–brown, and rarely blue–black (because of large amount of hemosiderin), firm, flat papule or nodule. Lateral compression produces a characteristic 'dimple'

## DERMATOFIBROSARCOMA PROTUBERANS

Red or purple indurated plaques or nodules, often with a purulent exudate and ulceration, which looks like an **infected keloid**. Most common on the trunk of middle-aged patients

## DERMATOMYOSITIS

### Pathognomonic Findings
Gottron's papules
Flat-topped, violaceous papules over the knuckles
Gottron's sign
Symmetrical erythematous–violaceous patch with or without edema on the dorsal interphalangeal joints of the hands, olecranon process of elbows, patellas, and medial malleoli

### Characteristic Findings
Periorbital edema and heliotrope and violaceous erythema
Periungual telangiectasia and associated dystrophic cuticles
Red–violaceous patches on the dorsum of the hands, extensor aspect of the arms and forearms, deltoids, posteriod shoulders, V of the neck and upper chest and forehead

## DERMATOPHYTOSIS

Red–brown, annular, arciform, circular, polycyclic, with scaling and central clearing; active border

## ECCRINE POROMA

Slow growing, 2–12 mm, usually solitary and on the soles of the feet or the palms of the hands (but may occur anywhere), sessile or slightly pedunculated, rather firm, reddish tumor which bleeds easily upon slight trauma. Frequently a cup-shaped, shallow depression is noted from where the tumor grows and protrudes

## ECCRINE SPIRADENOMA

Deep-seated, often tender, 1–2 cm solitary intradermal nodule with a normal-appearing or blue or pink overlying skin. Occurs most frequently between the ages of 15–35; may occur anywhere in the body. Multiple lesions may occur in a linear or zosteriform pattern. **Painful paroxysms** may be a characteristic finding

## ECTHYMA GANGRENOSUM

Grouped, tense vesicles surrounded by a narrow pink to violaceous halo. The vesicles soon become hemorrhagic and rupture and form round ulcers with necrotic black centers. Usual site is on the buttocks and the extremities

## ECZEMA

In general, lesions are ill-defined, polymorphous, and pruritic

### Clinical Variants
Asteatotic eczema (eczema craquele)
Dry skin with **red fissures** and slight scaling; lesions are diffuse with irregular reticulation, and sometimes with lichenification

Atopic dermatitis
**Chronicity and pruritus**. Usually symmetrical, red to brown, slightly scaly, poorly circumscribed, often with

lichenification, excoriation, and crust, but no vesicles

Contact dermatitis
Acute and subacute: irregular, poorly outlined patches studded with vesicles, bullae; diffuse erythema, edema, oozing and crusting
Chronic: erythematous patches with scale, excoriation, and lichenification

Dyshidrotic eczema (pompholyx)
Bilateral, roughly symmetric weeping patches containing clusters of **deep-seated vesicles**, most pronounced at the sides of the fingers. Often accompanied by pruritus, burning, and excessive perspiration

Juvenile plantar dermatosis
Plantar surfaces of feet are **symmetrically** red, painful, and fissured. It almost exclusively occurs in the 3–14 year age group

Lichen simplex chronicus (neurodermatitis)
Lichenified, excoriated, poorly circumscribed, slightly scaly red-brown plaque; no vesicles

Nummular eczema
Fairly well-demarcated, coin-shaped, erythematous, edematous patches/plaques studded with vesicles, erosions or crust

Seborrheic dermatitis
Greasy, yellow, pinkish or brown patches, papules or plaques with fine scaling and various shapes and sizes; characterized by exacerbations and remissions

Clinical Variants
cradle cap
dandruff (pityriasis sicca)
erythema desquamativum (generalized seborrheic dermatitis, Leiner's disease)
pityriasis steatoides
seborrheic (marginal) blepharitis

Stasis dermatitis
Thinned epidermis, red–purple to brown hyperpigmented patch with scales and dilated superficial veins; associated pitting edema and varicosities

Sulzberger–Garbe syndrome (exudative discoid and lichenoid dermatitis)
Very pruritic eruption with some features of nummular eczema, lichenification, and exudation. **Penile and scrotal lesions** commonly occur and are almost **pathognomonic**

## EHLERS–DANLOS SYNDROME

In general, skin is hyperextensible (recoils **promptly** to normal position after stretching; cf. cutis laxa), fragile, with impaired wound healing which results in atrophic scars. Joints are hypermobile and may dislocate (see also under Diseases and their features)

## ELASTOSIS PERFORANS SERPINGINOSA

Skin-colored to erythematous keratotic papules (0.2–0.5 cm) usually in a symmetrical **circular or serpiginous** pattern, and usually confined to one anatomic site (most commonly nape and sides of the neck, face, and the upper extremities). Lesions last from 6 months to 5 years and then spontaneously resolve, leaving a superficial scar. Koebner phenomenon is usually present

## EOSINOPHILIC CELLULITIS (Wells' Syndrome)

Sudden and recurrent episodes of painful or pruritic erythematous swellings which become indurated in 2–3 days and resolve in 4–8 weeks; peripheral blood eosinophilia is often present

## EOSINOPHILIC FASCIITIS (Shulman's Syndrome)

Often involves the extremities with tenderness, diffuse swelling, and bound-down skin. **Coarse peau d'orange**, erythematous and edematous skin (cf. scleroderma, skin is **smooth** and **taut**). Involved skin may show surface irregularities, depression or ridges giving a cobblestone appearance, or irregular dimpling

## EOSINOPHILIC PUSTULAR FOLLICULITIS

Erythematous patches with mostly follicular papules and pustules, often with an annular or serpiginous arrangement and a tendency toward central healing with peripheral extension. Most commonly involves the face, trunk, and arms

## EPIDERMAL (Sebaceous) CYST

See sebaceous cyst

## EPHELIS (Freckle)

Brown, non-scaly macule, more prominent with **sun exposure** (cf. lentigo maligna/lentigo simplex)

## EPIDERMAL NEVUS

Grayish to yellow–brown, velvety, granular, warty, or papillomatous papules arranged in a linear fashion in continuous or broken streaks, bands or patches

## EPIDERMOLYSIS BULLOSA ACQUISITA

Blisters with predilection for traumatized areas, heal with scars and milia. Adult onset and skin fragility are other features; however, other bullous disorders need to be ruled out

## ERUPTIVE VELLUS HAIR CYST

AD, yellowish to reddish brown, 1–2 mm follicular papules, some of which have a crusted or umbilicated surface. Most commonly seen on the chest and proximal extremities

## ERYSIPELAS (St Anthony's Fire)

Characteristic asymmetrical, **tense, hot, painful, shiny bright red, brawny, infiltrated plaque** with a highly characteristic **raised, indurated border**

## ERYSIPELOID

Erysipelas-like eruption after exposure to fish, crabs, shellfish or pork. Painful swelling with sharply demarcated and often polygonal patches of bluish–purplish erythematous lesions. **Migratory, new** purplish–red patches at nearby areas are **characteristic**

## ERYTHEMA AB IGNE

Persistent bown–red, reticulated, non-scaly, **non-blanchable** patches (cf. livedo reticularis). Occurs in areas exposed to heat; more common in the female

## ERYTHEMA ANNULARE CENTRIFUGUM

Chronic and recurrent annular or serpiginous lesions that often occur on the trunk and extend peripherally in the course of several weeks. The border is red, raised, and firm

## ERYTHEMA DYSCHROMICUM PERSTANS (Ashy Dermatosis)

**Sharply demarcated gray–blue** patches with some violaceous hues and a fine erythematous slightly infiltrated border, and minimal to no scales

## ERYTHEMA ELEVATUM DIUTINUM

Symmetrical, usually painful, brown–red to purple papules, nodules, and plaques, (0.5 to a few centimeters), with preferred location over the joints (characteristically on the wrists, forearms, ankles, thenar and hypothenar eminences). Vesicles and bullae may be present

## ERYTHEMA GYRATUM REPENS

Wave-like parallel bands of slightly elevated erythema with an annular or serpiginous arrangement, like the **grain of wood**. Bands of erythema move at a rate of about 1 cm per day

## ERYTHEMA INDURATUM

Usually symmetrical, painless but somewhat tender, deep nodules and ulcers with irregular, steep, and undermined edge. Most commonly affects the **calves**, and is more common in females

## ERYTHEMA INFECTIOSUM

Characteristic '**slapped cheek**' appearance and subsequent **lacy, reticulated, marble-like** pattern on the upper arms and thighs

## ERYTHEMA MARGINATUM (Rheumatic Fever)

**Very evanescent**, arciform and oval, pink to red, non-scaly, urticaria-like lesions; eruption may move hourly

## ERYTHEMA MULTIFORME

Multiform lesions, including macules, papules, vesicles, and bullae, persistent urticaria or purpua. The lesions may have an annular or circinate configuration. Hemorrhagic crusting of the lips is a characteristic finding; as is **target lesion** on skin, which represents macules or papules with a **central vesicle** (cf. toxic epidermal necrolysis)

### Clinical Variants
Bullous erythema multiforme
Large hemorrhagic bullae on an erythematous base, usually sparing the trunk
Maculopapular erythema multiforme
Bright bluish-red, well-defined macules or flat-topped papules which are edematous and tend to spread peripherally into polycyclic patches

## ERYTHEMA NODOSUM

Bilateral, asymmetrical, red to blue, **painful**, 1–5 cm nodules, most commonly on extensor aspect of legs, without ulceration, which last a few days or weeks

### Clinical Variants
Erythema nodosum migrans
Chronic form of erythema nodosum, usually unilateral, and less tender

## ERYTHEMA TOXICUM NEONATORUM

Macules, papules, and large irregular erythematous patches and occasionally pustules occur in 40–50% of all newborns, usually within the first 48 hours and last 2–3 days. Blood eosinophilia and eosinophils in the smear preparation are notable (cf. transient neonatal pustular melanosis)

## ERYTHRASMA

Sharply delineated, dry, reddish-brown (light brown), slightly scaly even patches with polycyclic borders in intertriginous areas (primarily in the groins, in the axillae, and between the toes); under Wood's lamp examination, diagnostic **coral red** fluorescence is noted

## ERYTHROPLASIA OF QUEYRAT

Bowen's disease of the glans penis. Similar to Bowen's disease. Sharply demarcated, bright red, shiny, slightly infiltrated plaque on the penis of uncircumscribed men

## ERYTHROPOIETIC PROTOPORPHYRIA

### Acute
Edematous plaques, erythema, purpura (severe cases), or urticarial eruption; smarting, stinging or burning sensations of the face and hands during or immediately after sun exposure (cf. polymorphous light eruption, solar urticaria)

### Chronic
Shallow scar and waxy thickening of the skin of the nose and cheeks. Also, weathering of the knuckles (thickening of the skin), circumoral linear scars. Rims of ears may be atrophic and a persistent violaceous erythema may be present

## EXTRAMAMMARY PAGET'S DISEASE

Pruritic, reddish, slowly enlarging patch with a **sharp, irregular border**, with oozing and crusting. Vulva is most commonly affected; less commonly perianal area, male genitalia, and axillae

## FACTITIAL DERMATITIS/ULCER

**Geometric, or linear** configuration

## FAVRE–RACOUCHOT SYNDROME (Nodular Elastosis With Cysts And Comedones)

Multiple open and dilated comedones on the face, particularly lateral to the eyes

## FIBROUS PAPULE OF THE NOSE (Solitary Angiofibroma)

Solitary, skin-colored or pigmented, firm, dome-shaped, small (5 mm) papule on the nose or face

## FIXED DRUG ERUPTION

Sharply circumscribed, oval or annular dusky red, violaceous, erythematous (solitary or few) plaques (urticaria and bullae may occur as well), which **recur** in exactly the same spot upon **rechallenge**. After resolution, post-inflammatory hyperpigmentation occurs which may last for months or years

## FOCAL DERMAL HYPOPLASIA

Linear and often serpiginous, reddish tan areas of hypoplasia of skin resembling striae distensae. Also, yellowish nodules (fat herniation) most commonly seen on the buttocks, axillae, and thighs. Characteristics X-ray finding of long bones, osteopathia, are fine, parallel, vertical striations in metaphysis

## FOCAL EPITHELIAL HYPERPLASIA (Heck's Disease)

Sessile or pedunculated papules of a few millimeters in diameter; ovoid or round; usually soft or rough and firm, with a smooth or slightly corrugated surface. The lesions are discrete, clustered or confluent, irregularly distributed in the oral mucosa

## FOLLICULITIS

Grouped pustules in hair follicles on an erythematous base

## FORDYCE'S DISEASE (Condition)

Tiny (pinhead-sized) orange or yellowish globoid papules or macules on the vermilion border of the lips or on the oral mucosa; seen in 70–80% of the elderly (ectopic sebaceous glands)

## FOX–FORDYCE DISEASE (Apocrine Miliaria)

Very pruritic, flesh-colored or grayish, discrete follicular papules which occur after puberty (most commonly in females) in areas of apocrine glands (axillae, breast, perineum)

## FURUNCLE (Boil)

Acute, erythematous, round, **tender**, circumscribed, **deeply indurated perifollicular** (staphylococcal) abscess

## GEOGRAPHIC TONGUE

Sharply circumscribed, ringed or gyrate red patches with a narrow yellowish white border; usually affect the dorsal aspect of the tongue. Tongue resembles a map which changes its appearance on a daily basis

## GLOMUS TUMOR

Two types:
Solitary
Skin-colored to purple or dusky blue, 1–20 mm, firm nodule with a **paroxysmal pain**. Most frequent location is subungual
Multiple (glomangioma)
Widely distributed over the body, and usually non-tender. May have autosomal dominant inheritance

## GRAFT VERSUS HOST DISEASE – ACUTE

Extensive maculopapular, erythematous eruption on the face and upper trunk, and occasionally follicular papules simulating folliculitis. Extensive erythematous to violaceous scaling eruption with bullae formation seen in severe cases, and may progress to exfoliative erythroderma

## GRAFT VERSUS HOST DISEASE – CHRONIC

Early lichenoid stage resembles lichen planus.
Late sclerotic stage: firm and inelastic skin with atrophy and reticulate pigmentation. Dyspigmentation, alopecia, and 'parrot-beak' deformity of the nose develop

## GRANULOMA ANNULARE

Flesh-colored, annular eruption; **border is composed of closely set small nodules**; usually occurs near joints

*Clinical Variants*
Actinic granuloma
familial
Generalized granuloma annulare (hundreds of discrete or confluent papules)
Granuloma multiforme (arcuate dermal erythema)
Linear
Localized
Macular granuloma annulare
Nodular granuloma annulare (subcutaneous granuloma annulare), especially seen in children
Perforating granuloma annulare (umbilicated lesions which occur in a localized distribution)

## GRANULOMA GLUTEALE INFANTUM

Few millimeters to few centimeters, reddish blue, round or oval, smooth nodules with an irregular distribution in the diaper area

## GRANULOMA INGUINALE

Soft, usually non-tender, button-like papule(s) or subcutaneous nodule(s) form an irregular ulcer with a beefy-red, friable base and a border that is **raised and 'rolled'**. True inguinal adenopathy is rare; instead, perilymphatic granulomatous lesions produce inguinal swelling

*Clinical Variants*
cicatricial
hypertrophic (rare)
nodular
ulcerovegetative (most common)

## GRANULOSA RUBRA NASI

Erythema and **hyperhidrosis** on tip of the nose

## GROVER'S DISEASE (Transient Acantholytic Dermatosis)

Pruritic, discrete papules or papulovesicles and rarely vesicles or bullae which most commonly occur on the chest, back, thighs; most common in middle-aged or elderly men. Lesions **last two weeks to three months**, but can persist for several years

## HAILEY–HAILEY DISEASE (Familial Benign Pemphigus)

Recurrent, localized eruption of vesicles/bullae on an erythematous base with a predilection for the intertriginous areas of the axillae and the groins. Lesions appear in crops and last several weeks, and spread peripherally, producing a circinate configuration

## HEMANGIOMA

Red to purple–black **blanchable** papules, plaques, or nodules

## HERPANGINA

Six to ten lesions which characteristically occur in the posterior oral and throat area (tonsils, faucial pilars, posterior pharyneal wall, soft palate, uvula). Gray–white papulovesicles (1–2 mm) soon rupture and leave a shallow ulcer with a typical erythematous areola

## HERPES SIMPLEX

Recurrent bouts of acute, self-limited, grouped, umbilicated vesicles on an erythematous base which occur most frequently at or near the mucocutaneous junctions (cf. herpes zoster)

### Clinical Variants
congenital herpes simplex
eczema herpeticum
genital herpes simplex
herpes gladiatorum (sports-related, e.g. wrestling)
herpes in the immunocomprised; three forms are noted:
  chronic ulcerative herpes simplex
  generalized acute mucocutaneous herpes simplex
  systemic herpes simplex
herpes simplex encephalitis
herpes simplex in homosexual males (herpes analis, herpetic pharyngitis)
herpes simplex pneumonia
herpes vulvovaginitis
herpetic gingivostomatitis
herpetic keratoconjunctivitis (most common cause of blindness in the USA)
herpetic sycosis (herpetic folliculitis of the bearded region)
herpetic whitlow (deep seated vesicles restricted to the paronychial or volar sides of the distal phalanx of the fingers)
intrauterine and neonatal herpes simplex
oro-facial herpes simplex
primary inoculation complex
recurrent herpes simplex

## HERPES ZOSTER

**Unilateral**, painful, grouped, umbilicated vesicles on an erythematous base in a **dermatomal distribution**

## HIDROCYSTOMA (Apocrine)

Solitary bluish or brownish (0.5–1.5 cm) dome-shaped, smooth-surfaced, translucent nodule with a cystic quality. When it is pierced with a needle, a clear or brownish fluid is expressed. Most commonly located on the face

## HISTIOCYTOSIS X

See section on 'Some diseases and syndromes highlighted'

## HYDROA VACCINIFORME

Vesicles and papulovesicles on an erythematous base in sun-exposed areas, most common in prepuberty; improves by adolescence. Vesicles later become necrotic, umbilicated, and then crusted. Lesions can be reproduced by **UVA**

## ICHTHYOSIS

### Epidermolytic Hyperkeratosis (Bullous Congenital Ichthyosiform Erythroderma) (AD)
Generalized erythema at birth. Few days after birth, thick grayish-brown **verrucous scaling**, with **marked** involvement of the **flexural** extremities. Superficial, tender **bullae** are characteristic. Frequently, a **fetid odor** is present. Normal-appearing skin in the middle of a hyperkeratotic area is a highly diagnostic finding

### Ichthyosis Linearis Circumflexa (AR)
Extensive erythematous scaly lesions which are polycyclic and migratory. A characteristic **double-edged** scale may be present at the periphery

### Ichthyosis Vulgaris (AD)
Large and adherent scales on the **extensor** surfaces of the extremities, resembling **'fish-scale'** or 'pasted-on' appearance. Flexor surfaced are spared. Hyperkeratosis of palms and soles present; keratosis pilaris often associated

### Lamellar Ichthyosis (AR)
Generalized (mucous membrane and lips spared), **large** (5–15 mm), grayish-brown scales. Moderate hyperkeratosis of the

palms and soles. Infants often born encased in collodian membrane

### X-Linked Ichthyosis (XR)

Generalized, large, yellowish-brown to black scales, having a **dirty** appearance. Scales **spare** the **flexural** areas, palms and soles, and central face; lateral face and neck are commonly involved

## IDIOPATHIC GUTTATE HYPOMELANOSIS

Multiple well-demarcated 2–8 mm off-white or porcelain-white macules with a circular or angulated outline. **No scales or atrophy**. Most commonly on the extensor aspect of the arms and legs

## IMPETIGO CONTAGIOSA

Discrete thin-walled vesicles rapidly become pustular and rupture. A thin straw colored seropurulent discharge remains. The dried exudate leaves a **honey-colored** (golden-yellow), superficial crust, on erythematous base

## INCONTINENTIA PIGMENTI

Bands of slate–brown to blue–gray splashes, lines, streaks, whorls, splattered Chinese-figure-like patches on trunk and extremities
Stages:
I   Starts with **inflammatory vesicles or bullae** that develop in crops over the trunk and extremities. Present during the first two weeks of life, and last for weeks to months
II  **Irregular, linear, warty or verrucous** eruptions on the extremities follows the vesicular stage and lasts several months

III  The **most characteristic** stage. See the general description above. Lasts into adolescence or early adulthood
IV   Depigmented or hypopigmented lesions are noted

## INCONTINENTIA PIGMENTI ACHROMIAS (hypomelanosis of Ito)

Unilateral or bilateral hypopigmentation, 'negative picture' or incontinentia pigmenti

## INSECT BITES

Grouped **urticaria with central punctum**

## INTERTRIGO

Pink to red patch with erosions and slight scaling in intertriginous areas

## KAPOSI'S SARCOMA

Reddish, violaceous, or bluish-black macule, patch, plaque, or nodule with a rubbery consistency

### Clinical Variants
classic (sporadic)
endemic (African)
epidermic (AIDS related)

## KELOID

Raised, firm, irregularly shaped, pink or red (initially), brown (later stages) with smooth, glossy, thinned surface; cf. **hypertrophic scar**; keloids have **claw-like** projections and extend beyond the original wound

## KERATOACANTHOMA

Elevated, firm, dome-shaped nodules with **keratin plug** in the depressed center (volcano-like); **rapid evolution**. Most commonly seen on sun-exposed areas

*Clinical Variants*
**Keratoacanthoma (solitary)**
Giant keratoacanthoma
Reaches a size of 5 cm or greater, most commonly on the nose and eyelids
Keratoacanthoma centrifugum marginatum
May reach 20 cm in diameter and show no tendency to spontaneous resolution. Most commonly involves **the dorsa of the hands and the legs**
Subungual keratoacanthoma
Tender, does not regress spontaneously
**Keratoacanthoma (multiple)**
Ferguson Smith
Self-healing (often with scar) epitheliomas which begin to appear in childhood or adolescence. Usually in sun-exposed areas, but occasionally involve genital or nailbed. Occasional familial occurrence; male predominance
Gryzbowski (eruptive keratoacanthoma)
Generalized, **pruritic** papules and nodules which occur rapidly. Palms, soles, oral mucosa and larynx may be involved. Onset later in life, and heal with pitted scars
Witten Zak variant
Large, self-healing and multiple miliary type keratoacanthomas

## KERATODERMA CLIMACTERIUM

Thickening of palms and soles in women during or after **menopause**

## KERATOSIS PILARIS

Perifollicular, grouped, tiny pinkish papules give the appearance of gooseflesh or plucked chicken skin

## LARVA MIGRANS

Bizarre, serpent-like, thread-like red eruptions

## LEIOMYOMA

*Multiple piloleiomyoma*
Painful, brownish or red, **grouped or linearly arranged** 2–20 mm intradermal nodules. Most commonly located on the trunk

*Solitary angioleiomyoma*
Painful subcutaneous nodules (up to 4 cm) most common on the lower extremities of middle-aged females

*Solitary genital leiomyoma*
**Painless**, intracutaneous or subcutaneous nodules on the scrotum, labia majora, and rarely on the nipples

*Solitary piloleiomyoma*
Intracutaneous, freely mobile, painful 2–20 mm nodules with a reddish or violaceous overlying skin

## LEISHMANIASIS

*Cutaneous*
Acute leishmaniasis
Primary lesions last ten years or less. Start as papules, grow into nodules that usually ulcerate and heal with a depressed scar

Chronic leishmaniasis
Primary lesions last more than two years. Elevated red plaques, 'apple jelly' nodules

Leishmanasis recidivans
Reactivation after several months to many years after healing of the primary infection. Circinate papules are noted at or near the periphery of old scars

Disseminated anergic cutaneous leishmaniasis
Widespread nodular or plaque-like lesions

### Mucocutaneous

### Visceral (kala azar)
May see one of the three types of cutaneous lesions; erythematous patches, hypo- or hyperpigmented patches, nodules

## LENTIGO MALIGNA

**Unevenly pigmented brown macule/patch with variation in color, and irregular, jagged border** (cf. lentigo solaris)

## LENTIGO SIMPLEX

Evenly (uniformly) brown to black pigment macule (usually few millimeters in size), **without predilection to areas of sun exposure**: clinically indistinguishable from junctional nevus (cf. ephelis)

## LENTIGO SOLARIS

**Uniform dark brown** macule/patch with **irregular outline** which commonly occurs on sun-exposed areas

## LEPROSY

Thickening and hardening of nerves are most typical of leprosy

### Borderline Lepromatous Leprosy
Symmetrical circinate maculopapules, nodules or plaques with **ill-defined** borders

### Borderline Tuberculoid Leprosy
Similar to tuberculoid leprosy, but more numerous lesions, and border is less distinct

### Indeterminate Leprosy
Small, **ill-defined** macules, slightly hypopigmented in dark skin, hypopigmented or pinkish in light skin

### Lepromatous Leprosy
Numerous small **ill-defined** macules with little or no loss of sensation, also widespread symmetrical plaques, nodules, or diffuse infiltrations which are commonly anesthetic. Usually no nerve thickening and no changes in sweating are noted

### Tuberculoid Leprosy
**Sharply defined** and elevated border; hypopigmented or erythematous macule/patch (few millimeters to many centimeters) or plaque. Annular, arciform or circinate patterns with variable thickness of borders are noted as the lesions clear

## LICHEN NITIDUS

Flesh-colored, flat-topped, pinpoint (2–3 mm), closely grouped, non-scaling papules, most common on the penis, arms and abdomen

## LICHEN PLANUS

'5 P': papular, planar, purple, polygonal, pruritic. **Violaceous–purplish**, flat-topped, shiny, dry, polygonal papules, with scanty scales, lying between and defined by the natural skin lines. Grayish puncta or streaks, **Wickham's striae**, are caused by a focal increase in thickness of the granular layer and of total epidermis. White lacy pattern, **net-like, reticulated lesions in oral mucosa**

### Clinical Variants
Acute (widespread) (lichen planus)
Annular lichen planus
    Characteristically involves penis and scrotum, more common in Blacks. A typical papule enlarges peripherally with a central clearing
Bullous lichen planus
Chronic (localized) lichen planus
Erosive and ulcerative lichen planus
    Bullae, erosions, and ulcerations develop on the **feet and toes** and result in atrophy, scar, and loss of toenails. There is high incidence of carcinoma in foot ulcers

Hypertrophic lichen planus (lichen planus verrucosus)
Symmetrical **purple to gray or black or bluish patches** which thicken and become verrucous plaques, often occurring on the shins

'Invisible lichen planus'
Lesions not apparent to the naked eye, but may be noted using Wood's light. Pruritus is a premonitory sign

Lichen planopilaris (follicular lichen planus, Graham Little syndrome)
Often affects the scalp. In the beginning, **perifollicular erythema**, or follicular papules are noted. Later, irregular patches of alopecia, similar to pseudopelade of Brocq develop

Lichen planus atrophicus
Atrophy in the center of the papules

Lichen planus–lupus erythematous overlap syndrome
Bluish-red or reddish-purple violaceous discoid lesions with central atrophy and hyperpigmentation, which most commonly occur on the acral parts of the extremities

Lichen planus erythematous
Discrete erythematous (deep red), soft papules of 5–10 mm in diameter which blanch on pressure, and occur singly on the trunk and extremities

Lichen planus pemphigoides
Bullae arise from papules of lichen planus, and from normal-appearing skin

Lichen planus pigmentosus (actinicus, tropicus)
Annular lesions with a pigmented center, and a well-defined, pale border. Most commonly occur in **Middle Eastern** countries, and on the exposed body parts, especially on the face

Linear lichen planus

## LICHEN SCLEROSIS ET ATROPHICUS

Early lesions are flat-topped, grouped papules with black follicular plugs and an erythematous to violaceous halo around white papules. Later, one finds well-circumscribed, **ivory white** (bone white), flat papules or plaques which are atrophic, hairless, slightly scaly, with comedones and dell formation; sclerotic white ring at preputial opening is diagnostic; skin is wrinkled

### Clinical Variants
Lichen sclerosis et atrophicus of vulva
Balanitis xerotic oblisterans
Involves glans penis and prepuce. White, atrophic, slightly edematous patches

## LICHEN STRIATUS

Sudden appearances of unilateral, continuous or interrupted, linear, flat-topped and lichenoid papules which are flesh-colored, red or purple with a grayish scale, commonly on the extremities and sides of the neck, and mainly in children. Usually non-pruritic, and spontaneously involute

## LIPOMA

Well-defined, moveable, soft, rounded or lobulated subcutaneous mass

## LIVEDO RETICULARIS

Red–blue, *blanchable*, net-like mottling, ("fishnet") in a reticular pattern (cf. erythema ab igne)

## LUPUS ERYTHEMATOUS

### Discoid Lupus Erythematous
Well demarcated, dull red papules or plaques with telangiectasia, **follicular plugging ('carpet tacks'), atrophy, scarring**, and hypo- or hyperpigmentation

### Lupus Profundus
Rubbery–firm, usually non-tender, but painful, deep dermal or subcutaneous, 1–4 cm nodules. Commonly involve scalp, face, upper arms, trunk (especially the breasts), thighs, and buttocks

### Subacute Cutaneous Lupus Erythematous

Psoriasiform or polycyclic, annular lesions with thin easily detachable scale, and telangiectasia. Absent follicular plugging or scarring. Lesions commonly occur on the sun-exposed areas, shoulders, extensor surface of arms, dorsum of hands, upper back, V of neck, upper chest, and rarely the face. Uncommon in Blacks or Hispanics

### Systemic Lupus Erythematosus

Red papules or plaques with atrophy, fine scales, hyper- or hypopigmentation, and telangiectasia, especially butterfly distribution on face. Other lesions may include discoid papules on the face and arms, as in discoid lupus erythematous; urticarial lesions; urticarial lesions with purpura (urticarial vasculitis); and bullous lesions which are often hemorrhagic

## LUPUS VULGARIS

Groups of reddish brown nodules with central scarring. When blanched by a glass slide, a **pale, brownish yellow or 'apple-jelly'** color is notable. 'Apple-jelly' lesions are also seen in lupus miliaris disseminatus faciei, and in cutaneous leishmaniasis

## LYMPHANGIOMA CIRCUMSCRIPTUM

Blood-filled, deep yellow vesicles, scaly and wart-like papules, grouped together, giving the appearance of '**frog-spawn**'. Most commonly noted around and within the mouth (especially the tongue), axillae, and abdomen

## LYMPHANGITIS

**Red streak** extending from a purulent lesion from an extremity

## LYMPHOGRANULOMA VENEREUM

Herpetiform vesicles or erosions which soon become shallow ulcers. The ulcer is characteristically **evanescent and is rarely seen**. Groove's sign is pathognomonic (seen the second subsection). Tender inguinal adenopathy, unilateral (66%) and bilateral (33%), in a chain, which may fuse into a large mass, and the overlying skin is violaceous

## LYMPHOMATOID PAPULOSIS

Continuous appearance of papulonecrotic (with a tendency to coalesce), nodular, and plaque-like lesions lasting more than 10 years with a 10–20% chance of developing lymphoma (cf. pityriasis lichenoides et varioliformis acuta)

## MASTOCYTOSIS

### Generalized Mastocytosis

*Diffuse Cutaneous Mastocytosis*

The entire skin may be thickened and result in a peculiar yellowish-orange **'doughy' or 'leathery'** appearance. Bullae may appear spontaneously or following trauma, thus bullous mastocytosis. It may also present as generalized erythroderma, where the skin has a leather-grain appearance the term erythrodermic mastocystosis is applied

*Generalized Cutaneous Mastocytosis (Urticaria Pigmentosa)*

Usually begins during the first week of life. Yellowish brown to yellowish red macules and papules (but nodules or bullae, too) 5–15 mm in diameter. When lesions are rubbed (vigorously) they urticate (Darier's sign); dermographism is usually present; 10–30% of patients have systemic involvement

*Telangiectasia Macularis Eruptiva Perstans*
Usually in adults, hundreds of lentigo-like macules with a slightly reddish tinge on the trunk* and extremities. Lesions may be confluent and often little or no telangiectases evident. Darier's sign and dermographism may be present

### Localized Mastocytoma
Almost exclusively in infants, often solitary, round or oval, flesh-colored to light brown macule, papule, plaque or nodule with a smooth or a slightly warty/pebbly (peau d'orange) surface, 1–5 mm in diameter. Most common on the arms (especially near the wrists), also on the neck and trunk. Most lesions involute spontaneously by age 10; Darier's sign present

### Malignant Mastocytosis
Mast-cell leukemia more commonly develops in adults. Overwhelming infiltration of mast cells in the various organs

### Systemic Mastocytosis
Most frequently bones, liver, spleen, lymph nodes, and peripheral blood involved. Up to 50% of patients have no skin manifestations

### Malignant Melanoma
Brown–black, blue, variegated, irregularly pigmented with white or red pigmentation. The border is irregular and sometimes notched. Surface irregularities are present as well

### Acral Lentiginous Melanoma
Commonly seen in Blacks, Hispanics, Chinese, and Japanese. Occurs in palms and soles and the ungual and periungual regions, but most commonly occurs on the soles

### Lentigo Malignant Melanoma
Like lengtigo maligna, but is indurated with one to several intradermal blue–black nodules

### Nodular Melanoma
An elevated, deeply pigmented blue–black (blueberry-like) nodule which grows rapidly (4 months to 2 years); may become polypoid, and often ulcerates

### Superficial Spreading Malignant Melanoma
Slightly elevated, variegated color (brown, black, pink, blue–gray) papule/plaque (usually 2.5 cm), with an irregularly irregular, partly arciform or scalloped border

### Clinical Variants
Amelanotic melanoma
Lacks pigment. It may be pink, erythematous or flesh-colored. Typical in albinos
Desmoplastic melanoma
May be a primary tumor, but often occurs in a recurrent malignant melanoma, most commonly in lentigo malignant melanoma
Inflammatory melanoma
Associated with a poor prognosis
Mucosal melanoma
Metastatic melanoma
Most commonly metastatic to the skin
Neurotropic melanoma
Possibly a variant of desmoplastic melanoma
Polypoid melanoma
A variant of nodular melanoma
Verrucous melanoma
The lesion is hyperkeratotic with a relatively uniform pigmentation and sharp demarcation

## MELASMA

Patchy, hyperpigmented, non-scaly macules, usually sharply demarcated. Typically on malar areas, forehead and upper lip

## MELKERSSON–ROSENTHAL SYNDROME (Cheilitis Granulomatosa)

Consists of a triad of (1) non-pitting edema of the lips, (2) furrowed, 'scrotal' tongue, and (3) recurrent facial paralysis or paresis (cf. Ascher's syndrome). At times, swelling of the forehead, the eyelids, the cheeks, the chin, or the tongue may occur as well

## MILIA

Multiple 1–2 mm white, globoid, firm lesions. A **white core** is expressed upon nicking (cf. comedo, sebaceous cyst)

## MILIARIA CRYSTALLINA

Seen in sunburned areas or after profuse sweating; lesions consist of small, superficial, clear, **non-inflammatory** vesicles resembling dewdrops; asymptomatic and self-limited

## MILIARIA RUBRA (Heat Rash, Prickly Heat)

Multiple uniformly distributed, very pruritic, flesh-colored to red, small papules or papulovesicles at the orifice of sweat glands. These lesions may become confluent later and form a bed of erythema. In severe cases, pustular lesions may be noted

## MILIARIA PROFUNDA

Flesh-colored, **non-pruritic** vesicles, usually follow a severe course of miliaria rubra and are only noted in the tropics

## MOLLISCUM CONTAGIOSUM

Flesh-colored to pink, smooth, dome-shaped papule with central umbilication

## MONGOLIAN SPOT

Uniformly blue to blue–black, non-infiltrated, round or ovoid, **poorly defined** patch, which resembles a bruise; most commonly on the trunk and buttocks (sacrococcygeal region); present from birth, and usually

disappears spontaneously by age 3 to 4. Commonly seen in Blacks and Orientals

## MULTICENTRIC RETICULOHISTIOCYTOSIS

Few to a hundred firm, red, brown and yellow nodules, 2–10 mm wide, which occur most commonly on fingers and hands. 'Coral bead' appearance when lesions are arranged about nailfolos. Periungual papules are pathognomonic

## NECROBIOSIS LIPOIDICA DIABETICORUM

Well-circumscribed, hard, depressed, **atrophic**, waxy, brown–red–yellowish plaque with **telangiectasia**. The border is broad and violet-red to pink in color. Scale, crust or ulceration may occur

## NEUROFIBROMATOSIS

**Cafe-au-lait spots** are hallmark of neurofibromatosis; 6 or more of these lesions at least 1.5 cm in diameter (Crowe's sign) in adults; in children, a minimum diameter of 0.5 cm is diagnostic
**Lisch nodules**: glassy, clear to tan, dome-shaped, translucent papules up to 2 mm in iris of 94% of post-pubertal patients with neurofibromatosis
**Neurofibroma**: smaller lesions may be invaginated into an underlying dermal defect using a moderate digital pressure – 'button-holing'

## NECROTIZING FASCIITIS

Starts with redness, pain, and edema, and within 24 to 48 hours quickly progresses to patches of **dusky blue** discoloration. Serosangiuneous blisters may or may not be present (cf. cellulitis)

## NEVUS (Melanocytic)

Sharply circumscribed, round or oval shaped, uniform brown, black or flesh-colored macule or papule (usually < 10 mm)

### Nevus Achromicus (Nevus Depigmentosis)
Usually **unilateral** (most often on the trunk). Congenital irregularly shaped macular lesions, **bands** or **bizarre streaks of hypopigmentation**

### Nevus Anemicus
Hypopigmented patch with a sharply demarcated, jagged border that **does not become red** after rubbing (unlike ash-leaf spots). It presents as an area of pale skin

### Nevus Araneus (Spider [Nevus] Angioma)
A telangiectasia characterized by a central (sometimes elevated) punctum with symmetrically radiating thin legs (branches). Diascopy of the central punctum produces blanching

### Nevus, Blue
Well circumscribed, dome-shaped nodule, blue–black or slate–blue in color and usually less than 1 cm in diameter (common blue nevus). Cellular blue nevus is usually 1–3 cm in diameter with a smooth or irregular surface

### Nevus Comedonicus
Band-like or linear grouping of slightly elevated papules with central **keratinous plugs**, resembling comedones. Most commonly occur on the trunk. Secondary lesions, such as cysts, abscesses, fistulas and scars may form

### Nevus, Connective Tissue
Light yellow to orange papules which may be grouped and form plaques, 1–15 cm in

diameter, and my show zosteriform arrangement. Characteristically occur on the trunk, especially in the lumbosacral area

### Nevus Depigmentosus
**Well-circumscribed** hypomelanosis with irregular, serrated, feathered, or geographic borders, present at birth and **stable**. Most commonly seen as a single lesion on the trunk and the proximal portion of the extremities

### Nevus, Dysplastic
Like melanocystic nevus but with irregular, frequently angulated, indistinct borders, with a macular component almost always present. 'Fried egg' appearance is characteristic. Most commonly seen on the back, and usually 5–12 mm in size

### Nevus, Epidermal
Congenital gray to yellow–brown, papillomatous, granular, warty or velvety plaques with a unilateral or bilateral, often dermatomal distribution, favoring the extremities

### Nevus, Epithelioid and Spindle Cell (Benign Juvenile Melanoma, Spitz Nevus)
Dome-shaped, pinkish or red–brown, brown or dark-brown, firm, smooth or verrucous-surfaced papule/nodule with surface telangiectasia. At times it mauy have a polypoid or pedunculated shape. The borders may be irregular and/or not well demarcated, or smooth and well-demarcated. Lesions usually spare palms, soles, and mucous membranes

### Nevus, Halo (Sutton's Nevus)
A pink or brown central nevomelanocytic nevus with a regular sharply demarcated border, surrounded by a symmetrical round or oval depigmented zone or halo. Most commonly occurs in the trunk; usually in teenagers

### Nevus of Ito

Brown to slate–blue speckled discoloration of partially confluent macular lesions, usually not infiltrated. They are commonly unilateral and are located in the scapular, suprascapular, and deltoid areas

### Nevus of Ota

Like nevus of Ito, but located in the periorbital, forehead, temple, malar, and nose regions

### Nevus Sebaceus

Yellow or yellow–brown to orange or pink, **hairless**, usually solitary plaque, with a flat, velvety surface. During puberty, the lesions become nodular and verrucous. As a rule, the lesions are located on the scalp or the face

### Nevus Spilus

Present at birth or may appear later. Solitary, brown, non-hairy patch containing darker brown or black–brown freckle-like macules or papules of 1–2 mm in diameter

## OCHRONOSIS

Black cerumen and black urine seen in patients with ochronosis
**Osler's sign**: pigmented macule on sclera and cartilage of ear in early ochronosis

## ORAL FOCAL EPITHELIAL HYPERPLASIA

Numerous discrete, some confluent, white, soft, 2–4 mm papules of oral mucosa; most commonly on the lower lips

## ORAL LEUKOPLAKIA

A white patch or plaque that will not rub off (cf. erythroplakia of the oral mucosa; red appearance)

## PAGET'S DISEASE, EXTRAMAMMARY

Commonly pruritic, reddish patch with oozing and crusting which enlarges slowly and resembles an eczematous eruption; however, its border is **sharp and irregular**

## PAGET'S DISEASE OF THE BREAST

Unilateral, well demarcated, slightly infiltrated, erythematous patch with scaling, oozing, and crusting, which starts in the nipple or the areola of the breast

## PAPULAR ACRODERMATITIS OF CHILDHOOD (Gianotti–Crosti Syndrome)

Monomorphous, erythematous papules (1–5 mm) which erupt suddenly (over a few days) over the face, buttocks, and extremities, and usually last about three weeks

## PARAPSORIASIS

### Large Plaque Parapsoriasis

Similar to small plaque papapsoriasis, but the patches are 5–15 cm in diameter, more **irregular in shape, and less sharply defined**, with variegated color. In the atopic type, mottled hyperpigmentation and telangiectasias are noted

### Small Plaque Parapsoriasis

Symmetrical, non-indurated, brownish or yellowish red, or yellowish (xanthoerythroderma perstans), oval to round, often fingerprint-like patches of 1–5 cm in diameter with a **sharply defined, regular border**. A fine scale typically produces a **wrinkled appearance**. Lesions commonly occur on the trunk and the proximal extremities

## Variegate Parapsoriasis

Extensive brown–red scaling papules in a **net-like or zebra-like pattern**. As atrophy develops, telangiectasias and mottle pigmentation appear

## PEMPHIGOID

### Bullous Pemphigoid

Large, tense bullae on erythematous or normal skin, with predilection for the groin, axillae, and the flexor surfaces of the forearms. After the rupture of the bullae, the denuded areas show **no** tendency to peripheral extension (unlike pemphigus vulgaris), but heal spontaneously. Often, erythematous patches and urticarial plaques with a tendency to central clearing are noted

*Clinical variants*
Localized
Most common on the lower extremities
Vegetating
Verrucous vegetations in the groin and axillae
Vesicular
Small, tense blisters, occasionally grouped

### Cicatricial Pemphigoid (Benign Mucous-Membrane Pemphigoid)

A chronic disease with evanescent vesicles which occur on the mucosal surfaces (especially the oral mucosa and conjunctiva) and heal with **scarring**, and little tendency to remission

*Clinical variants*
Brunsting–Perry pemphigoid
Recurrent crops of blisters occurs on one or several circumscribed erythematous patches, which usually occur on the head and neck, and eventually result in atrophic scarring. **No mucosal lesions**

### Herpes Gestationis (Pemphigoid Gestationis)

**Very pruritic** with onset during pregnancy (most commonly second trimester) and puerperium. Usually starts with urticarial papules and plaques around the umbilicus and extremities and later spread over the abdomen, back, chest, and extremities. Annular or polycyclic, tense blisters develop within the erythematous plaques

## PEMPHIGUS

### Paraneoplastic Pemphigus

Painful mucosal (oral, pharyngeal, esophageal) ulcerations and a polymorphous and blistering eruption on trunk and extremities. They may include erythema multiforme-like annular and targetoid lesions

### Pemphigus Erythematous (Senear–Usher Syndrome)

Erythematous, thickly crusted patches, bullae, follicular hyperkeratosis (facial lesions), with clinical similarities (location and morphology) to lupus erythematous and seborrheic dermatitis. It represents either an abortive form or an early stage of pemphigus foliaceus

### Pemphigus Foliaceus

Flaccid, superficial bullae, which break easily and leave **shallow erosions**, (not denuded areas as in pemphigus vulgaris) usually on an erythematous base. It commonly occurs on the scalp, face, and trunk, and may spread symmetrically leading to a moist, red, edematous, crusted (localized or generalized) exfoliative eruption. Oral lesions rarely occur. Nikolsky's sign is present

*Clinical Variants*
Brazilian pemphigus (fogo selvagem)
An endemic form of pemphigus foliaceus, most commonly found in Brazil (also in the tropical regions), in children and young adults

### Pemphigus Vulgaris

Flaccid, thin-walled bullae that may appear on an erythematous base or the normal skin and mucous membrane. The bullae break easily and leave **denuded areas** with a tendency to show **peripheral spreading and extension**. Nikolsky's sign is present. The bulla fluid is initially clear but may become hemorrhagic or seropurulent. Most commonly involve mouth (where it may appear first), then the scalp, neck, axillae, groin, or genitals

*Clinical variants*
Pemphigus vegetans
  Hallopeau type (pyodermite vegentante)
    Like pemphigus vulgaris, but the primary lesion is a **pustule**. Denuded areas heal with vegetation or papillomatous proliferations, especially in body folds. Direct immunofluorescence is **negative**
  Neumann type
    Like pemphigus vulgaris, but the denuded areas heal with vegetation or papillomatous proliferations, especially in body folds. Direct immunofluorescence is **positive**

## PERNIO (Chilblain)

Painful or tender violaceous/purplish plaques on acral body parts (fingers and toes)

## PIEBALDISM

Symmetrical white (depigmented) patches with **jagged or geographic borders**. Often associated with a white forelock (poliosis) (cf. albinism, vitiligo). Hyperpigmented macule within areas of hypomelanosis or hyperpigmented macules in the normal skin are **characteristic**

## PIGMENTARY PURPURIC ERUPTIONS

### Doucas and Kapetenakis disease (Itching Purpura)
Possible variant of Schamberg's disease; scaly purpuric lesions with lichenification and secondary **eczematous** changes; involves the trunk, upper and lower extremities

### Gougerout and Blum Syndrome (Pigmented Purpuric Lichenoid Dermatitis)
Tiny, rust-colored, **lichenoid papules** which coalesce and form plaques with an indistinct border; most common on the lower trunk, legs and thighs

### Majocchi's Disease (Purpura Annularis Telangiectodes)
Symmetrical, bluish red, **annular patches**, with dark red telangiectatic puncta within them; occur on the lower legs

### Schamberg's Disease (Progressive Pigmentary Dermatitis)
Pinhead-sized, reddish brown puncta, resembling a **'salt and pepper'** pattern on legs (shin and ankles)

## PILOMATRICOMA

Usually **solitary**, deep-seated, firm nodules of 0.5–3 cm, cove **tent sign** red by normal blue–red or pink skin. Stretching of the skin may elicit the ' ', with multiple facets and angles. Most commonly occurs in the first two decades of life and on the face and upper extremities

## PITYRIASIS ALBA

Hypopigmented, scaly, pale pink or light brown macule/patch (0.5–3 cm) with a **poorly defined, circular or oval** border (cf. tinea versicolor). Most commonly seen on the face and neck

## PITYRIASIS LICHENOIDES CHRONICA

Insidious appearance of erythematous, yellowish, scaly macules and recurrent crops of brown–red, lichenoid papules on the trunk, thighs, and arms. Lesions persist indefinitely. A diagnostic feature is that if scales are present, they can be detached by gentle scraping to reveal a **shiny brown surface**

## PITYRIASIS LICHENOIDES ET VARIOLIFORMIS ACUTA

Characterized by sudden appearance of crops of macules, papules, or papulovesicles that tend to develop central necrosis and crusts

## PITYRIASIS ROSEA

**Herald patch** (mother patch), seen in 50–90% of patients, is an oval or round plaque with a central, salmon-colored, wrinkled area and a darker red peripheral area; when the plaque is irritated, it will have an eczematous appearance. Salmon-colored, oval or circinate macules/patches or papules follow the **lines of cleavage** and have a **Christmas-tree pattern** of distribution

## PITYRIASIS RUBRA PILARIS

Characteristic islands of uninvolved skin. **Follicular papules** on the dorsal aspect of the fingers are pathognomonic. A characteristic finding in pityriasis rubra pilaris is 'sandal', hyperkeratosis of the palms and soles, extending up the sides of feet or hands

## POLYMORPHOUS LIGHT ERUPTION

Pruritic papules, papulovesicles, plaques or erythematous patches, **occur 2 hours to 5 days** after sun exposure, and subside over 7 to 10 days. UVA is implicated in most cases. The eruption is usually **monomorphous** in a **single patient** (cf. erythropoietic protoporphyria, solar urticaria)

## POROKERATOSIS

See 'Some diseases and syndromes highlighted'

## PORPHYRIA CUTANEA TARDA

**Fragility** of skin (dorsa of hands), crusts, **scar**, milia, vesicles and bullae, **thypertrichosis** of the face, especially on cheeks and temples

## PRURIGO NODULARIS

Discrete, firm, erythematous or brownish hyperkeratotic nodules (5–12 mm), often in a linear arrangement on the extensor surface of the extremities. Pruritus is characteristically **severe, paroxysmal and confined to the lesions alone**

## PSEUDOXANTHOMA ELASTICUM

Closely grouped clusters of pebbly, yellowish or cream-colored papules in a reticular pattern at sites of considerable movement of skin (the neck, axillae, antecubital, groins, facial and body folds). Soft, thickened and lax skin which hangs in folds. Angioid streaks in the retina are characteristic

## PSORIASIS

Sharply defined, red papules or plaques. Hallmark: silvery micaceous scales, generally present at the center rather than the periphery of lesions. Removal of scale results in fine, punctate bleeding (Auspitz sign). Nail dystrophy and/or nail pitting is common

### Clinical Variants
*Erythrodermic Psoriasis*
*Generalized Pustular Psoriasis (Von Zumbusch)*
Sudden onset, lakes of pustules form; most severe type with systemic involvement

*Clinical Variants*

Acrodermatitis continua of Hallopeau
(dermatitis repens)
Groups of shallow pustules on an
erythematous base which may be crusted,
eczematoid or psoriasiform. Occur
**asymmetrically** on the hands and feet
(especially acral portion of **fingers and
toes**)

Impetigo herpetiformis
During pregnancy, an acute, extensive
(usually febrile onset) eruption of grouped
pustules on an erythematous base. It begins
in the groin, axillae and neck

*Guttate Psoriasis*
Erythematous, scaly papules the **size of water
drops** (2–5 mm), that usually occur after
acute infections such as streptococcal
pharyngitis

*Inverse Psoriasis (Flexural Psoriasis)*
Involves flexural surfaces, folds, and recesses

*Lichen Planus-like Psoriasis*
Often affects areas favored by lichen planus
(flexor and extensor surfaces of the upper
extremities, the lower legs, and the inner
thighs)

*Nummular Psoriasis*
Oval or irregularly shaped plaques of varying
sizes (one to several centimeters)

*Ostraceous Psoriasis*
Lesions have thickened and tough lamellar
scales like the outside of an oyster shell

*Psoriasis Follicularis*
Small, scaly lesions located at the orifices of the
pilosebaceous follicles. More commonly
seen in children

*Psoriasis Rupioides*
Lesions resemble syphilitic rubia; limpet-like
lesions with a cone-shaped hyperkeratosis.
Commonly seen in the feet

*Psoriatic Arthritis*

*Pustulosis Palmaris Et Plantaris*
Small, deep-seated pustules within areas of
erythema and scaling with predilection for

**mid-palms and thenar eminences of
hands, heels, and insteps of feet** (cf.
acrodermatitis continua of Hallopeau; acral
portion of the fingers and toes involved)

*Seborrhiasis, Seborrheic Psoriasis*
Occurs in the retro-auricular fold or the
external auditory meatus

## PYODERMA GANGRENOSUM

Violaceous, boggy, undermined ulcer 1–2 or up
to 30 cm. Initial lesion is usually a pustule.
Border is raised and tender. The base of the
ulcer is irregular, rough, and purulent. **Pain**
is a prominent feature, as is **pathergy**

### Clinical Variants

*Bullous Pyoderma Gangrenosum (Atypical Pyoderma
Gangrenosum)*
Lesions are more superficial, border is bullous,
and blue–gray in color. Found often on the
face and the upper extremities. Occurs in
patients with preleukemia or leukemia

*Malignant Pyoderma*
No undermined border and no erythema
around ulcers. No associated systemic
disease. Atypical location head and neck

*Pyostomatitis Vegetans*
Chronic, pustular, vegetative lesions involve
oral mucosa, scalp, axillae, or groins. Almost
all associated with inflammatory bowel
disease

## PYOGENIC GRANULOMA

Dark red, soft or slightly firm, 0.5–2 cm nodule
with a smooth surface, which often shows
superficial ulceration and crusting.
Hemangioma-like or granulation-tissue
appearance; **rapid growth**. Many lesions
have a collarette scale around their base.
May bleed profusely if traumatized. Often,
trauma precedes the onset of lesions

## RADIODERMATITIS

### Early
Within about a week of radiation, erythema develops which may heal with desquamation and pigmentation. Occasionally, blisters develop, which heal with atrophy, telangiectasia, and painful, irregular pigmentation

### Later
After a few months to many years, **well demarcated atrophy**, depigmentation, hyperpigmentation, loss of hair, telangiectasia, keratoses, ulceration

## REITER'S DISEASE

Skin lesions are present in two thirds of patients; start as small yellowish vesicles which break and form superficial ulcers. On glans penis, a brownish red patch with central clearing, **balanitis circinata** is noted. On the palms and soles, lesions start as pustules which become crusted and hyperkeratotic. Subungual hyperkeratosis is also commonly seen

## RELAPSING POLYCHONDRITIS

**'Beefy red'** pinnae or ear **only**; tenderness and swelling of other involved areas. Cauliflower shaped ear

## ROCKY MOUNTAIN SPOTTED FEVER

Small, red macules or small purpuric lesions, which **start in wrists and ankles** and spread (cf. atypical measles and coxsackievirus infections, which have identical eruptions. However, in typhus, a similar eruption **starts** from the **trunk and spread peripherally**)

## ROSACEA

Mainly affects central face; no comedones.
Three types:

### Erythematous–Telangiectatic
Erythema, telangiectasia, follicular pustules

### Glandular Hypertrophic
Rhinophyma, enlarged nose

### Papular
Many 1–3 mm papules, usually in association with erythema

### Clinical Variant
*Lupus Miliaris Disseminatus Faciei (Acne Agminata)*
Solitary or groups of discrete, red papules on the face

## SARCOIDOSIS

Papules, nodules, plaques, or subcutaneous nodules; elastic and firm, with dull tints of brown, purple, red or yellow (according to the developmental stage of the lesion). Overlying skin may be thinned, with discoloration, scale or telangiectasia

### Clinical Variants
*Erythrodermic Sarcoidosis*
Red, scaling patches which may extend into an infiltrated brownish-red sheet

*Hutchinson's Plaques*
Symmetrical, large, lobulated, nodular plaques on the cheeks, nose, and arms

*Hypopigmented Sarcoidosis*
Earliest sign of sarcoidosis in Blacks

*Ichthyosiform Sarcoidosis*
Scaling patches, most commonly seen in the lower extremities

333

### Lichenoid Sarcoidosis
Sudden onset, eruptive, shiny, lichenoid papules, more common in females

### Lofgren's Syndrome
Erythema nodosum and sarcoidosis, frequently seen in Scandinavian patients, and associated with good prognosis

### Lupus Pernio
Smooth, violaceous, shiny plaques involve the acral body surfaces, ears, and nose

### Mucosal Sarcoidosis
Pinhead papules may fuse to form a plaque, most commonly seen on the hard palate

### Papular Sarcoidosis (Miliary Sarcoidosis)
Numerous papules on the face, eyelids, neck, and shoulders, which eventually involute to faint macules

### Psoriasiform Sarcoidosis
Well demarcated plaques with psoriasiform scales on the trunk and extremities

### Scar Sarcoidosis
Develop in old scars and resemble **keloids**

### Subcutaneous Sarcoidosis
A few, deep-seated, 1–3 cm nodules on the trunk and extremities

### Ulcerative Sarcoidosis

### Verrucous Sarcoidosis
Verrucous lesions, only seen in Blacks

## SCABIES

Papules (due to temporary invasion of the larval stage), vesicles (due to sensitization of the host) and characteristic **burrows** (home of invading **female** mite) which may be straight or S-shaped. **Extremely pruritic, especially at night**. In men, pruritic papules on the scrotum and penis, and in women, pruritis of nipples associated with a generalized pruritic eruption

### Clinical Variants
*Nodular Scabies*
One to three persistent, dull red nodules for weeks or months after scabies has been treated

*Norwegian (Crusted or Hyperkeratotic) Scabies*
*"like heaps of beige sand"*
Heavily scaly and crusted eruption that may also involve scalp and face; most common in immunosuppressed patients and people with Down's syndrome

## SCLERODERMA

### Early
**Poorly defined indurated, thickened**, hard, smooth, shiny, ivory-colored skin. May see mottled hyper- and hypopigmentation, and loss of hair. **Round finger pad** is an early sign of scleroderma

### Late
Skin is tense, smooth, hardened, and bound down

### Clinical Variants
*CREST Syndrome*
Calcinosis, Raynaud's phenomenon, esophageal dysmotility, sclerodactyly (always present), telangiectasia

*Generalized Morphea*
Widespread, indurated plaques with hypo- and hyperpigmentation

*Guttate Morphea*
Chalk-white, flat or slightly depressed macules

*Linear Scleroderma*
Called 'en coup de sabre' when occurs on the forehead

*Morphea (Localized Scleroderma)*
Yellowish white or ivory-colored, sclerotic, rigid, **atrophic** plaque surrounded by a **violaceous or lilac-colored** inflammatory **border**. Follicular orifices may be unusually prominent

*Morphea Profunda (Pansclerotic Morphea of Children)*
Sclerosis extending to the subcutaneous tissue, fascia, muscle (and sometimes bone) results in disabling limitation of motion

*Progressive Systemic Sclerosis*
Fibrous thickening of skin and blood vessels and thus Raynaud's phenomenon

*Vinyl Chloride Disease*
Acrosclerosis and Raynaud's phenomenon in workers cleaning vinyl chloride polymerization reactors

## SCLEREDEMA

Erythematous induration, hardening and stiffening of the subcutaneous areas (feels woody or cartilaginous); **non-pitting edema**, no hair loss, no atrophy, no pigmentary change

## SCLEROMYXEDEMA (Lichen Myxedematosus, Papular Mucinosis)

Generalized or widespread, symmetric, lichenoid papules. Characteristic **fibrous, sclerotic, woody**, skin. Infiltrated papules in the forehead accentuate the folds and creases; as a result, a vertical swelling at the root of the nose is formed

## SCURVY

**Perifollicular petechiae** (capillary hemorrhages surrounding hyperkeratotic follicular papules). **Curled up hairs in keratotic plugs**

## SEBACEOUS (Epidermal) CYST

Commonly fluctuant and tense, freely mobile, 0.5–5 cm nodule with smooth and shiny overlying skin which is often **attached** to it. **Cheese-like** material can be expressed. A central pore is often noticeable (cf. comedo)

## SEBACEOUS HYPERPLASIA

One or more, commonly several, 2–3 mm, soft, multilobulated, yellowish papules with a central depression. Lesions occur on the face, and most commonly, past middle age

## SEBORRHEIC DERMATITIS

Scale has an oily consistency & a tan-yellow color

## SEBORRHEIC KERATOSIS

Well-circumscribed, brown to black papules or small plaques with a **'stuck-on appearance.'** Surface is rough, scaly and irregular with friable consistency. With a magnifying lens, characteristic pits and furrows may be noted

### Clinical Variants
#### Dermatosis Papulosa Nigra
Small, smooth, pigmented (brown–black) papules seen in 35% of all Blacks, most commonly on the malar region of the face

*Stucco Keratosis*
Symmetrical, small (1–5 mm), gray–white, loosely attached and thus easily scratched-off papules. Most commonly in men over the age of 40, and on the distal portion of the extremities, especially the ankles

## SMALLPOX

Tense, sharply demarcated, at times hemorrhagic, umbilicated vesicles, in **the same stage of development** (cf. varicella)

## SOLAR (Actinic, Senile) LENTIGO

**Uniform**, dark brown macule/patch, irregular outline, non-scaling (cf. lentigo maligna/simplex)

## SOLAR URTICARIA

Pruritic urticarial (evanescent) eruption **within minutes** of sun exposure (cf. erythropoietic protoporphyria, polymorphous light eruption)

## SPOROTRICHOSIS

Linear nodules along lymphatics on an extremity. Most commonly seen in florists, gardeners, people injured by thorns of plants or by straw

## SQUAMOUS CELL CARCINOMA

Dull red, telangiectatic, plaque-like nodule with shallow, centrally crusted ulcerations, and a wide, elevated, indurated border

### Clinical Variants
*Adenoid (Acantholytic) Squamous Cell Carcinoma*
Seen almost always in sun-damaged skin of the elderly

*Mucin-Producing Squamous Cell Carcinoma*
Has the most aggressive clinical course

*Verrucous Carcinoma*
Clinical Variants
  Plantar verrucous carcinoma (epithelioma cuniculatum)
  An exophytic mass which penetrates deeply and results in numerous deep cysts, filled with horny material and pus
  Verrucous carcinoma of genitoanal region (giant condyloma accuminata of Buschke and Loewenstein)
  Papillomatous growth on the glans penis and foreskin (mostly of uncircumcized men), and vulva and anal areas in women
  Verrucous carcinoma of oral cavity (oral florid papillomatosis)
  Oral mucosa affected with white, cauliflower-like lesions

## STAPHYLOCOCCAL SCALDED SKIN SYNDROME (Ritter's Disease)

Most commonly seen in neonates and young children. Begins abruptly, with fever and tender skin and scarlatiniform eruption, and within 24–48 h progresses to spontaneous wrinkling of skin, followed by large, flaccid bullae (superficial epidermal necrosis, separates immediately below the granular layer) in axillae, groin, neck and body orifices and later spread in a generalized fashion in which skin exfoliates in sheets. **The mucous membrane is spared**. Nikolsky's sign is present (cf. toxic epidermal necrolysis)

## STEATOCYSTOMA MULTIPLEX

Multiple, yellowish, moderately firm, cystic nodules (2–6 mm in diameter) that are adherent to the overlying skin and which often contain a **syrup-like**, odorless, yellowish, oily material and occasionally clusters of hair. Most commonly seen in the sternal region; axillae and arms, as well

## SUBCORNEAL PUSTULAR DERMATOSIS (Sneddon–Wilkinson Disease)

Symmetrical, annular, circinate, or bizarre serpiginous patterns formed by coalescence of pustules, with predilection for the axillae, groin, abdomen and sub-mammary areas. Pus characteristically accumulates in the **lower half** of large pustule

## SWEET'S SYNDROME (Acute Febrile Neutrophilic Dermatosis)

Large (2–10 cm, but usually 0.5–2 cm), tender, dark-(blue)red plaques or nodules which rapidly extend and coalesce to form irregular plaques. Surface may be mamillated, appearing like a "relief of a mountain range". Commonly involve the face, neck, and extremities. In one third of cases, the plaques are studded with pustules (cf. Wells' syndrome)

## SYNOVIALMYXOID CYST

Dome-shaped, smooth-surfaced opalescent and shinny. On dorsal aspect of the distal phalanges or proximal nailfolds. **Milky fluid** may be expressed

## SYPHILIS

### Prenatal Syphilis
Early congenital syphilis
Late congenital syphilis

### Primary Syphilis – Chancre
Usually a solitary lesion. Few millimeters to few centimeters in diameter, most commonly on penis (extra-genital on tongue), painless, round or oval induration with surface **erosion**, serous fluid exudation, and **cartilage-hard** consistency, and a dark, velvety, red appearance. Bilateral lymphadenopathy is usually present (cf. chancroid)

### Secondary Syphilis – Syphilids
Skin manifestations of secondary syphilis:
*Alopecia Syphilitica*
Characteristic 'moth-eaten' appearance
*Annular syphilid*
Common in Blacks
*Condyloma latum*
Soft, red, often mushroom-like, 1–3 cm papule/plaque with a smooth, moist, weeping surface. Commonly occurs on folds of moist skin, especially the anal and genital areas
*Corymbose syphilid*
A large central plaque surrounded by a group of minute satellite papules
*Follicular or lichenoid syphilid*
*Leukoderma colli*
Commonly occurs on chin and neck. Small, round or oval, ill-defined, depigmented macules surrounded by hyperpigmented areolae. Lesions persist indefinitely.
*Lues maligna*
Severe pustules and ulcers
*Mucosal lesions*
Mucous patch
  Macerated papules with a flat, grayish appearance; very infective
Syphilitic sore throat
  Most common mucosal lesion; a diffuse pharyngitis
Ulcers
*Papular syphilid (and split papules)*
Papulosquamous syphilid
Pustular syphilid
Rupial syphilid
Superficial ulcer is covered with a pile of crust resembling oyster shell

### Latent Syphilis
Begins with disappearance of secondary syphilis

### Tertiary Syphilis

Cutaneous lesions are in general more localized and asymmetric in distribution. They occur in groups and patterns, and are more destructive, and heal with scar

*Gumma*

May be isolated, single or disseminated or in serpiginous pattern

*Noduloulcerative (tubercular)*

Reddish brown or copper-colored firm papules or nodules with a serpiginous, circular or kidney-shaped pattern

## SYNRINGOMA

Skin-colored, yellowish, brownish, or pinkish, 2–3 mm, soft, translucent, discrete and closely set papules. Most frequently seen in women after puberty. Most commonly seen in (lower) eyelids and upper cheeks

## TELOGEN EFFLUVIUM

Hair density is uniformly decreased

## TINEA CORPORIS

Circular, sharply circumscribed erythematous and scaly patch, with an elevated border; central clearing often noted

## TINEA VERSICOLOR

Brownish, yellowish or hypopigmented, guttate or nummular macules/patches (**borders not completely round**, cf. pityriasis alba) with fine, furfuraceous scales

## TOXIC EPIDERMAL NECROLYSIS

**Tender**, moist, raw, crusted, red erosions ('wet dressing' appearance); **positive Nikolsky's sign**. Targetoid (target-like) lesions (cf. erythema multiforme). More than 90% of patients develop oral erosions or ulcerations (cf. staphylococcal scalded skin syndrome, absence of painful skin and abscence of mucosal involvement)

## TRANSIENT NEONATAL PUSTULAR MELANOSIS

Flaccid vesiculopustules, almost always **present at birth** (commonly in Black newborns), which rupture in 1–2 days and develop into hyperpigmented macules, which themselves perist for weeks to months (smear of the pustule reveals **neutrophils** and rare eosinophils; cf. erythema toxicum neonatorum)

## TRICHILEMMAL (Pilar) CYST

Morphology is similar to epidermal cysts; however, less common, and 90% occur on the scalp. Often an autosomal dominant mode of inheritance

## TRICHOEPITHELIOMA

Many rounded, flesh-colored, 2–8 mm, firm papules and nodules. Most commonly located in the nasolabial folds; may occur on the nose, forehead, and the upper lip

### Clinical Variants

*Desmoplastic Trichoepithelioma*

Not heritable, most commonly seen in females, and almost always on the face. A solitary, indurated lesion (3–8 mm in diameter) with a raised, annular border and a depressed, non-ulcerated center

*Giant Solitary Trichoepithelioma*

Several centimeters in diameter, most commonly on the thighs and perianal regions

*Multiple Trichoepithelioma*
AD, located primarily in the **nasolabial folds**. Small, rounded, shiny papules and nodules of 2–8 mm in diameter, most frequently grouped, but discrete; appear in childhood

*Solitary Trichoepithelioma*
Not heritable, less than 2 cm in diameter. Onset in childhood or early adulthood

## TRICHOFOLLICULOMA

Small (5 mm), skin-colored, dome-shaped nodule, frequently with a central pore. Most commonly seen on the face and scalp. **Tuft of (wool-like) white (often immature) hairs** emerging from a central pore is a characteristic finding

## TRICHOTILLOMANIA

Focal area of thinned hairs of irregular length

## TUBERCULOSIS

### Endogenous
*Acute miliary tuberculosis (tuberculosis cutis miliaris disseminata)*
In the low immunity state, rare, acute, generalized, brownish red, acuminate papules which become necrotic and form small ulcers

*Lupus Vulgaris*
In the high or low immunity state, most common type of cutaneous tuberculosis. F : M ratio 2–3 : 1. 90% occur in head and neck; on diascopy, 'apple jelly' color (brownish-yellow); different forms: hypertrophic (tumorous), papular and nodular, plaque (plain), ulcerative and vegetating

*Metastatic Tuberculous Abscess (Tuberculous Gumma)*
In the low immunity state, hematogenous spread; non-tender, subcutaneous abscess on scalp, trunk, and extremities

*Orificial Tuberculosis (Tuberculosis Ulcerosa Cutis et Mucosae)*
In the low immunity state, more in men; most commonly on the tongue; reflects advanced internal disease and unfavourable prognosis

*Scrofuloderma (Tuberculosis Colliquativa Cutis)*
In the high immunity state, the second most common cutaneous tuberculosis; spreads via contiguous involvement. Common in parotidal, submandibular and subclavicular areas. Keloidal scars are characteristic

### Exogenous
*Primary Inoculation Tuberculosis (Tuberculous Chancre)*
In the low immunity state, more common in males and in children. Painless ulcer with unilateral regional adenopathy

*Tuberculosis Verrucosa Cutis (Warty Tuberculosis)*
In the high immunity state, warty vegetations, usually seen on hands of previously infected and sensitized patients

### Tuberculosis Due to BCG Vaccination

### Tuberculids
### Facultative Tuberculoids
Erythema induratum
Erythema nodosum

*True Tuberculids*
Lichen scrofulosorum
  Lichenoid eruption
Papulonecrotic tuberculoid
  Necrotizing papules appear in crops in a symmetric distribution and heal with scar. Lesions have a predilection for the extensor aspect of the extremities

## TUBEROUS SCLEROSIS

### Adenoma Sebaceum
Multiple flesh-colored to red papules, usually bilaterally symmetrical, in nasolabial folds, cheeks and chin

### Ash-leaf Spots
Ash-leaf-like or confetti-like hypopigmented macules/patches; present at birth in 70–90% of patients

### Shagreen Patches
Raised, flesh-colored papules or plaques, with an 'orange-peel' or 'pigskin' appearance, most commonly on lumbosacral region

### Tooth Pits
Punctate, round or oval, 1–2 mm, randomly arranged. **Enamel defects** are a marker for tuberous sclerosis

## ULERYTHEMA RETICULOSIS

**Gridlike**, depressed scars; symmetrical involvement of the face

## URTICARIA

Annular, arciform, circular, geographic or polycyclic, non-scaly, well-circumscribed, erythematous eruption. Evanescent areas of edema involve the superficial portions of the dermis (in angiodema, the edema extends into the deep dermis or subcutaneous and submucosal layers). Frequently **very pruritic**

## URTICARIA PIGMENTOSA

Brown, non-scaly macules/patches (may consist of papules, plaques, nodules, vesicles, or bullae, as well). When firmly stroked or vigorously rubbed, urticaria with a surrounding erythematous flare develops (**Darier's sign**). (Also see under Diseases and their features, Mastocytosis)

## VARICELLA (Chickenpox)

Red papules give rise to umbilicated vesicles that develop into pustules and, later, crust.

**Lesions are seen in different stages of development** (cf. smallpox)

## VERRUCA

### Condyloma Acuminatum
Gray, pale yellow or pinkish, small, pointed or cauliflower-like projections, which may multiply and form large, vegetating clusters. Affect genital and anal areas

### Epidermodysplasia Verruciformis
AR, widespread, flat, wart-like lesions, and erythematous hyperpigmented or hypopigmented macules, which may resemble seborrheic dermatitis or pityriasis rosea, or plaques, which may resemble psoriasis. Palms, scalp, and mucous membranes are spared. Malignant degeneration may occur in sun-exposed areas

## VERRUCA VULGARIS

Flesh-colored to pink, discrete papules with verrucous surface. When pared down, multiple, **fine bleeding points** are noted

## VINCENT'S ANGINA (Acute Necrotizing Ulcerative Gingivitis)

Begins with rapid onset of painful gingiva, which bleed easily and lead to characteristic 'punched out' ulceration on the **interdental papillae and marginal gingiva**. There is a characteristic **foul–fetid** odor and a **metallic taste**

## VITILIGO

Ivory-white non-scaly macule or patch with **complete loss of pigment**; border is **convex** and may have three different presentations; (1) intermediate level of color (trichrome vitiligo) (normal brown, light tan and white); (2) erythematous halo (inflammatory vitiligo); (3) hyperpigmented rim (cf. albinism, piebaldism)

## WARTY DYSKERATOMA

Solitary, brownish red papule or nodule with a soft, yellowish keratotic, umbilicated center. Most commonly seen on the face, neck, scalp, or the axilla

## WELLS' SYNDROME (Eosinophilic Cellulitis)

Recurrent, sudden onset of erythematous, indurated, persistent, urticarial eruption or infilterated erythemas with annular borders; frequently with a central bulla with a border

which is sharp, rosy or violaceous. The size and number of the lesions are variable, but often pruritus and pain are present, as is peripheral blood eosinophilia (cf. Sweet's syndrome)

## XANTHOGRANULOMA

Yellow to reddish-brown papule or nodule with a discrete, firm or rubbery consistency

## XERODERMA PIGMENTOSUM

Dry, parchment-like, freckled skin. Actinic skin changes develop in childhood

# Eruptions trivialized

In this subsection, a collection of some common and some uncommon terms or conditions are presented, as they pertain to different diseases. An effort has been made to identify some characteristic findings that may aid the clinician in the diagnostic process

## ACHROMIA PARASITICA

A severe, rapidly spreading variant of tinea versicolor in dark-complexioned children

## ALBRIGHT'S HEREDITARY OSTEODYSTROPHY

dimple sign over knuckles when fist is clenched.

## AUTOINOCULATION

A characteristic of chancroid in its ability to infect opposing contiguous areas of the skin

## BABOON SYNDROME

Acute exanthematous eruption involving the anogenital area, the buttocks, and the flexural extremities. Diffuse light-red symmetrical erythema within hours of systemic exposure to allergens (e.g. Amoxicillin, Ampicillin, erythromycin, heparin, mercury, nickel, and food additives.

## BAZEX'S SYNDROME (Acrokeratosis Paraneoplastica)

Violaceous erythema and scaling of the fingers, toes, nose, and aural helices; secondary to gastrointestinal tract or pulmonary malignancies or metastatic carcinoma of the lymph nodes

## BLACK DEATH

Kala azar, because of the skin (especially face) pigmentation. Also refer to *Pasteurella pestis* infection (plague)

## CALABAR SWELLING

One or more, slightly inflamed, edematous, transient swellings about the size of a hen's egg in loaiasis, at the sites of migration of microfilaria

## CARPET TACKS (Langue Au Chat, Cat's Tongue)

Adherent scales (produced by retained follicular keratin spike) in discoid lupus erythematosus

## CASAL'S NECKLACE

Dermatitis affecting necklace area of patient with pellagra

## CAVIAR TONGUE

Dilatations of blood vessels on the undersurface of the tongue, in old age

## CLUSTERS OF JEWELS

Rosette or annular array of bullae in chronic bullous disease of childhood

## COCKARDE NEVUS

An unusual variant of acquired nevomelanocytic nevus. The lesion is **target-like**; there is a central nevus, an intervening non-pigmented zone, and finally a peripheral pigmented halo

## CULLEN'S AND TURNER'S SIGN

Periumbilical or flank purpura associated with hemorrhagic pancreatitis

## DARIER'S DISEASE

'Sandwich' of red and white lines with a peripheral notch or split is pathognomonic

## DECK-CHAIR SIGN

Seen in papuloerythroderma, where areas of skin creases are spared

## DIMETHYLGLOXIME

Used to test presence of nickel in an object

## DOLLAR PAPER MARKINGS

Almost exanthematic redness, like threads of paper money, in chronic liver disease

## DEWDROP ON A ROSE PETAL

The early vesicle in varicella is surrounded by an irregular area of erythema

## ELEPHANT SKIN

Thickened skin in onchocerciasis

## EPSTEIN'S PEARL

Milia in oral cavity of infants

## FABRY'S DISEASE

Maltese Cross: material seen on polaroscopy of urine of patients with Fabry's disease (angiokeratoma corporis diffusium). The characteristic spoke-like appearance of the posterior subcapsular cataracts are **pathognomonic** of Fabry's disease

## FINGERNAIL SIGN

Characteristic dust-like or furfuraceous scales in tinea versicolor which can be produced by lightly scraping the fingernail over the involved area

## FLAG SIGN

Alternating bands of pale and dark hair (poor nutrition periods) in kwashiorkor

## FOLLICULAR SPICULES OF NOSE

SEEN IN MULTIPLE MYELOMA (RESULT OF ACCUMULATION OF IgG DYSPROTEINS & CRYOGLOBULINS)

## FOOT PRINT IN SNOW OR SWISS CHEESE APPEARANCE

Seen in atrophoderma of Pasini and Pierini

## FORCHEIMER'S SIGN

In rubella, pinhead red spots, scattered over the soft palate

## FORME FRUSTE

Of basal cell carcinoma: palmar pits in nevoid basal cell epithelioma syndrome
Of stasis changes: chronic pigmented purpura
Of pemphigus foliaceus: Brazilian pemphigus

## FOUNTAIN-SPRAY SPLATTERS

Morphological pattern seen in incontinentia pigmenti

## GAUNT FACIES

Seen in progressive lipodystrophy

## GORLIN'S SIGN

50% of patients with Ehlers–Danlos syndrome can touch tip of the nose with their tongue

## GREAT WALL OF CHINA

Diagnostic feature of porokeratosis of Mibelli; raised hyperkeratotic peripheral ridge surrounded by a furrow

## GROOVE'S SIGN

Pathognomonic lymphogranuloma venereum. When femoral and inguinal adenopathy occur, a groove corresponding to Pauport's ligament separates the two; the overlying skin is violaceous. In eosinophilic fasciitis, when the affected limb is raised, collapsed veins resemble a system of merging brooks because of absent dermal fibrosis around the superficial veins

## HAIR COLLAR SIGN

ring of thick dark hair surrounding a membranous area of aplasia cutis congenita.

## HAMSTER-NECK OR HORSE-COLLAR

Seen in patients with benign symmetric lipomatosis

## HAND, FOOT, AND MOUTH DISEASE

Characteristic vesicles with elliptical football-shaped appearance, most frequently seen on the dorsal aspect of the fingers and toes, as well as the lateral borders of the feet

## HEBRA NOSE

Seen in infiltrative stage of rhinoscleroma; nose become similar to hippopotamus & rhinoceros.

## HERTOGHE'S SIGN

Thinning of lateral eyebrow in atopic dermatitis.

## HITZELBERGER'S SIGN

Hypesthesia of the postauricular & superior aspect of the external auditory canal associated with acoustic neuroma.

## HOURGLASS OR FIGURE-EIGHT

Terms applied to whitish, atrophic areas which form this characteristic configuration in the vulva and anus of patients with lichen sclerosis et atrophicus

## HUTCHINSON'S PLAQUES

Nodular symmetrical plaques on the cheeks, nose, and arms of patients with sarcoidosis

## HUTCHINSON'S SIGN

Vesicles on tip of the nose, indicate nasal nerve involvement of **herpes zoster**; a predictor of future ophthalmic involvement.

Also, periungual spread of pigmentation to the surrounding proximal and lateral nail folds in subungual malignant melanoma

## HUTCHINSON'S TRIAD

Pathognomonic of late congenital syphilis:
(1) Eight-nerve palsy
(2) Hutchinson's incisors
(3) Interstitial keratitis

## INFECTIOUS MONONUCLEOSIS

Eyelid edema is seen in 50% of all patients with this infection

## KAPOSI'S SIGN

One is able to pinch the skin on dorsum of the second toe, diagnostic aid for lympedema

## KATAYAMA DISEASE (URTICARIAL FEVER)

Fever, malaise, abdominal pain, diarrhea, arthralgia and hepatosplenomegaly with schistosomiasis (*Schistoma japonicum*++)

## LA MAIN EN LORGNETTE (OPERA-GLASS HAND, TELESCOPE FINGERS)

Telescopic shortening of the phalanges and digits seen in multicentric reticulohistiocytosis

## LEOPARD SKIN

Spotted depigmentation seen in onchocerciasis

## LILAC RING

Violaceous border of enlarging morphea lesion

## LIVER PALMS OR DAWSON'S PALMS

A bright red coloration of contact surfaces of palms and pulps seen in patients with rheumatoid arthritis

## LOVER'S HEEL

Designation for the calcaneus of patients with Reiter's syndrome

## LUMPY JAW

Cervicofacial type of infection with actinomycosis, where one notes chronic granulomatous and suppurative inflammation with multiple abscesses and sinus tracts

## MACULAE CERULAE

Bluish/slate-colored macules due to louse bites, saliva of louse changes bilirubin to biliverdin

## MARBLE CAKE CONFIGURATION

Seen in patients with incontinentia pigmenti achromians (AD)

## MARJOLIN'S ULCER

Refers to cancers (most commonly squamous cell carcinoma) that arise in chronic ulcers, sinuses, and scars of various etiologies

## MAZZOTTI'S TEST

After first dose of diethylcarbamazine for onchocerciasis, exacerbation of arthralgias, fever, pruritus occurs

## MEASLES

Pathognomonic finding, **Koplik's spots**: clusters of white papules (like a cluster of fine grains of sand) on an erythematous base appear on the buccal mucosa, near the upper molars or mucosa of the inner lip

## MENKE'S HAIR

Seen with copper deficiency

## MICKY MOUSE APPEARANCE

Large and protruding ears seen in patients with Cockayne's syndrome

## MOROCCAN LEATHER SKIN

Epidermal thickening in patients with diffuse cutaneous mastocytosis

## MOUSY ODOR

Characteristic of gas gangrene (clostridial myonecrosis)

## MYERSON'S NEVUS

A pigmented nevus surrounded by eczema.

## NUTMEG GRATOR (OR THORNY FEEL)

Flat to conical projections (1–3mm) with hair-like horny spines, seen in **Lichen Spinlosus**.

## OLLENDORFF'S SIGN

Seen in secondary syphilis; papules that are exquisitely tender to touch of blunt probe

## ONCHOCERCIASIS

'Skin snip' test: lift skin with a needle; snip; look at under microscope with a drop of saline; filariae wriggle out at the edges of the skin slice

## PEBBLING OVER SCAPULA

Mucopolysaccharidosis II (Hunter's disease)

## PERIAURICULAR PAPULE OR NODULE

Rarely, associated with **renal abnormalities**

## PHOTO–KOEBNER PHENOMENON

Noted in Darier's disease

## PINCH PURPURA

Amyloidosis (**periorbital purpura** is very characteristic of this disease)

## PLUCKED CHICKEN SKIN

Plaques of irregular yellow papules that may coalesce to form yellow reticular pattern in patients with **pseudoxanthoma elasticum**

## PROSECTOR'S WART

Results from infection arising from autopsies or handling of tuberculous meat; it is a prototype of tuberculosis verrucosa cutis

## PYOSTOMATITIS VEGETANS

Very rare non-infectious pustular disease that results in erythematous, vegetating papules along the lips and buccal folds. A marker for ulcerative colitis; may be seen with Crohn's disease

## RACCOON EYES OR OWL EYES

Characteristic periorbital erythema, strong clue to diagnosis of neonatal lupus erythematosus

## RACCOON-LIKE PERIORBITAL DEPIGMENTATION

May be caused by rubber edges of swim goggles

## RAMSAY HUNT'S SYNDROME

Involvement of geniculate ganglion with herpes zoster, involving facial paralysis and vesicles in the exterior auditory canal

## RAIN DROPS ON A DUSTY ROAD

Seen in arsenical hypopigmentation

## RED MAN SYNDROME

Caused by rapid infusion / overdose of Rifampin
or Vancomycin

## ROMANA'S SIGN

Edema and inflammation of lacrimal glands in
Chagas' disease (American trypanosomiasis)

## ROPE SIGN

prominent linear cutaneous bands on the trunk
in interstitial granulomatous dermatitis

## ROSE SPOTS

2–3 mm pink papules which blanch on pressure,
are non-tender, and are seen in **typhoid
fever** (*Salmonella typhi*)

## RUDDY COMPLEXION, ERYTHREMIA

Seen in patients with **polycythemia vera**

## SCHOOL OF FISH OR RAILROAD TRACK

Smear of an ulcer from a **chancroid** (stained
with methylene blue, Wright, Giemsa, or
Gram Stain) will show parallel chains of two
or more red organisms (bacilli of
*Haemophilus ducreyi*)

## RUMPEL–LEEDE TEST

In Rocky Mountain spotted fever, pressure
from sphygmomanometer may produce
petechiae

## SERUM SICKNESS

A purpuric band of erythema at the margin of
palmar or plantar skin is characteristic

## SPINDLING OF FINGERS

Highly characteristic finding in juvenile
rheumatoid arthritis. The spindle-shaped
deformity of the fingers develops because
the proximal interphalangeal joints are
affected more severely than the distal joints

## STEINBERG'S SIGN

In Marfan's syndrome, when thumb is opposed
across the palm, it extends beyond the ulnar
margin

## STEMMER'S SIGN

Thichening of skin over dorsal toes or fingers,
characteristic of Elephantiasis Nostrans

## STRAWBERRY GINGIVITIS

Early pathognomonic finding in Wegener's
granulomatosis

## STRING OF BEANS

Linear, waxy, slightly yellow papules on the
margin of eyelids, characteristic of lipoid
proteinosis

## SULFUR GRANULES

Discharged in actinomycosis and botryomycosis

## SYPHILIS, CONGENITAL

Cluton's joints (hydrarthrosis)
Higoumenahis's sign (sternoclavicular swelling)
Hutchinson's triad
  eight-nerve palsy

Hutchinson's incisors
interstitial keratitis
Mulberry (moon) molars
Sabre skin (periosteal thickening of tibia)
Saddle nose

## SYSTEMIC SCLEROSIS

Neck sign: seen in 90% of patients with systemic sclerosis. Ridging and tightening of skin of neck on extension of head. Symmetrical hypopigmentation of forehead, near hear line, the chest and the abdomen with perifollicullar pigment retention

## TANGIER'S DISEASE

Characteristic finding: large tonsils with orange–yellow striations

## THUMBPRINT PETECHIAE

Periumbilical purpura with 'thumbprint' petechiae are characteristic of **disseminated strongyloidiasis**

## TUFTSIN

Produced in spleen, allows neutrophil chemotaxis

## VARNISHED APPEARANCE

A shiny and waxy appearance of skin in lepromatous leprosy

## VOIGHT'S OR FUTCHER'S LINES

Represents abrupt dorsoventral pigmentary demarcation of about 10 cm around arms

## WALLACE'S LINE

Well demarcated line around margin of foot, dividing diseased from normal skin

## WATERBAG SIGN

In cutaneous focal mucinosis noted with deformation with a pen.

## WHITE DERMATOGRAPHISM

Development of a white line upon stroking of the skin, instead of a normal red response; seen in **atopic dermatitis**

## WILKINSON'S TRIANGLE

The area behind the earlobe spared from an eruption

## WINTERBOTTOM'S SIGN

Pronounced enlargement of the posterior cervical lymph node in **African trypanosomiasis**

## ZEBRA EFFECT

Alternate black and white bands seen under polarizing light microscopy of hair of patients with **trichothiodystrophy**